CLINICAL PSYCHIATRY

A. K. AGARWAL.

CENTRAL

CLINICAL PSYCHIATRY

A. K. AGARWAL. D.P.M., M.D.
Professor and Head, Department of Psychiatry,
King George's Medical College, Lucknow.

New Central Book Agency (P) Ltd.
8/1, Chintamoni Das Lane, Calcutta-700 009

CLINICAL PSYCHIATRY

First Published 1995

Publisher
New Central Book Agency (P) Ltd.
8/1, Chintamoni Das Lane,
Calcutta - 700 009

Typesetter
Barun Kumar Sasmal.
3, Garanhatta Street,
Calcutta - 700 006

Printer
Book & Allied (P) Ltd.
8/1, Chintamoni Das Lane,
Calcutta - 700 009

Technical Editor
Dr. Sujit Ghosh

Proof Reader
Subas Maitra

Cover Designer
Sandipan Bhattacharya

Supervisor
Usha Bhowmik

ISBN 81-7381-048-6

Price
Rs. 85.00 (Rupees Eighty five) only.

Caution

Though every effort has been made to provide standard dosage of drugs, yet it is recomended that the dosage and side effects may be checked from current literature.

About the author

The author of this book Dr. A. K. Agarwal is currently working as the Professor and Head, Department of Psychiatry, King George's Medical College, Lucknow. He has been teaching Psychiatry for nearly thirty years to under-graduate and post-graduates. He has published nearly eighty articles and had edited few books. He has been the Editor of Indian Journal of Psychiatry. He has been Chairperson of Ethics Commitee of Indian Psychiatric Society. He is the president of Indian Psychiatric Society for 1994.

ACKNOWLEDGEMENTS

The author wishes to put on record his indebtedness to his teachers, colleagues, students and various texts in Psychiatry which have been instrumental in shaping his thinking and thus, are largely responsible for the contents of this book.

I must acknowledge the help of Dr. Sudhir Kumar, Asst. Professor, Dr. J. Sahay, Scientist, C.D.R.I., Lucknow, Dr. Vimal M. Aga, Junior Resident in preparation of this book. Thanks are also due to Drs. Shalabh Jain, Pankaj Kishore, Vikas Jain, Srikant Srivastav for their help in proof reading. Km. Vandana Varma has been very helpful in the proof reading of this book. Dr. Sujit Ghosh, Psychiatrist, Calcutta has been involved in the final stages of this book for which the author is obliged. Mr. Gaurav Kishore and his group have been patient with the author and are responsible for typing the manuscripts. New Central Book Agency (P) Ltd. is responsible for the production of this book and the author is greatful to them.

The author wishes to specially acknowledge W.H.O. for permitting brief extracts from the I.C.D.-10 classification of mental and behavioural disorders. Clinical descriptions and diagnostic guidelines. Geneva, World Health Organization, 1992.

All diagnostic guidelines in this book have been reproduced from the above book. These have been marked to (I.C.D.-X) at appropriate places.

Lastly, I must acknowledge the help and encouragement provided by my wife and my family without which I could not have completed this book.

Lucknow.
October, 1994.

A. K. Agarwal

PREFACE

Mental disorders are quite common and most of the apidemiological studies conducted in different parts of the world reveal that nearly ten percent of the population suffer from these disorders. It has also been observed that more than one-fifth of the patients visiting general practitioners suffer from emotional disorders and as such minimal knowledge of human behaviour and psychiatric aliments is mandatory on the part of each and every medical practitioner. Unfortunately, the reality is just the contrary. Psychiatric training at the undergraduate level has been largely deficient in this country. Consequently, the majority of medical practitioners are grossly ill-equipped to provide reasonable treatment to the patients having emotional problems. The problem becomes of enormous significance in view of the fact that due to social stigma or other reasons a large chunk of psychiatric patients prefer to seek treatment only from general practitioners. Even in the countries having optimum psychiatric facilities, like United States, it has been reported that sixty percent of these patients never visit a psychiatrist and continue to consult primary care physician. Unfortunately, the situation is less likely to change in the coming time as well. Hence, proper training in psychiatry for the medical practitioner has been a long-felt need. Efforts should also be made to extend this knowledge to the specialists of other branches of medicine so that they could easily identify the associated emotional problems of their patients.

In the context of the exiting scenerio it is obvious that psychiatric teaching should be greatly strengthened at the undergraduate level and effort should be made to impart basic knowledge of the discipline to the practicing general physicians. But one of the major lacuna in achieving this objective has been non-availability of a simple text book of psychiatry which is concise and readily comprehensible. The present book is a step in this direction. Though a large number of Western and some Indian text books of psychiatry for undergraduate level are available, perhaps a majority of the students find it difficult to maintain their due interest in the subject either because of language problem or inability to empathize with clinical description of the patients belonging to alien culture. It is, therefore, hoped that if both these impediments could be overcome there is likely to be a greater involvement of medical students as well busy general practitioners. Keeping this aim in mind, the present book mainly incorporates the pattern of symptomatology of various disorders as observed in this culture.

International classification of Diseases of 1992 (ICD-X) has been used throughout the book. The strength of this classification lies in the fact that it has been field-tested in large number of countries of the world and as such, the classification is fairly reliable. The diagnostic guidelines of this classification have been used throught this book in describing various mental disorders.

This book could be used as a basic book by all medical men who are interested in psychiatry and should also be useful for practising psychiatrists and psychiatric residents for a quick update of knowledge.

The author welcomes suggestion for improvement in this book from the readers.

Lucknow. October, 1994.

A. K. Agarwal

CONTENTS

CONTENTS

CHAPTER 1

INTRODUCTION

Mental disorders have been known from ancient times. The epics of Ramayana and Mahabharata provide many examples of mental disturbances. King Dasaratha experienced two episodes of depression ; one after he accidentaly killed Shravana and second, when his son Rama went into exile. Similarly, the Mahabharata very clearly depicts the anxiety experienced by Arjuna at the battle-field and the Geeta is a classical example of psychotherapy. Ancient Greek and Roman literature also provide many examples of behaviour which could be called mental disorders today. Hippocrates (460-377/359 B.C.), the father of modern medicine described hysteria. He conceptualised that mental illnesses are caused by disturbances in four essential humours, eg. blood, phlegm, yellow bile and red bile. Many physicians and writers have, described the symptomatology of mental disorders from time to time.

However, it was only in the later part of the seventeenth century that the mentally ill were considered worthy of humane treatment. Phillip Pinel (1745-1826) in France, Benjamin Rush (1745-1813), in USA and William Tuke (1732-1822), in U.K. nearly simultaneously but independent of each other emphasised on the humane approach to the treatment of the mentally ill person. This led to various reforms in the management of these patients all over the world.

The second major development took place in psychiatry towards the end of the nineteenth century when two psychiatrists working independently of each other laid the foundation of modern psychiatry. Emil Kraepelin (1856-1926), after prolonged observation of mentally ill persons, divided mental disorders into dementia praecox and manic depressive psychosis. He observed that in one group of patients the illness starts in adolescence and they develop mental deterioration prematurely and he called such persons as suffering from dementia praecox. The label was later changed to schizophrenia by Eugene Bleuler (1857-1939) because he demonstrated that all such patients do not develop dementia. Kraepelin also described manic depressive psychosis as a circular illness with remissions and relapses. Kraepelin laid the foundation of modern psychiatry.

Sigmund Freud (1856-1939) developed the principles of psychoanalysis. He emphasised on the psychological causation of mental disorders and on their psychological management. He influenced not only psychiatry but also literature and other social sciences. Freud's theories have been modified and improved by many of his illustrious followers.

The early part of the current century was mainly devoted to psychological explanation of psychiatric disorders. When many patients did not show benefit with these psychological treatments, many workers started looking for organic treatments for mental disorders.

Wagner von Jauregg (1917) described malarial treatment for general paralysis of insane which was strongly criticised as unethical because a sick person was being inflicted by another disease. Manfred Sakel (1933) described insulin coma treatment for schizophrenia. It produced benefit in some patients. Von Meduna (1937) noted that schizophrenia and epilepsy do not occur together and he produced epileptic fits in schizophrenia by injecting metrozol which produced remarkable improvements in some patients. Later, Cerletti and Bini (1937), produced epileptic fits by electric current. This treatment is still used in psychiatry. Major changes started occurring in psychiatry in the fifth decade of the current century when Delay and Deniker used Chlorpromazine to treat schizophrenia. Few years later A. Janssen (1952), described iproniazid as an antidepressant. Cade (1949), described lithium in the treatment of mania which was only rediscovered later.

The last four decades have seen a tremendous change in the following :

a) Diagnostic methods in psychiatry has been standardized and new classifications have been developed. The latest are International Classification of Diseases (X) (WHO 1992), and DSM-IIIR (American Psychiatric Association).

b) Etiology of psychiatric disorders has been studied with more precision, both from biological and psychological view points.

c) Newer drugs and other treatment methods have been developed and scientifically evaluated.

d) Mental disorders are being treated as any other disease or disorder without considering them as signs of moral or psychological degradation.

EPIDEMIOLOGY OF PSYCHIATRIC DISORDERS

Psychiatric disorders are prevalent all over the world and in all socio-economic status. It was previously thought that psychiatric problems are a result of affluence and modernisation but the etiological studies done over the world have shown that psychiatric disorders are equally present all over the globe. There may be certain areas where a particular disorder is more prevalent than others. Indian workers have done a number of epidemiological studies on small samples. Surya, El Nagar, Dubey, Sethi, Nandi and Verghese are some of the prominent workers in the area. General conclusions are :

– Severe mental disorders (schizophrenia, depression and other psychosis) are prevalent in 2% population.

– Another 10% population suffers from minor disorders like anxiety, mild depression, obsessions, hysteria, etc. It appears to be an estimation towards the lower side.

– 20% to 30% persons coming to primary health care have psychiatric problems.

– Mental disorders are more common in elderly people.

– Suicide rate in India is approximately 10/100,000.

ETIOLOGY OF PSYCHIATRIC DISORDERS

Psychiatric disorders have been conceptualised according to the prevalent thinking of the time. In the earlier period, psychiatric disorders were considered to be due to moral deprivation, or due to antireligious activities. Later, they were considered as due to degeneration of the brain. In earlier part of this century all psychiatric disorders were considered to be caused by psychological or social disturbances.

The last four or five decades have been productive in etiological research and now psychiatric disorders are considered to be multifactorial in origin. The following factors are important in etiology of these disorders.

BIOLOGICAL FACTORS

It is now accepted that large number of psychiatric disorders are associated with aberrations in neurophysiology. These disturbances could be at cellular receptor or at biochemical level. Recent methods of research by brain imaging techniques, have produced wealth of data regarding regional cerebral blood flow and various biochemical changes in different areas of the brain. Though there is as yet no complete consensus regarding the abnormalities in various disorders it is expected, that we may be able to unravel the mystery of psychiatric disorders in the near future.

These disturbances could be due to the following :

a) Genetic factors. Certain genes may be responsible for specific neuro-chemical changes which may lead to a disorder.

b) These changes may be a result of injury or disease of brain, e.g. in drug intoxications, epilepsy and CNS disturbances.

GENETIC FACTORS

Large number of psychiatric disorders show a definite evidence of inheritance, e.g. schizophrenia, manic depressive psychosis and panic disorders.

Evidence for genetic factors is studied in the following manner :

a) To study the prevalence of psychiatric disorders in the first degree relatives of psychiatric patients and compare it with the general population. If the illness has a hereditary influence, then the prevalence should be more in first degree relatives.

b) Twin studies — Monozygotic twins have the same genetic material. If a disorder is purely genetic, then both the monozygotic twins should have hundred per cent similar illness (concordance rate). Dizygotic twin will show similar concordance as seen in brothers and sisters of the proband.

c) Study of adoptees — Many investigators felt that high prevalence of an illness in the brothers and sisters of a patient could be due to similar psychosocial factors. To exclude the effect of similarity of environment, we should study the prevalence of the disorder in the biological and adoptee parents of a sick proband. If the prevalence is higher in biological parents then the role of genetic factors is established ; if it is higher in the adoptee parents, then the role of psychosocial factors is indicated.

d) Linkage studies — Currently linkage studies are being done to identify if the disease gene is linked with certain known genetic markers like blood groups, colour blindness etc.

e) Recently, efforts are being made to identify the specific gene/genes. It is likely to succeed in the near future ; human genome has already been mapped and the chances of identifying specific genes are bright.

Brain Anatomy — Recent brain imaging techniques have produced useful data regarding brain structure in various disorders. There is some evidence of disturbances in brain structure in schizophrenia.

Neurophysiology — Cerebral blood flow and brain metabolism is being studied in various disorders. There is good evidence of changes in brain physiology in various disorders.

BIOCHEMICAL FACTORS

Brain neurones pass messages to each other with the help of certain chemicals, which are called neurotransmitters. Following are common neurotransmitter systems :

i) Acetylcholine.

ii) Monoamines (Noradrenaline, adrenaline, dopamine, 5 Hydroxytryptamine, histamine).

iii) Amino-acids (Gamma Aminobutyric acid (GABA) glycine, glutamate, etc.

iv) Peptides (Encephalins, endorphines etc.).

These neurotransmitters may show abnormality in their production, metabolism or there may be changes in the sensitivity of the receptor system.

These days abnormalities in second order messenger system are also being studied (Cyclic AMP).

Toxin and Poisons — There is also some evidence that certain toxic substances may be generated in the body which may give rise to some disorders, e.g. abnormal proteins in Down's Syndrome. The psychiatric disorder could also be a result of external intoxicant, such as alcohol, opioids, antihypertensives and other drugs acting on brain.

Factors relating to physical disorders — Any disorder which directly or indirectly affects the function of brain may lead to a psychiatric disorder :

a) Infection or trauma to brain.

b) Systemic disorders like uraemia, metabolic disorders, etc.

PSYCHOSOCIAL FACTORS

Psychosocial factors can be divided into the following :

a) Personality.

b) Psychosocial environment.

Personality — Each individual is endowed with a unique personality constellation. Personality is formed by the following :

a) Genetic endowment — Each newborn child has specific genes which determine the range of developmental possibilities. Newborn children have different temperament, few will be quiet, others will be hyperactive. As they grow up, some may easily adapt to grown ups others may show fear of strangers, etc. The genes provide a range of possibilites but their expression will depend on the environment.

b) A child's personality development will also depend upon consistency of parenting, exposure to stress and strains, availability of supports and on his achievements and failures.

A child develops a stable personality by the late adolescence (16-18 years of age) For instance if a child gets proper support from his parents and performs well in school then he is likely to develop a stable and mature personality. While a child who is inconsistently treated by his parents and whose performance in school, is also not good, may develop an anxious personality.

Psychosocial Environment — Many psychiatric disorders may be precipitated by psychosocial disturbances. Some disorders are directly caused by such disturbances when the stress is very severe, as seen in post traumatic stress disorders (e.g. after earthquakes or as seen in Bhopal Gas Tragedy). If stresses are minor but persistent then they can give rise to various adjustment disorders.

In other disorders the role of stress or psychological disturbances may not be so direct but it may only be an associated factor. In many of the psychiatric disorders role of psychosocial environment is of this nature. The effect of these stresses are directly related to the personality of the individual. The personality strength will decide whether a particular stress will precipitate a disorder or not.

Following are the investigative techniques to study the role of psychosocial factors :

1. Personality measurement — Many tests and questionnaires are available to ascertain the type of personality, e.g. 16 Personality factor inventory, Eysenck personality inventory, etc.

Psychological conflicts — These can be studied by various projective tests. The individual projects his problem through these tests. Rorschach ink blot test, Thematic apperception test, Sentence completion test, etc.

Life Event Inventories — Holmes and Rahe adjustment inventory.

SCOPE OF PSYCHIATRY

One of the biggest problems that confronts psychiatry is to define mental health and disorders. However, no universally acceptable definition of either is available. Health can be perceived as absence of disease but the World Health Organisation specifically defines health as the state of complete physical, mental and social well-being and not merely the absence of disease. Other workers try to define health as an average function of people in a group or society. The average functioning may be considered a cultural norm but may not denote health.

Mental health may be defined as a state of creative adjustment with self and others. This definition emphasises adjustment within the self that would imply contentment and satisfaction and a state of harmony with others. The key element is creativeness. The individual should produce something new or novel to be really mentally healthy. This is again an idealistic definition which may not be acceptable to many.

Most of the symptoms of mental disorders may also be present in normal people. Thus the differentiation between illness and normality is basically dependent on the frequency and duration of symptoms. Some symptoms which are only seen in mental disorders like hallucinations and delusions can easily indicate a disorder. In most other situations mental disorders are diagnosed on the basis of the following :

1. The symptoms are too frequent and are out of proportion to the situation, e.g. a person may feel anxious all the time on losing or misplacing an inconsequential object.

2. The symptom should affect the individuals personal life or occupational life, e.g. in the former example, due to anxiety a person may become irritable and may not do his job properly.

3. The duration of symptoms should be prolonged than expected in normal people, e.g. sadness or depression is common after any loss or bereavement, but if it continues to persist for many months, then it will be considered a disorder.

For diagnosis of psychiatric disorders all of the above symptoms should usually be present.

Problems of society, like violence, corruption, discrimination are not the subject matter of psychiatry. Though some psychiatrists may develop expertise on these issues, that is because of their own personal interest and expertise. Similarly, marital problems, problems of criminals or the elderly may require expertise from other fields like sociology, psychology, lawyers etc. and the psychiatrist could be a member of the team.

Psychiatry is primarily concerned with the identification of mental disorders and their treatment and prevention.

METHODS USED IN PSYCHIATRY

Psychiatry primarily relies on psychiatric interview of the patient and his relatives for identifying the disorder. Physical examination is done to find out if there is any evidence of physical impairment or disorder.

Investigation — These could be biological or psychological.

Biological investigation — Includes all investigations done in other branches of medicine with a special emphasis on brain related investigations, e.g. computerised axial tomography of brain, and other recent brain imaging techniques.

Psychological Investigation — There are large number of standardized tests to study intelligence, personality, psychosocial conflicts and signs and symptoms of various disorders.

Treatment — The treatment includes both pharmacological and psychological management. Some patients may require other specialised treatments like elctroconvulsive therapy, brain surgery or occupational and rehabitational methods. The methods of treatment differ from patient to patient.

FUTURE OF PSYCHIATRY

Psychiatry has made rapid strides in the last few decades and the improvement rate in all psychiatric disorders has increased tremendously. Nearly 70% to 80% of these patients show a very good response to this treatment. It is hoped that new researches will be able to unravel the etiology of many of these disorders by which we will be able to plan effective treatment and preventive strategies.

CHAPTER 2

DEFINITIONS OF TERMS USED IN PSYCHIATRY

This chapter provides a comprehensive list of terms used in psychiatry. These terms are repetitively used in this book, as well as in most of the discussions among professionals regarding mental disorders. It is essential for a student in this field to be aware of these terms for proper understanding of this book, as well as to participate in any discussion of diagnosis and management of psychiatric disorders.

I GENERAL TERMS

Psychiatry — A medical speciality concerned with the study of etiology, diagnosis and management of mental disorders.

Psychology — The science which deals with the study of human behaviour in relation to individual's environment.

Clinical Psychology — Application of psychological principles in the understanding of diagnosis, management and prevention of mental disorders.

Psychoanalysis — Psychoanalysis is a system of understanding human behaviour enunciated by Sigmund Freud. It includes :

a) Theory of human psychological development.
b) Method of study of human behaviour.
c) Method of treatment of mental disorders.

Psychopathology — It refers to the precise description of various psychological processes, signs and symptoms of mental disorders.

Psychodynamics—This refers to the description of various intrapsychic forces responsible for the development of a mental disorder. This was primarily emphasised by the psychoanalysts. Currently, this term is also used for describing both intrapsychic as well as interpersonal and social forces responsible for development of mental disorders.

Psyche — It is derived from Greek that means soul. It is used interchangably with mind.

Mind — Mind refers to the functional capacity of the brain. It includes all mental functions : Cognition, Conation and Affect.

Cognition — This refers to the functions of the brain which are concerned with knowledge about the self or the world. This includes intelligence, memory and perception.

Conation — It refers to those functions of mind that are responsible for initiation, continuation and stoppage of all activities. It is also called volition or willing to act.

Affect — It refers to state of feeling which is experienced by the individual all through his waking life. Affect can be of any of the following types — Happy, sad, angry, fearful, irritable, perplexed, etc.

Personality — It refers to the characterstic way of thinking, feeling and behaving of an individual. Each individual has certain unique features in his personality, so that no two individuals have absolutely identical personalities. Yet people can be divided into different personality types. Persons having similar personality types will have predominantly similar behaviour.

Personality Traits — Trait is defined as a generalized predisposition to certain behavioural consistencies. These refer to a group of behaviour which tend to occur together and are usually persistent e.g. shyness, aloofness, assertiveness, etc.

Mental Disorder — This refers to some alterations in psychological functions like thinking, feeling, intelligence or memory which adversely effects an individual's personal, social or occupational life. Social deviance alone without personal dysfunction is not included in mental disorders.

Psychosis — This is defined as a mental condition in which the person is unable to distinguish reality from fantasy. He may act, think and feel in a manner which is not in accordance with reality. A person may walk naked on the road, may feel he is poor while he may have plenty of money, or may feel happy when there is no real reason to do so. Earlier, mental disorders were divided into psychosis and neurosis. It is not done so now because psychosis appears to be related to severity of illness rather than to its etiology.

Neurosis — This term referes to those mental disorders which were characterised by the following :

a) The reality testing is intact and the general behaviour follows social norms.

b) There was also an etiological presumption that such disorders primarily develop due to disturbances in psychological development, mainly due to intrapsychic or interpersonal difficulties.

Mental Health — This is conceptualised in one of

the following ways :

— Absence of mental illness

— Person feels, thinks and behaves like an average person in his group

— Mental health is conceptualised as a state of moral, social and psychological well-being which is associated with the ability to adjust with self and environment in a creative manner.

Syndrome — When a group of symptoms occur together but may be due to different etiologies ; such a cluster of symptoms are called syndromes, (e.g. nephrotic syndrome). Most psychiatric disorders are indeed syndromes.

Disorders — This is a term of convenience. This refers to a group of signs and symptoms occurring together. These may or may not have the same etiology.

Symptoms — Subjective complaints of the patient.

Signs — These are objective findings elicited by clinicians. However, in psychiatry there is an overlap between signs and symptoms because many phenomena can be listed both as symptoms and signs. A patient can complain of hearing voices which is a symptom, while, when a clinician elicits hallucinations during the mental state examination, it becomes a sign. Signs and symptoms of psychiatric disorders can be subdivided into the following :

General Appearance and Motor Behaviour — Motor behaviour of the person is the external expression of his wishes, motivations, drives and instinctual needs. It also indicates his will power (ability to initiate an act or to control it). The following symptoms and signs are included :

1. **Psychomotor agitation** — The person shows excessive motor activity. He cannot sit still and is all the time moving from one place to another. He may show aggressiveness or impulsive behaviour.

2. **Restlessness** — The patient is not as active, as in psychomotor agitation but shows signs in the form of eyes darting, rubbing of his palms or repetitive moving of the limbs. When such symptoms arise in response to intake of phenothiazines, it is called akathisia.

Psychomotor Retardation — This refers to slowing of psychomotor activity. The patients are slow in their speech; spontaneous motor movements are reduced. This may (in extreme form) lead to stupor.

Catatonic Symptoms

Catatonic Stupor — Marked slowing of motor activity leading to complete immobility and inability to speak (mumbles slowly). However, the eyes are open and the patient may show movements of the eye- balls.

Catalepsy — Maintenance of an immobile posture for long time. The patient may continue standing in a place for hours.

Catatonic Excitement — Purposeless motor activity may lead to violence or destructiveness.

Catatonic Posturing — Maintenance of bizzare postures for long periods of time, e.g. a patient used to lie on the bed with his head raised few inches above the pillow for long periods of time. (Psychological pillow).

Waxy Flexibility — The patient's limbs can be put in odd postures and the patient does not revert to a comfortable position. The body may be moulded like wax. Since wax can be moulded into any shape, this condition is known as waxy flexibility.

Echopraxia — The person repeats the movements performed by other person, e.g. if doctor takes out a handkerchief and wipes his face, the patient will repeat the same action.

Echolalia — Repetition of words spoken by the other person, e.g. the doctor asks the patient to tell his name. The patient will put the same question to the doctor.

Cataplexy — Temporary loss of muscle tone leading to slumping down of the person, with no impairment of consciousness.

Stereotypy — Spontaneous and repetitive performance of an act without any purpose.

Perseveration — Repetitive performance of an induced act, e.g. the patient is asked to show his tongue once but he repetitively does the same.

Mannerisms — These are repetitive, goal directed, unusual activities. The person may show unusual movement of hands or face repetitively whenever he initiates conversation. Some workers do not differentiate it from stereotypy.

Automatic Obedience — The person follows the commands of the other even when he is given an option not to follow and even when they are unnecessary or painful, e.g. patient may be asked to show his tongue and the examiner tells him that he is going to prick it with a pin. Ordinarily, people will withdraw the tongue but patients with automatic obedience will not do so.

Mutism — The patient does not speak, though the motor speech functions are normal.

Negativism — The patient does the opposite of what he is told to do. If the examiner asks the patient to open his mouth, he shuts it tightly.

Tics — Spontaneous twiching of a small group of muscles repetitively. These are usually associated with expressive function, e.g. winking of eyes, furrowing of forehead, clearing of throat, raising of shoulders, etc.

Disorders of Consciousness and Orientation

Disorientation — The person is not able to recognise people, place or to identify the hour of the day, date, weekday, month or year.

Clouding of consciousness — The level of consciousness is variable and the patient is not fully oriented and cannot perceive stimulus clearly.

Stupor — This is really not a disturbance of consciousness, as the patient can recall the events which occurred during this state. Stupor is included under the disturbances of consciousness because the patient does not respond to external stimuli.

Delirium — This is a state of variable level of consciousness associated with hallucinations and affective changes.

Coma — The patient is fully unconscious and does not respond to any stimuli.

Somnolence — The patient shows excessive sleepiness but he can be woken up into full consciousness.

Sleep Drunkenness — The patient remains in a half asleep state for long periods of time even after waking up.

Disturbances of Attention and Concentration

Inattention — The patient is not able to attend to a stimuli.

Distractibility (poor concentration) —

The patient is not able to maintain attention on a given task because irrelevant stimuli distracts him (Tested by serial subtraction of 7 from 100).

Hypervigilance and Scanning —

These patients will exhibit rapid shifting of attention and scanning movements of eyes. This state is seen in acute fear and anxiety.

Disturbances in Suggestibility

Suggestion implies uncritical acceptance of an idea or command.

Increased Suggestibility — These patients can accept any suggestion uncritically. Commonly seen in dissociative disorders and organic patients.

Hypnosis — This is a method by which one person can make the other perform activities by suggestion. The second person is totally under the influence of the other. It is due to heightened suggestibility.

Disturbances in Speech

1. **Pressure of Speech** — Rapid flow of speech which may be difficult to interrupt.

2. **Volubility** — Excessive speech which is coherent and logical.

3. **Poverty of Speech** — Patient speaks only few sentences and replies in monosyllables.

4. **Non-spontaneous Speech** — Patient replies only when questions are asked.

5. **Dysprosody** — Loss of normal speech melody.

6. **Stuttering** — Frequent repetition or prolongation of a sound or syllable leading to slow and incomprehensible speech.

Aphasia

Motor Aphasia — The patient understands speech but cannot put the thoughts into word (lesion in Broca's area).

Sensory Aphasia — The patient is unable to understands spoken words. The motor speech functions are normal but the speech becomes incoherent and un-understandable because the patient is not able to understand as to what he is saying (lesion in Wernicke's area).

Nominal Aphasia — The patient is unable to name objects but can tell their use, e.g. if shown a pen he will say it is something to write with.

Thinking — Normal thinking is a goal directed sequential flow of ideas (process) or the content of throughts could become unrealistic.

Disturbances of Thought Process

This group is characterized by disturbances in

association of ideas or intrusion of unrelated material.

Loosening of Associations —

Two segments of thoughts lose their association with each other. This find expression in various ways like incoherence, tangentiality, circumstantiality, derailment etc.

Incoherence — The thoughts are incomprehensible. The sentences are poorly formed and convey no meaning, e.g. A patient describes his problems as, "stars are falling, Ram dead, dog...."

Irrelevance — When the patient's answer is not relevant to the question asked, e.g. what is your name ? Ans. "The world is a wicked place".

Circumstantiality — The patient includes unnecessary details in his answer, though he completes the answer correctly, e.g. "what is your occupation." ? Ans. "There is no point in working these days. Everybody is corrupt. I work in Railways, but the work gives me no pleasure".

Thought Block — The patient stops abruptly in the middle of a sentence or an idea. After a few seconds he may start a new chain of thought. He does not remember what was being said earlier.

Tangentiality — The patient's answer hovers around the correct response but does not reach it. E.g. "what is your income" ? Money is immaterial, why should we work for money ? "Money is the cause of all evil".

Peresveration — The answer to previous question is repeated in response to a new question. E.g. "what is your name" ? "Ans. Shyam". "What is your age" ? "Ans. Shyam".

Derailment — Gradual or sudden shift in the train of thinking. The patient shifts to a new topic.

Verbigeration — Meaningless repetition of a phrase or words "Everyone is dead"' being repeated again and again.

Neologisms — The patient coins new words which have no meaning.

Word Salad — Incoherent mixture of words and phrases.

Flight of Ideas — This is characterized by continuous, excessive speech. The thoughts are connected with each other not by logic but by similarity in meaning, sounds or the patient may respond to unrelated external stimuli. The speech may appear meaningless but close attention can reveal some connections. E.g. one patient saw a rose and said " Roses are beautiful. They have thorns too, the world is full of thorny problems, Hanuman is the saviour. Jai Hanuman". This statement shows shifting of ideas from rose to thorn, thorn to problems in life and then to the saviour.

Clang Association — When words of similar sound are associated. They usually do not have any logical connection.

Shy, try, fry.

Rhymimg — Let us go to bazaar, Eat Achar etc.

Disorders of Content of Thinking

1. Poverty of Thought — Thoughts provide very little information because there are very few thoughts or there are vagueness or meaningless repetitions.

2. Delusions — False beliefs not based on external reality cannot be corrected by reason and are not consistent with patient's socio-cultural background. E.g. If in a village everybody believes that there is a spirit on a peepul tree, it will not be called a delusion as it is a shared belief. On the contrary, if a person believes inspite of all persuasion that a group of people are trying to kill him while no one else in his family or social group shares this idea, will be called a delusion. Delusions can be divided into various types according to their contents.

Paranoid Delusions — These include delusions of reference, persecution and grandiosity.

1. Delusions of Reference — These are fixed beliefs where a person feels that the actions of others have meaning for him. These must be differentiated from the ideas of reference where a person feels that others are looking at him or talking about him, but he at the same time retains insight that it may not be so, while in delusions the person is convinced that others are talking about him. E.g. programmes in T.V. or radio discuss him, everyone on the road stares at him, etc.

Delusions of Persecution — The patient feels that other people are planning to harm him, or harm people close to him. E.g. a patient believed that people belonging to other castes were trying to kill him and his family.

Delusion of Grandeur — These persons believe that they have immense wealth, power or they hold positions of importance. E.g. one patient held a fixed belief that he is the prime-minister designate of India and he has to go to New Delhi to take the oath.

Delusion of Infidelity — The person believes that his spouse is unfaithful to him and has an illicit relationship. E.g. A patient accused his wife of having illicit relationship with every male person she came in contact with, including her own father.

Erotomania — Delusional belief that other person is deeply in love with him or her. This other person usually belongs to higher socio-economic status.

Bizarre Delusions — These persons have unusual and fantastic beliefs, e.g. men from the moon have invaded the earth ; or all mankind will turn into dogs, etc.

Delusions of Guilt — The person falsely believes that he has done some thing wrong and sinful act for which he is being punished.

Nihilistic Delusions — These persons believes that the self or the world is non-existing or is going to end. One female patient believed that she was already dead.

Somatic Delusions — These persons believes that functioning of certain parts of their body have become defective. They may believe that their brain is rotting, their abdomen is empty, etc.

Delusions can also be divided into mood congruent/incongruent. When the content of delusion is in harmony with the mood of the individual, these are called congruent, and when not so, they are called mood incongruent, eg. a sad patient may have delusions of guilt or poverty. These will be called mood congruent.

If a sad patient had delusions of grandeur that he has lots of money then these will be called mood incongruent.

Over Valued Ideas — One particular idea or group of thoughts become all important for a person, though the person is aware of his excessive concern with these ideas, eg. an unmarried girl became sc preoccupied with the idea of will happen to her parents after she got married, that she refused all marriage proposals. The marriage was being arranged by her parents themselves and there was no real problem for them.

Preoccupation — The person is preoccupied with a group of ideas for long periods. This may be a suicidal, homicidal or any other thought and the person is aware of the realistic situation and may try to control this preoccupation.

Delusion of Control (Thought Alienation) — These patients feel that their thoughts, actions or moods are not their own, and are being controlled by other forces external to them.

Thought Withdrawal — The patient feels that his thoughts are being removed or stolen by other forces. One patient felt that his thoughts are being stolen by his former teacher who wanted him to marry his daughter.

Thought Insertion — The patient believes that some of the thoughts are not his own but are being implanted in his mind by some external agency, e.g. one patient believes that thoughts are being implanted in his mind through the help of transmitters. He even went to a neuro-surgeon to get this transmitter removed.

Thought Broadcasting — The patient feels that all his thoughts become known to others by some means. A female patient firmly believed that all her past is known to everyone in town. Due to this fear she could not attend any social gathering.

Thought Control — The person believes that his thoughts are being controlled by an external agency. It could be an evil spirit, CBI or some such other force.

Hypochondriasis — Preoccupation with somatic symptoms of disease but the patient maintains insight and the preoccupation with somatic symptoms is not of delusional intensity.

Obsession — These are characterized by :

a) Recurrent irresistible thoughts coming to one's mind ;

b) The person knows that they are his own thoughts, and that they are wrong ;

c) He cannot control them by logic and any attempt at doing so leads to anxiety.

E.g. a patient used to get repetitive obscene ideas whenever he saw pictures of goddesses. He knew these thought was wrong but could not stop them and felt very distressed at having such thoughts.

Compulsion — These are characterized by ;

a) Repetitive acts ;

b) The person performing it knows that it is wrong, but does so to avoid some future anxiety or bad happenings ;

c) Any attempt to stop these acts leads to severe tension and anxiety.

Coprolalia — Compulsive utterance of obscene words or abuses.

Phobia — This is defined as pathological dread of some object or situation resulting in attempts to avoid them (fear of going out, of heights, lizards, stage, etc.)

a) Simple Phobia - Fear of some discrete objects (e.g. spiders, lizards, etc.)

b) Social Phobia - Fear of rejection or humiliation in social situations (meeting a small group of people, member of opposite sex, etc.)

c) Acrophobia — Fear of heights.

d) Agoraphobia such — Fear of going out.

e) Claustrophobia — Fear of closed spaces.

f) Zoophobia — Fear of animals.

Disturbances of Perception — Perception is a process by which an individual gives meaning to a sensory stimulus. Common perceptual disorders are :

a) Hallucination — These are perceptions without an external stimulus. Hallucinations can be divided according to the sense modality involved.

Auditory Hallucinations — False perception of voices or sounds.

Visual Hallucination — False perception of images or figures.

Olfactory Hallucinations — False perception of smell. Common in organic disorders.

Gustatory Hallucinations — False perception of taste.

Tactile Hallucinations — False perception of sensation on the skin, e.g. insects crawling on skin.

Synesthesia — One sensation trigger of perception in other sense modality. E.g. person may experience that he can see voices or feel that he can hear a scene.

EMOTIONS

There are feeling states like happiness, sadness, anger, fear, etc. When one state feeling of persists for sometime, it is called mood.

Mood is a persistent state of feeling. The person usually describes it as happy or sad. A person with a sad or happy mood can show other emotions also but these are usually transitory, e.g. a depressed person may be able to laugh at a joke. This laughter is usually transitory. Mood can be of the following types :

Dysphoria — An unpleasant mood may be associated with sadness, apprehension or fear.

Euthymia — Normal range of mood.

Expansive Mood — The person expresses his feeling vividly and without restraints. This feeling is usually of happiness.

Irritability — Person gets annoyed repetitively on trifles.

Euphoria — Feeling of intense happiness and grandeur.

Ecstasy — Person feels intense pleasure of divine or heavenly experiences.

Depression — Persistent feelings of sadness which are excessive to situation.

Anhedonia — Inability to feel pleasure. It is experienced as painful by the person, e.g. patients usually complain that they are not able to enjoy anything.

Grief — Normal reaction of sadness or mourning following a severe loss (death of near ones).

Alexithymia — Person is unable to experience feelings.

Anxiety — Feeling of apprehension caused by anticipation of difficulty or danger, usually unknown.

Fear — Anxiety caused by a specific situation or object.

Agitation — Severe anxiety associated with motor restlessness.

Tension — Increased muscular tension of presumably psychological origin.

Panic — Acute anxiety associated with a feeling of impending death or disaster associated with autonomic symptoms.

Apathy — Lack of emotional response.

Ambivalence — Existence of two opposing feeling states towards the same person at the same time, e.g. loving and hating the father at the same time.

Affect — This is the external experience of emotions which is inferred from facial expressions, body movements and speech.

Appropriate Affect — When the affect is in harmony with thoughts and actions of the individuals, e.g. patient is talking of happy events and shows affect of happiness.

Inappropriate Affect — The affect is not in harmony with the thought process or activities, e.g. a person is talking of sad things but smiling.

Constricted Affect — The range and depth of emotion is decreased. The person does not exhibit normal joyfulness or sadness but gives restricted and superficial responses.

Flat Affect — The experience of emotions is severely restricted. Patient shows very little emotional response.

Labile — The affect swings rapidly from one state to another. The patient who was laughing a moment back, suddenly starts crying. It is typically seen in organic brain diseases.

Diurnal Variation — The mood may show worsening either in the morning or in the evening.

ORGANIC BRAIN FUNCTIONS

Memory — This is the ability to register, store and recall events when desired.

Memory disturbances can be of the following types :

Amnesia — The inability to recall past events, completely or partially.

Anterograde Amnesia — The inability to remember current events.

Post-traumatic Amnesia — Amnesia following head injury. It includes memory loss after the injury.

Retrograde Amnesia — This refers to loss of memory of events prior to the head injury and may extend from few minutes to months.

Confabulation — Filling up memory gaps with false material.

De ja vu — A new situation appears to be familiar as if he has experienced it earlier.

Jamais vu — Feeling of unfamiliarity with a situation which has been experienced earlier.

Intelligence — It refers to the person's ability to utilize previous learning for constructively adapting to new situation. The disorders of intelligence are as follows :

Mental Retardation — When intelligence has not been either developed properly or the development has been retarded due to some organic or psychological factor. This develops before 16 years of age. These patients are unable to accomplish tasks which are appropriate to their age.

Levels of retardation :

Mild — I.Q. 50 - 69
Moderate — I.Q. 35 - 49
Severe — I.Q. 20 - 34
Profound — I.Q. less than 20

Intelligence Quotient

This is a ratio derived by the following formula

$$\frac{\text{Mental age}}{\text{Chronological age}} \times 100$$

if Mental age = 4

$$\text{E.g.} \quad \frac{4}{8} \times 100 = 50$$

and Chronological age = 8

I.Q. = 50

* Chronological age above 16 years is always taken as baseline, to find the Intelligence Quotient.

Dementia — Deterioration of intelligence after normal development. Dementia is always caused by neuropathological changes.

Pseudo-dementia — Some patients of depression may clinically exhibit signs of intellectual deterioration though there is no pathological change in brain.

Dyscalculia — Inability to calculate.

Dysgraphia — Inability to write properly.

Anosognosia — Inability to recognise that one has an illness.

Autotopognosia — Inability to recognise ones own body parts.

Concrete Thinking — The patient is not able to abstract concepts and can only speak in concrete terms.

Abstract Thinking — Patient is able to abstract commonness or differences between objects and can draw inference from proverbs.

The insight — Ability to understand that one is ill.

The judgement — Ability to take appropriate decision in a given situation.

CHAPTER 3

PSYCHIATRIC HISTORY AND EXAMINATION

Psychiatric evaluation primarily consists of history and mental status examination of the individual. Psychiatric history is of crucial importance as the majority of the patients would have exhibited many symptoms during the course of the illness which might not be present at the time of the examination. Many a times, the diagnoses may solely rest on history. Thus, it is of fundamental importance to learn to obtain psychiatric history systematically.

The Interview :

Psychiatric consultation or the interview is different from other medical disciplines because we wish to obtain information about the patient's problems, both physical and psychological, his life-long experiences, interests, hobbies, problems, interpersonal or intrapersonal difficulties, job stresses and other miscellaneous problems and assets, which may contribute towards the development or maintenence of the problem and may be useful for management.

Setting of the Interview :

The interview should be conducted in a separate room, where repeated interruptions should not take place, e.g. telephone ringing, persons and patients coming in, etc. All these interruptions will disrupt the flow of interview. The people outside the room should not be able to overhear the conversation. This will ensure confidentiality. The seating arrangement could be around a table. It is better to seat the patient on the righthand side of the table so that the doctor can restrain the patient, if need arises. The table should not have loose objects which could be used by the patient as missiles. The chairs should be comfortable. If any recording devices are used, the patient should be informed, e.g. "I am tape recording this interview, do I have your permission? or, I will be taking notes of this interview, I hope you will agree to it". If the patient refuses the use of recording devices he must be convinced of its need. He should be told that it will help the doctor to remember his problems later and will also help in planning proper treatment.

Interview process involves the following :

a) Doctor

b) Patient

c) Relatives and friends.

a) **Doctor** — The doctor will require training for becoming a skilled interviewer. Interviewing skills involve the following :

i) **Personality of the Doctor**

The doctors should have same kinds of personalities that are seen in the general population and they will also have their emotional problems, prejudices and preferences. Due to these personality problems, doctors may react inappropriately to the patient. The training should include learning about their own reactions and to develop certain therapeutically conducive temperamental qualities. These qualities are

Learn to understand that different people can approach a problem in different ways and each of these approaches may be correct for the given individual, e.g. the therapist may like to respond to a minor insult by retaliation, while one patient may like to tell the involved person quietly that his behaviour was not correct, another may withdraw and yet another may store the insult for future retaliation. All these responses can be appropriate depending on who is insulting, what the situation is, and what is the personality type.

The doctor should learn about his own prejudices and moral stance and should not evaluate others on his personal scale, eg. his prejudice can be against other religions, against people who tell lies, or steal, etc.

The doctor should learn to respect his patients, their beliefs and life styles.

He should develop the capacity to empathise with the patient and be able to put himself in the patient's place and should be able to understand their thoughts, feelings and actions.

He should be able to understand his own countertransference towards the patient (countertransference means that the doctor is not really reacting to the patient but he is reacting to his own earlier experiences with similar people in the past. E.g. If his father had been punitive, or wife nagging, he may transfer these qualities to every elderly man or married woman.)

He should have the patience to listen and should not interrupt needlessly. Humour or jokes should be avoided till such time a good relationship has been established.

The Patient — The patients can be divided into the following categories :

a) The patient who has sought consultation himself ;

b) Who has been brought by his family members against his wish ;

c) Referred by other agencies like the police, employer or by other doctors ;

d) Violent and stupurous or non-communicative patients.

a) Patient who has sought consultation himself :

This patient considers himself to be psychologically disturbed and is usually prepared to discuss his problems with the doctors. However, the following questions usually bothers him.

What he should tell which can help him ;
What he should not tell ;
Will the doctor have enough time to listen to him ;
Is the doctor reliable and will he maintain confidentiality ;
His anxiety, fear or depression may not allow him to communicate freely.

His personality will influence his narrative, e.g. the obsessive may go in excessive details, and paranoids may try to be secretive. The doctor has to guide the patient regarding the content of his communications. He should be able to tell the patient that, not everything in the minutest detail need to be told but, typical examples of his problem, the antecedent events and the outcome only. If any further information is required, the interviewer will ask questions. He must also tell the patient how much time he can spare for this interview and it is not essential that everything should be told in the first interview. He should also assure the patient regarding the confidentiality of the communication.

If the patient is anxious or fearful or depressed, it is always useful to try to put him at ease and he can be informed that he should not worry if he cannot recall everything because other things could be discussed later.

b) Patients who are brought against their wishes by the family members :

Such patients will usually be hostile or suspicious and may not volunteer information. They should be clearly told that the doctor will like to hear their side of the story and no decision regarding the treatment would be taken without hearing them in detail. Such patients should be interviewed alone (in the absence of relatives). It is good practice to interview them first and then talk to the relatives.

c) Referred by other agencies (Police, Employers, Courts and other Doctors) :

Such persons are usually apprehensive. They may often have a feeling that they are not mentally sick but the referring agency and the consulting doctor may declare them insane. These fears of the patients have to be put at rest. They must be informed that they will be examined only with their consent and the result of the examination will be communicated to them. They should also be informed that, every patient seen by a psychiatrist is not necessarily insane and the majority of the patients have only minor anxieties, fears or depressions.

However, patients referrred by courts or police may have to be examined against their will. The examination report has to be sent to the concerned authorities.

d) Violent, stuporose or noncommunicative patients :

These cannot be interviewed in the normal manner. These patients have to be observed and the observations recorded.

(Details described later)

Relatives — Most of the patients are brought by their relatives in India. The relatives are usually decisive in treatment acceptance. The relatives should be interviewed either alone or in the presence of the patient. The information rendered by the relatives should be checked by asking counter questions and the effort should be made to develop a consistent sequence of the events. The relatives may sometimes suppress information or exaggerate certain aspects, and the doctor has to be cautious and must understand the motives of the informants.

Reliability of the Information :

This is assessed by the following :

a) The intelligence and observational consistency of the informants ;

b) The duration of the stay with the patient. The informant can give reliable account of the period when he was living with the patient. The account of other periods will depend on hearsay.

c) Motivation — One will have to look at the motivation of the informant. If he is concerned about the patient, he is likely to give a correct account. If he is prejudiced or fed up with the patient, then he may exaggerate the negative points.

d) If the accounts of two different informants are consistent then the information is likely to be reliable. If the accounts of two different informants is divergent then both the versions are recorded separately.

Plan of History Taking

History taking is divided into the following sections :

Identifying Data :

Name, Age, Sex, Education, Occupation, Income, Residential Address, Office Address, Type of family (Nuclear/Joint/Extended) Case No.

a) Name of the informants and their relationship with the patient.

b) Chief complaints.

The patient should be asked the reason for consultation. His complaints should be recorded in chronological order, i.e. the longest duration first and shortest duration last. It is advisable to record the complaints in the vernacular, i.e. in the patient's own words. In case the patient emphasises on one or two complaints as the most important or as the main reasons for seeking help, they should be specified by underlining.

If the patient says that he has no complaints, this should also be recorded. The complaints should also be asked from the relatives or other informants and these should be recorded separately. They should also be recorded with duration and in the chronological order. The most distressing complaints should be specified.

History of Present Illness — It can be divided into the following :

Time and type of Onset — The patients and the relatives should be asked the exact time of onset of disorder. If they are not able to pinpoint a date, then they may be asked to grossly specify when was the patient fully well. The onset is divided into the following :

Acute Onset — When the illness starts acutely and florid clinical picture develops within two weeks.

Subacute Onset — When the illness has developed within 4 weeks but exact date cannot be specified.

Insidious Onset — When the illness has developed imperceptibly and the patient or the relatives are not able to pinpoint the time in days or weeks but state that the illness has gradually developed over a period of few months.

The present episode of illness should have been clearly separated from other episodes by a period of 3 months of symptoms free period or minimal symptoms.

Prodromal Symptoms :

Often the patient and the relatives notices abrupt changes in behaviour and minor disturbances prior to the onset of distinct symptoms which are ignored. It is always good clinical practice to specifically ask whether the patient showed some minimal changes in his behaviour prior to the development of clearcut symptoms, e.g. changes in daily routine, poor appetite, disturbances in sleep, lack of interest in work or studies, irritability, etc. Many patients will exhibit prodromal symptoms for weeks or months prior to the onset of florid illness.

Precipitating Factors :

Many psychiatric disorders are associated with stressors at the time of the onset of the disorders. These stressors could be psychological or biological. It is essential to elicit whether any such factors were operating within 3 months prior to the onset of illness. Quite often, the patients and the relatives are defensive and suppress information in this area. It is always better to ask about these problems after the history of present illness has been obtained and while personal and family history is being asked for. The questions could be framed differently. Rather than asking whether there were some difficulties/problems at the time of onset, one should enquire who all were living at home at that time, what was the routine of the family, where the patient was working, how was his job performance and so on. The aim is not to emphasise the association between illness and psychological factors but to try and elicit their quality independently.

Development of Symptoms :

Recent diagnostic approaches are based on symptom, severity, duration and amount of distress it produces to the individual. Therefore, it is essential to clearly identify each symptom for its quality, frequency, duration and distress caused by it. For instance, if a patient complains of sadness of mood, then the interviewer should ask the following questions :

Since when has the sadness started ;

Was it the first symptom to occur or did some other problem lead to it ;

Does it remain everyday and its frequency ;

How severe is the sadness — tolerable, can do some work ; no work is possible, stays secluded and so on ;

How it affects his personal/social life ;

Are there any day to day variations.

Similar questions should be asked for every symptom.

It may be difficult for a beginner to ask all the relevant questions to each patient but experience and familiarity with psychiatric illnesses will help the individuals to develop proficiency in this area.

Quite often the presenting symptoms could be a manifestation of other psychiatric disorders, so it is mandatory to rule out other disorders by asking the following questions :

Organic Disorders

Does the patient have difficulty in remembering, whether it is only for recent events or is global or for a specific period ;

Can the patient do various intellectual tasks as efficiently as earlier ;

Were there any periods when the patient was confused or disoriented (could not recognise people, place or time, was in altered state of consciousness);

Any other neurological problem.

Drug Abuse

Does the patient use any drugs or intoxicant ? If so, what is the nature of the drugs/intoxicants, frequency of use, amount and effect ;

Duration of use ;

Any evidence of drug- related physical or psychological problems.

Schizophrenia and Related Disorders

Does the patient feel people are conspiring against him, or are talking about him ;

Is he suspicious of others ;

Does he show repetitive episodes of purposeless excitement or withdrawl ;

Is he fearful or depressed without any cause ;

Can he think clearly and respond adequately to questions ;

Does he feel that his thoughts are being stolen/ implanted by other agencies?

Mood Disorders

Does the patient feel elated, happy and excited ;

Does he make wild schemes and plans ;

Does he spend excessively and purposelessly (or there may be very little purpose) ;

Talks excessively ;

Feels he is very rich or powerful ;

Does he feel depressed most of the time without much cause ;

Are there feelings of hopelessness and worthlessness ;

Suicidal ideation and attempts.

Phobic and Other Stress Related Disorders

Does the patient have excessive fear of situations such as going out of home, travelling, heights, dark places, stage and meeting people etc.

Does the patient feel anxious and apprehensive and if so, how often. Is it due to some other condition or is it independent of other problems.

Does the patient get some recurrent ideas or doubts in mind which he feels are wrong but cannot resist, e.g. fear of dirt, contamination, repetitive checking of locks, bolts, etc.

Multiple Somatic Symptoms Persisting for Long Periods Without Any Physical Basis.

Excessive or reduced appetite.

Vague bodily symptoms, which do not conform to any diagnostic pattern.

Any sexual difficulty or problem, like homosexuality.

Lack of interest or decreased desire for sex.

Difficulty in erection or ejaculation.

Difficulty in obtaining orgasm in females.

These are some of the questions which may indicate the presence of other disorders in addition to the presenting symtoms. In case there is any evidence of these disorders then one should ask further questions to confirm whether this is an additional disorder or basic disorder.

Treatment Taken and Response

Obtain details of treatment taken and response to treatment; whether allopathic or some other system of medicine including faith healing have been used. Ask for drugs, dosage, duration of treatment and patients compliance and response.

Always ask for history of weight loss, menstrual difficulties. Obtain pattern of sleep. There may be difficulty in falling asleep, difficulty in remaining asleep or early morning awakening. There could also be distortion in sleep-wake cycle, e.g. delayed cycle. Patients sleep at 1-2 AM and sleeps till 11 AM, or there could be a phase reversal, the patient is awake at night and sleeps in the day.

Past Medical and Psychiatric History

Information must be obtained about any prolonged physical illness, neurological illness, head injury or other illnesses which may have associated psychiatric dysfunctions.

Patients should also be asked for any history of mental illness in the past, either of similar nature or of any other symptomatology. Questions given under present history may be asked to elicit symptoms. If there is history of psychiatric disorder available, the following information should be obtained :

Time of onset and duration.

Symptomatology.

Treatment and response.

Also obtain the information about the interval period—whether the patient was completely normal, or were there some residual symptoms ; whether the patient has shown any change in social or occupational functioning.

Family History

This includes the family of origin, i.e. the patient's parents, siblings, grandparents, etc.

The information should be obtained about the following :

a) Pedigree chart showing the patient his siblings, parents and grandparents on both sides.

b) Any evidence of mental illness in the family . The same questions can be repeated as given under present history.

Family History and Support System

Is the family nuclear or joint. Most of the families in India now have a nuclear living but with close dependence on joint family for economic and social decision making. It is essential to find out whether the joint family is :

Supportive.

Censoring and disruptive.

Neutral.

What was the family interaction when the patient was a child and current interactional patterns.

What is the nature of family support available now

Any familial assests.

Personality of parents and significant others who are interacting with the patient.

Socio-economic status.

Income (total).

Occupation of employed members of the family.

Any other relevant information.

Personal History

The aim of the personal history is to obtain developmental information both for psychological and physical development. For sake of convenience the history is divided into subsections.

PERSONAL HISTORY — DEVELOPMENTAL INFORMATION

Physical	Psychological
Prenatal and birth :	
H/O any disease during pregnancy, drug intake or exposure to radiation	Planned and wanted pregnancy or not
Any attempt at termination of pregnancy	Any psychological problem during pregnancy
Delivery normal or by Caesarian section and whether labour was prolonged	Response to sex of child.
	Neutral/feelings of regret

PERSONAL HISTORY — DEVELOPMENTAL INFORMATION

Child cried soon after birth, was the child blue

Birth weight

Infancy

Milestones of development
Head holding — 3 months
Sitting — 6 months
Walking — 12 months
Speaking few words —18 months
Full sentences — 24 months

Quiet/fretful
Smiles at mother at age of 3 months
Responds to family members with happiness/shows poor response

Early Childhood
Stable sleep pattern

Weaning (initiation to solid food)
Easy / difficult

Toilet training, at what age
Physical health during childhood
Repeated illnesses

Persistent maladaptive behaviour
Temper tantrum
child becomes excessively disturbed if his wishes are not fulfilled, lies down on the ground and starts crying or shouting - (occasional is normal, persistent may indicate adjustment difficulties)
Bed wetting beyond 5 years of age
Nail biting
Night terror (sudden awakening at night with marked fear, may cry and shout, goes to sleep afterwards)

Childhood and Adolescence
General Health
Development of secondary sexual characteristics
Menarche in women and menstrual cycle
Changing voice, growing of beard and increase in size of penis in males

Age at schooling/whether it is normal for that group
Reaction to school
Relationship with teachers, school mates
Interest in extracurricular activities
School performance
Excellent/Average/Poor/ deteriorating/fluctuating/steady.

Highest level of education achieved
satisfied with

PERSONAL HISTORY — DEVELOPMENTAL INFORMATION

Menstrual history
Pain or difficulty in coitus
Health of the spouse

Middle Age
Physical health-any diseases

Achievement/frustration
Did use unfair means in examination
Any evidence of fear of examination
Psychological response to success or failure

Adolescent Sexuality
Did the patient accept his gender role (masculinity/femininity) or he/she behaved opposite to her gender role

What sexual practices he or she performed (Masturbation, homosexuality, heterosexual relations)
Any guilt or anxiety associated with it
How knowledge of sex was obtained.

Occupation
What job he or she has,
Satisfied/dissatisfied
Steady job/frequent changes
Relationship with superiors, colleagues and inferiors

Marital and Sexual History
Age at marriage — age of spouse
Arranged by parents with consent of the patient/against his consent by self-choice with parental consent or without it

Marital relationship
Sexual relationship satisfactory/ if not what are the problems

Children — Their ages and sex
Parent-child relationship
Problems with children

Religion
Level of faith/
Obvious prejudices

Reaction to middle age
happy and satisfied/worried
causes of worries

PERSONAL HISTORY — DEVELOPMENTAL INFORMATION

Old Age

Physical health	Level of family and social supports
Sensory deficits	Economic status
	Attitude to old age
	Active and occupied
	Passes time aimlessly

Premorbid Personality

The aim is to find typical personality profile of the patient prior to the onset of his illness. If his illness has started in childhood or adolescence, then one can only describe temperament, as personality crystallizes only after maturity. For finding out about the personality one should always confirm the patient's statement from the relatives. Many times, when illness has been long, the relatives and patient may contaminate premorbid personality description by including post-illness behaviour. The following traits should be enquired for delineating the personality of the individual. If these traits are minimal or mild, it will then be called a **personality** but if they have affected his social or occupational activities it should then be called a **personality disorder**. Generally, each person may have a combination of various personality traits.

These patients will show the following traits :

Paranoid Personality

Excessive sensitiveness to insults
Excessive suspiciousness
Excessive feelings of self-importance

Schizoid Personality

Emotional indifference with limited capacity to express warmth or anger
Likes to stay aloof
Only has one or two friends, avoids social contacts

Dissocial Personality

Unconcern for the feelings of others
Incapability to maintain long-term relationships
Antisocial behaviour — (persistent lying, repetitive stealing, promiscuous sexuality, etc.)
Does not feel guilty or anxious
Does not learn from experience

Emotionally Unstable (Borderline Personality)

-Acts impulsively without consideration of consequences — patient's aims are unclear

Feeling of emptiness, may have multiple intense, unstable and unsatisfactory relationships.

Histrionic Personality

Dramatization and exaggerated expression of emotions
Wants to be the centre of attraction
May show seductive behaviour
Dresses flashily and takes extra care of physical appearance
Cannot form stable relationships

Anankastic (Obsessive) personality

Preoccupation with details, perfectionist
Very cautious in all activities
Markedly concerned with work and performance
Rigidity of time
Excessive cleanliness and orderliness.

Anxious (avoidant) personality

Persistent feeling of anxiety or apprehensiveness
Feels he is inferior and will not be liked by others
Therefore avoids social contacts unless certain of being liked

Dependant personality

They feel secure only if involved in a dependant relationship

They may give in to other person beyond normal requirements because of fear of being abandoned

All decisions are taken by the person on whom the patient is dependant

Feels anxious if the relationship breaks.

Most patients will show a mixture of personality traits from different personality types, e.g. a person may show some avoidant personality traits and minimal dependant personality traits.

Check List

Check whether all items of history have been

adequately covered. If there are any deficiencies, then write them here for completion or confirmation subsequently.

Physical Examination

Patients should be thoroughly examined to find out the presence of organic diseases.

General Examination

Cardiovascular system examination
Gastro intestinal system examination
Respiratory system examination
Neurological examination
Bones and joints
Skin

Mental Status Examination (MSE)

The aim of the mental status examination is to find out disturbances in any of the psychological functions of the patient. Though disturbance in one area can effect functioning in the other, this schemata is used to identify disturbances in different areas without reference to etiology. Generally, the M.S.E. should include only the findings at the time of examinations but quite often, symptoms experienced earlier are also included. Generally, one should include all signs exhibited in the past seven days, it is sometimes extended to the past one month or for the period of the current episode. The duration of observations included should be specified.

General Appearance and Behaviour

This should be described in short sentences which will make it easily understandable.

Appearance

Describe the patient's physical appearance (approximate height, weight, looks). How is he dressed, (describe his dress, its neatness and appropriateness to socio-economic level). Describe posture (way of standing, walking, sitting and lying)

Behaviour and Psychomotor Activities

Motor behaviour — He may show slowness of motor movement, or there could be excessive motor activity. He may show certain abnormal motor movements, e.g.

Tics — sudden, repetitive, purposeless movements of small group of muscles usually associated with initiation of an act, e.g. winking of eyes, repetitive contraction of shoulders, repetitive coughing

Grimacing — making inappropriate facial movements

Stereotypy — These are a spontaneous repetitive abnormal movements.

Perseveration — It is senseless repetition of goal directed movement, e.g. the patient is asked to stretch his hands and he repetitively does the same.

Relationship with the Examiner

How does the patient relate with the examiner (cooperative, hostile, suspicious, fearful, etc.). Can the examiner establish rapport with the patient (Rapport refers to the examiner's ability to share the feelings and thinking of the patient).

Consciousness

Whether the patient is fully alert and conscious. Consciousness implies awareness of the surroundings and ablity to interact with others. Few patients may show fluctuating consciousness — they may be fully aware and alert at one moment and may show inattentiveness in the next. Other patients may be fully unconscious (not responding to any stimuli), few may be partly unconscious, e.g. responding to painful stimuli or responding to a loud command.

Orientation

Is the patient aware of the time, place and person? He should be asked which place is this, what is the time now, which day, date, month or year. He should be asked to name and identify his relatives and the doctor (if familiar). Disturbances in orientation are usually seen in organic illnesses.

Attention and Concentration

Attention is defined as the ability to attend to an external stimulus. The patient should be able to respond, whenever a question is asked. If he can respond, one will conclude that attention is arousable. Patient's with organic illness, severe depressive disorder, dissociative disorder and stuporous conditions may not respond to external stimuli.

Concentration

This is defined as the ability to attend to a given task for a given period of time. It is usually tested by asking the patient to serially subtract 7 from 100 till the lowest number is reached. The norms for this test are not available. Intelligence, education and previous training will affect the performance. A normal individual should be able to perform this task in approximately 2 minutes with 2 mistakes.

Patients who cannot do this test because of poor education can be asked to do one of the following :

a) Serial subtraction of 3 from 20
b) Naming days of the week backwards
c) Counting from 20 backwards.

A conclusion can be drawn by the number of mistakes and time taken.

Mood and Affect

Mood refers to a sustained feeling state. A person may feel anxious, happy or depressed in response to a situation. If the state of anxiety, fear or depression, etc, persists for a period of time then it is called mood. This is the subjective experience of the patient. The patient will usually volunteer statements like, 'I feel sad most of the time, or anxious, fearful, irritable, angry, feel empty or feel no emotions at all.

Affect

This is the external expression of feeling state. It is inferred from facial expression, speech, body movements, etc. Affect is observed by the examiner as happy, sad, fearful, irritable, angry or hostile, etc. The affect can be congruous to the mood, e.g. the patient says he is sad and appears to be sad or incongruent to the mood, e.g. the patient says he is sad but he is smiling. Affect can be labile when it swings from one extreme to another within moments with or without any stimuli.

Affect is also described as within the normal range, i.e. normal changes of emotions are seen during interview.

Constricted Affect — When the range and intensity of emotional experience is reduced.

Blunted or Flat Affect — These patients show reduction of emotional expression. The sadness and happiness appear restricted in range and intensity.

Flat Affect — It implies virtual absence of emotions. The patient may neither express any feeling verbally or by expression.

Appropriateness — One has to observe whether the patient's emotional responses are appropriate to his thinking and situation. The patient may start laughing when talking of sad things.

Perceptual Disturbances

Perception refers to the process of giving a meaning to an external stimuli. Perception includes sensation and its interpretation. Common perceptual disorder is hallucination.

Hallucination — It is defined as perception without a stimuli. The person may hear a voice when no one is speaking, or see things when the thing is not present, smell nonexistent odours, feel taste when nothing is being eaten, or feels sensation on the skin when nothing is there.

Hallucinations should be described under the following heads.

Location	—	Sense modality and whether unilateral or bilateral
Elementary	—	Flashes of light, unformed voices
Content	—	Content of hallucination should be described
Level of	—	Fully conscious, or hallucination occur only while patients are going to sleep or waking up from sleep or in altered states of consciousness , e.g. during drug intoxication, delirium.
Frequency	—	How often do they occur
Any precipitaing stimulus		
Patients Response	—	Do they appear fearful or enjoy them/or are indifferent

Hallucination should originate from outside the body and should not be under patients voluntary control.

Illusions

It refers to misinterpretation of existing stimuli due to environmental conditions or the patients mental state. A rope in the dark may be mistaken as a snake. An apprehensive person walking in the night may mistake shadows for persons following him. Illusion is a normal phenomenon.

Speech

Describe the motor aspects of speech. Speech can be slow, fast, excessive, monotonous, loud, whispered or ununderstandable. Stuttering or stammering should also be included here.

Thought

Normal thinking is a sequentially connected stream of thought which leads to a goal. Thoughts are divided into thought process ; and content of thinking.

Thought Process

It refers to the way in which thoughts are organized and are associated with each other. Disturbances in thought process are the following :

Incoherent and irrelevant thinking
Flight of ideas
Tangentiality
Circumstantiality
Word salad
Neologism
Thought blocking
Vague thinking
Punning and clang associations

These are described in detail in chapter on definitions of terms.

Content of Thought

This refers to what the patient is thinking about. Common disorders are :

Delusions
Over valued ideas
Obsessions
Phobias
Suicidal or homicidal thoughts
Ideas of reference and influence
Poverty of content

The details of these are described in chapter on definition of terms.

The examiner should note the predominant content of the patient's thought.

For description of thought, one should record verbatim account of the question asked and the patient's response to it. One should infer disorders of thinking from these verbatim examples.

Memory

The patient's ability to recall previous and current experiences is evaluated here. Memory is traditionally recorded in the following areas.

Remote Memory

Can the patient recall events of the past life correctly or not. The patient could be asked about personal information like year of marriage, year of passing high school, etc., if an informant is available. If no informant is available then major local or national events could be asked depending on the education, intelligence and interest of the patient, eg. when was the last general election held, or when was the last Kumbh Mela held and so on.

Recent Past Memory

It is checked by recalling events in the past few months. (Same method can be used as described in remote past memory).

Recent Memory

This refers to the events in past 24-48 hours. The patient could be asked about what he ate in breakfast or who came to see him at his home or in the hospital. These will need to be checked with informants.

Immediate Recall

It is tested by giving the patients a digit forward and backward test. The patient should be able to recall 6-7 digits forward and 5-6 digits backward.

The patient may be given a list of five objects and he should be told that he will be asked to remember them later. He could be asked to repeat them immediately for testing immediate recall and may be asked to recall them after five minutes of interference for delayed recall.

Few patients may exhibit confabulation. They may fill in the memory gap with imaginary material.

General Information and Intelligence

While assessing intelligence one should keep in mind the patient's education, socio-economic background and interests.

Educated patients may be asked about the current political problems. They may also be asked about their ability to deal with normal day-to-day tasks and problems.

Less educated and rural patients could be asked questions like :

Name of the president, prime minister of India, chief minister of your state, headman of your village
Five major rivers
Five major cities
How many rupees will be left with you if you pay Rs. 12 from a 20 rupees note.
Other simple calculations could be asked.

This should give a rough idea about the patient's intelligence. Whether it is same as prior to the onset of the illness or it has deteriorated.

Abstract Thinking

This is tested by asking the patient to tell similarities

or differences between two objects, e.g. similarity between an apple and orange (both are fruits, both are round, etc.) or difference between a chair and a table (one is used for sitting and the other is used for keeping things or writing). The patient can also be asked to give meaning of common simple proverbs familiar to the patient.

One has to infer whether the patient is able to abstract the concept.

Impulse Control

Can the patient control his impulses or shows sudden outbursts of impulsive behaviour, e.g. sudden aggressiveness, meaningless sexual assault, etc.

Judgement

It refers to the capability of the individual to distinguish the right from the wrong whether the patient makes right decisions or not. It is asessed in two areas.

Test Judgement

The patient is provided with a hypothetical situation and he is asked to give his response to the situation, e.g. A stamped, addressed post card is lying on the road, what will the patient do. The correct response will be that he will post it in the nearest letter box. The incorrect could be, that he will read the address and deliver it to the person, etc. If he sees a house which has caught fire what will he do (the correct response will be to inform the fire brigade in the city and to call for help from the villages, an abnormal respone will be that he will try to extinguish it himself or let it burn).

Social and Personal Judgement

Can the patient make correct decisions for himself. He may be asked what he will do when he gets well (The correct response will be that he will do his work and look after his family, an incorrect response could be that he will raise a new force to uproot corruption, etc).

Insight

It refers to the patient's awareness of his illness, e.g. does he know that he is ill, or does he know that he has a mental illness and his thinking and actions are inappropriate.

Insight is divided into following the grades

1. Complete denial of illness, the patient does not feel that he is ill.

2. The patient is uncertain whether he is ill or not, may accept it at the moment and deny later.

3. The patient accepts that he is ill but blames it on the external events or on the organic factors.

4. The patient accepts that he is ill but cannot pinpoint the factors responsible for it.

5. Intellectual insight — The patient accepts that he is ill and feels that the illness is due to psychological factors but cannot alter them.

6. Emotional Insight — The patient is emotionally aware of his inappropriate feelings or thoughts. This emotional awareness is conducive to behavioural change.

Differentiation of the last two grades of insight is largely due to the influence of psychoanalysis and this concept is not very relevant today, as the majority of mental disorders are considered to be the last result of genetic/environmental interaction. Emotional awareness is neither necessary nor a sufficient condition for improvement.

Psychiatric Evaluation of Violent/Uncooperative/ **Stupurose Patients**

These patients will not cooperate in their history taking or examination yet the examination should not be deferred to a later time because some valuable information might later be lost.

a) To obtain the history of the patient from the relatives or the accompanying persons, e.g. policeman, or even if the patient has been brought by a casual acquaintance. The name and address of the informants should be noted and the history provided by them should also be separately noted. They should be asked whether the patient has attempted violent acts against himself or others. Do they suspect that he has a weapon, Does he show unpredictable violent behaviour, etc.

Basing on these informations one will need to decide whether the patient needs to be frisked for any dangerous weapons, or should be kept in restraints or not.

If the patient is assaultive, his weapons should be removed and he may be kept in restraints. The examination is mainly dependant on the observations.

The examiner should talk to the patient in a calm and pleasant manner. He should inform the patient that he wishes to examine him to find out whether he has any problems. He will do so only if he permits him self for the same. The doctors should not appear apprehensive. Adequate help should be necessary so that the patient can be restrained if required.

General Appearance

Note how the patient is dressed. Does he show any apparent injury marks. What is his posture ? Does he move his body parts voluntarily or are they loosely hanging ?

Does he show abnormal postures or does he maintain body parts in abnormal positions for longer periods?

Behaviour Towards Doctors and Relatives

Is he quiet, angry, hostile, boastful, unpredictable?

Facial Expression

Does the patient show happiness, anger, fear or vacant expression?

Eyes

Does he keep eyes open or closed. Does he show hypervigilance (eyes darting in every direction) does he follow the examiner by his eyes or eyes show a vacant look.

Speech

Does he speak spontaneously. Note the content.

Response to Commands

Does he follow instructions, ignore them or shows oppositional behaviour. His answers to questions should be noted.

Body Musculature

Does he show rigidity, flaccidity, resist movement. Shows waxy flexibility, i.e. maintain limbs in uncomfortable positions.

Do a physical examination if possible. The blood pressure and the pulse rate should be noted. If there are injury marks, look for fractures.

These patients should also undergo basic investigations to rule out other organic disorder :

Hb, TLC, DLC
Urine examination for sugar,
Blood sugar random
Serum electrolyte.
X-ray, if fracture is suspected
Fundus examination
E.E.G. and CT scan of head if head injury, epilepsy or other brain disorder are suspected.

Formulation

After obtaining the history and conducting the examination, one should write a formulation. It has following parts :

a) Diagnostic formulation
b) Psychodynamic formulation
c) Differential diagnosis
d) Further investigations
e) Management
f) Prognosis

Diagnostic formulation should contain identification data like age, sex, and occupation. It should summarize the main complaints, important aspects of history which should indicate the duration and frequency of the various symptoms : Any other positive or negative finding in history. Relevant past history, relevant points in family and personal history and positive findings on mental and physical examination. All these points should help one to reach a diagnosis. There could be only one clear cut diagnosis. There could be one main diagnosis or one could not make a definite diagnosis but may provide only differential diagnosis. The most probable diagnosis should be given the first and the least probable the last.

If further investigations are required for confirming the diagnosis, they should be mentioned. They may include the following :

More observation or information
Psychological tests
Physical investigations

Psychodynamic Formulation

In case the history and examination provides evidence of psychogenicity, it is good practice to formulate psychological development of the illness.

Management

A management plan should be made.

Prognosis

Possible prognosis of the patient should also be noted.

Investigations

If any organic disease is suspected relevant investigations should be done.

Specific Investigations Used in Psychiatry

Unfortunately there are no specific tests or investigations which can confirm or rule out a psychiatric disorder except in organic brain diseases and substance use disorders.

The following tests can be helpful :

1. Psychological tests

There are standardized instruments and the responses are obtained in a standard manner.

Intelligence Tests

These tests can measure the patient's intelligence or may be able to give an idea whether any deterioration has taken place due to the illness. The commonly used tests for asessing intelligence are given below :

1. Bhatia's battery of intelligence.
2. Wechsler adult intelligence scale.
3. Raven's Progressive Matrices for adults and children.
4. Binet Kamath test.

Tests to Find Out Involvement of the Brain (Organicity)

1. Bender Gestalt test.
2. Luria-Nebraska battery.

Test for asessing personality

Eysenck's Personality Inventory.
16 Personality factor inventory.
Minnesota Multiphasic Personality Inventory.
Multiphasic Personality Questionnaire.

Projective Tests

These tests give us some idea about personality dynamics and can also help in diagnosis.

Rorschach ink blot test.
Thematic appreception test.
Sack's sentence completion test.

Structured Psychiatric Interview Technique :

1. Schedule for clinical asessment of psychiatric disorders (SCID).

2. Schedule for clinical asessment in neuropsychiatry (SCAN).

Both these schedules are standard instruments for obtaining psychiatric history and examination. They are very helpful in making correct diagnosis.

Life Events Scale

Presumptive stressful life event scale.
Holmes and Rahe life event scale.

Screening Questionnaires to Identify Mentally Sick Individuals :

Cornell medical index health questionnaire.
Symptom check list.
General Health Questionnaire.

The above list is not comprehensive and only commonly used test are given.

Pentothal Interview

Some patients who are not able to provide enough information or who are too inhibited may be given sodium pentothal intravenously slowly.

This will reduce their inhibitions and they may be able to provide meaningful psychological information. This procedure is useful in dissociative disorders.

CHAPTER 4

CLASSIFICATION IN PSYCHIATRY

Classification of all phenomena and objects is essential for communication as well as for appropriate understanding of the phenomenon. Classification can be done on the basis of one or more qualities e.g. race, colour, intelligence, income, education etc. The quality of classification largely depends on the stability of the concept used for this purpose. One of the most scientific classifications is the periodic table where all elements are classified according to their atomic weight.

Psychiatric disorders have been differently classified for the last few centuries. Unfortunately psychiatric disorders have varying symptomatology as well as multiple etiology due to which classification is not very stable. Earlier, the main classifactory concepts were :

a) organic/functional disorders

b) neurotic/psychotic disorders.

Organic/functional dichotomy emphasised that there are a group of disorders which have a demonstrable organic pathology while others do not have any such disturbances; hence they were called functional disorders. However, this dichotomy has been proven false as recent methods of investigations have shown that many of the disorders which were earlier considered functional do exhibit changes at cellular/biochemical level. Yet, mental disorders which have a demonstrable organic pathology are kept in a separate category of organic mental disorders.

NEUROSIS AND PSYCHOSIS

This dichotomy implies different symptomatology as well as aetiology. Neurotic disorders were considered milder and these patients did not show disturbances in appreciation of reality. Their behaviour generally was appropriate to the demands of life. The distortions in psychological development were thought to be responsible for development of neurosis. Psychosis, on the other hand, showed behaviour which was inappropriate to reality. However, it was seen that psychotic behaviour is a function of severity of illness. Some illnesses when mild may show reality appropriate behaviour and when severe may show psychotic behaviour. For this reason this dichotomy is also not accepted these days.

World Health Organisation has been actively involved in developing classification. International Classification of Diseases has one chapter for Mental and Behavioural disorders. It has been revised in 1992 (ICD-X). This is a major revision. American Psychiatric Association has been also revising psychiatric classification from time to time. Currently, DSM-III-R is applicable in United States but shortly the American Psychiatric Association is likely to come up with DSM IV which is likely to be nearer to ICD-X.

The present book is solely based on ICD-X. Following are the basic features of this classification. This classification is based on symptomatolgy and syndromes of similar symptomatology has been kept together. The strength of this classification is that it has been tested extensively all over the world and found generally applicable.

This classification uses the term disorder instead of disease or illness because a particular disorder connotes a group of symptoms which may have same or different aetiology.

The classification divides all mental disorders into the following groups :

Organic, including symptomatic, mental disorders

Mental and behavioural disorders due to psychoactive substance use

Schizophrenia, schizotypal and delusional disorders

Mood (Affective) disorders

Neurotic, stress-related and somatoform disorders

Behavioural syndromes associated with physiological disturbances and physical factors

Disorders of adult personality and behaviour

Mental retardation

Disorders of psychological development

Behavioural and emotional disorders with onset usually occurring in childhood and adolescence

ORGANIC, INCLUDING SYMPTOMATIC MENTAL DISORDERS

This group includes all those disorders where psychological and behavioural disturbances are the result of a disturbance in brain functioning due to disease or injury. Most of these disorders will show a demonstrable brain pathology or the brain disorder appears to be strongly associated with the presenting symptoms.

MENTAL AND BEHAVIOURAL DISORDERS DUE TO PSYCHOACTIVE SUBSTANCE USE

This group contains all those mental disorders which are directly related to the use of the substances which have direct effect on brain. They result in different types of disorders ranging from drug dependance to various personality problems and drug induced organic mental disorders.

SCHIZOPHRENIA, SCHIZOTYPAL AND DELUSIONAL DISORDERS

This group includes all those disorders where disturbances of thinking and feelings, hallucinations, and disorders of behaviour are predominant. It is possible that disorders like schizophrenia and delusional disorders may be etiologically unrelated.

MOOD (AFFECTIVE) DISORDERS

This group includes all those disorders where basic symptom is alteration of mood. The person may be depressed or euphoric and all other psychological symptoms are secondary to this basic disorder.

NEUROTIC, STRESS RELATED AND SOMATOFORM DISORDERS

This group contains all those disorders which were earlier considered to be neurotic but the present classification neither acccepts the premise that they are psychologically caused, nor that they are interrelated amongst themselves. Some of these disorders may be genetic in nature while others may have a predominantly psychological component. This group includes disorders like anxiety, phobias, dissociative disorders, adjustment disorders and somatoform disorders etc.

BEHAVIOURAL SYNDROMES ASSOCIATED WITH PHYSIOLOGICAL DISTURBANCES AND PHYSICAL FACTORS

This group includes all those disorders where physiological changes are associated with psychological disturbances. This group includes eating disorders, sleep disorders, sexual disorders and psychological symptoms associated with other physical disorders.

These disorders were earlier called psychosomatic disorders. That term has been given up because it presumed a definitive aetiology. In this group of disorders an association between psychological factors and physical disorders is assumed but no direct etiological relationship is emphasised.

DISORDERS OF ADULT PERSONALITY AND BEHAVIOUR

This group includes all those disorders which are not usually considered abnormal by the individual, but produce difficulty in his adjustment with others. These may be developmental in nature or may be acquired later in life.

MENTAL RETARDATION

This group includes all those conditions where mental development has been arrested at the time of birth or during developmental phase (up to 16 years). These patients present with intellectual retardation and they are not able to cope with ordinary demands of life.

DISORDERS OF PSYCHOLOGICAL DEVELOPMENT

This group includes all those conditions where psychological development has been retarded in one particular area e.g. language development, visuospatial skills and motor co-ordination. This delay is characteristically much more than any delay in the intellectual development. This delay is often related to maturity of central nervous system and often the symptoms improve with advancing age.

BEHAVIOURAL AND EMOTIONAL DISORDERS WITH ONSET USUALLY OCCURRING IN CHILDHOOD AND ADOLESCENCE

This group includes a miscellaneous group of behavioural disorders which specifically arise during childhood. Adult neurotic disorders which may have early onset are not included in this group. The disorders may be induced both by organic and psychological factors.

GENERAL REMARKS ABOUT I.C.D.-X

I.C.D.-X is a futuristic classification and each category has scope for addition of newer disorders.

Each group also has two subheading of other and unspecified disorders. **Other disorder** — include all those conditions which do not fulfil criteria described earlier. This can include conditions which could not be included in other categories.

Not otherwise specified

This include those conditions, where the condition does not fulfil criteria for specific disorders or when full details are not available.

I.C.D X has also developed a research version which is more restrictive and should be used in research.

I.C.D X primary care version is under field trials. So that a simple classification could be developed for use by the primary care physicians.

This classification is a step forward in making the diagnosis universally uniform yet the biggest flaw of this classification is its dependance on improperly defined clinical criteria. However, most of these disorders have shown reasonable stability across time and in different parts of the world. It is hoped that future researches will make it more precise.

CHAPTER 5

ORGANIC, INCLUDING SYMPTOMATIC, MENTAL DISORDERS

These group of disorders includes all those conditions where mental symptoms develop because of demonstrable or possible brain pathology. This nomenclature is a legacy of the past, when mental disorders were divided into organic and functional groups. Organic mental disorders included conditions where brain pathology was demonstrated or was highly probable. Functional disorders were presumed to have developed because of psychological factors and no brain pathology was expected. Recent researchers have shown that many of the so-called functional mental disorders do have alterations in neuro-physiological activity of the brain. Thus, one should not assume that other psychiatric disorders do not have any organic pathology.

Organic brain disorders could be primary or secondary.

Primary disorder includes all those conditions where the brain is the site of pathology while secondary disorder includes all those conditions where brain involvement is secondary to a systemic disease.

The symptomatology in this group disorders can be of the following types :

a) Dementia—There is gradual decline in memory and intelligence.

b) Delirium — This usually develops acutely and it is characterized by confusion, hallucinations and delusions.

c) Amnestic syndromes — These conditions have predominant memory loss and the other cognitive fucntions are intact.

d) Psychological symptoms — Some patients may primarily present with affective symptoms like anxiety, depression and fear. Others may present with delusions and hallucinations. In all such situation, it is apparent that these psychological symptoms are secondary to organic brain pathology.

This section, however, does not include conditions which arise because of psychoactive drug abuse. These are included in next section.

CLASSIFICATION

Dementia in Alzheimer's Disease

Dementia in Alzheimer's Disease with early onset
Dementia in Alzheimer's Disease with late onset
Dementia in Alzheimer's Disease — atypical or mixed type
Dementia in Alzheimer's Disease — unspecified

Vascular Dementia

Vascular dementia of acute onset
Multi-infarct dementia
Subcortical vascular dementia
Mixed cortical and subcortical vascular dementia
Other vascular dementia
Vascular dementia, unspecified

Dementia In Other Diseases Classified Elsewhere

Dementia in Pick's Disease
Dementia in Creutzfeldt-Jakob Disease
Dementia in Huntington's Disease
Dementia in Parkinson's Disease
Dementia in Human Immune Deficiency Virus (HIV) Disease
Dementia in other specified disease classified elsewhere

Unspecified Dementia

Dementia may be specified as follows :
Without additional symptoms.
Other symptoms, predominantly delusional.
Other symptoms, predominantly hallucinatory.
Other symptoms, predominantly depressive.
Other mixed symptoms.

Organic Amnesic Syndromes, Not Induced By Alcohol And Other Psychoactive Substances

Delirium, not induced by alcohol and other psychoactive substances.
Delirium not superimposed on dementia, so described.
Delirium superimposed on dementia.
Other Delirium.
Delirium unspecified.

Other Mental Disorders Due To Brain Damage And Dysfunction And To Physical Disease

Organic hallucinosis.
Organic catatonic disorder.
Organic delusional (schizophrenia like) disorder.
Organic mood (affective) disorders.
Organic manic disorder
Organic bipolar disorder
Organic depressive disorder
Organic mixed affective disorder
Organic anxiety disorder
Organic dissociative disorder

Organic emotionally labile (asthenic) disorder

Mild cognitive disorder

Other specified, mental disorders due to brain damage and dysfuction and to physical disease

Unspecified mental disorders due to brain damage and dysfuction and to physical disease

Personality and Behavioural Disorders Due to Brain Disease, Damage and Dysfunction

Organic personality disorder

Post encephalitic syndrome

Post concussional syndrome

Other organic personality and behavioural disorders due to brain disease damage and dysfunction

Unspecified organic personality and behavioural disorders due to brain disease damage and dysfunction

Unspecified Organic Or Symptomatic Mental Disorders

DEMENTIA

Dementia is a chronic progressive disorder which is characterized by impairment in cognitive mental functions, e.g. memory, reasoning ability, attention and concentration, language functions, judgement and insight. They may also have symptoms of delirium, anxiety, depression and delusions. Dementia can sometime also be acute in onset. The etiology of dementia is varied.

Epidemiology

Dementia is a disorder of the elderly but it can occur in younger people due to brain trauma and infections. The prevalence of the disease increases with advancing age. In the United Sates of America, nearly 5 per cent of the people above sixty five years of age show significant symptoms of dementia while another 10% have milder symptoms. Our country has a very small population of elderly but this proportion is likely to change very soon due to longevity. The problem of dementia is going to increase with the passage of time. No large scale epidemiological studies are available from this country.

Etiology

Dementia can occur due to a number of causes. These are shown in accompanying table (1). Some types of the dementias are treatable if detected in time. Once neuronal degeneration has taken place, it cannot be reversed but further neuronal damage can be stopped or reduced.

Etiology of Dementia (Table No.1)

1. **Parenchymatous Diseases of the Brain**
   - Alzheimer's disease
   - Pick's disease
   - Huntington's disease
   - Parkinson's disease *
   - Multiple sclerosis
2. **Traumatic Disorder**
   - Head injury
   - Brain parenchyma injury
   - Subdural haematoma
3. **Infectious Diseases**
   - Tuberculous meningitis *
   - Other meningitis *
   - Viral encephalitis *
   - Cysticercosis *
   - Neurosyphilis *
   - H.I.V. disease
   - Creutzfeldt-Jakob disease
4. **Cerebrovascular Disorders**
   - Multiinfarct dementia *
   - Subcortical vascular dementia *
   - Cardiac arrythmias *
5. **Metabolic and Endocrinal Disorders**
   - Hypothyroidism *
   - Parathyroid disease *
   - Hypoglycaemia *
   - Wilson's disease
6. **Systemic Diseases**
   - Cirrhosis of liver
   - Renal failure
   - Respiratory encephalopathy *
7. **Deficiency Diseases**
   - Pellagra *
   - Folic acid deficiency
   - B_{12} deficiency *
8. **Toxic Encephalopathy**
   - Alcohol
   - Carbon monoxide
   - Lead poisoning *
9. **Neoplasms of brain** *
10. **Miscellaneous**
    - Hydrocephalus *
    - Sarcoidosis *

All the conditions which have been marked with

* are treatable to some extent.

Clinical Picture

The onset of this disorder is in the late 60s but may be earlier. Many of the early onset dementias develop due to brain infections, trauma, neoplasms, and deficiency states. Degenerative dementias usually develop after 65 years but, if the onset is early then they are called presenile dementias.

Patients usually give history of the following symptoms :

Memory impairment — This is often a prominent symptom. Generally, memory for recent events is lost. Patients start loosing keys or mislaying objects. They may not ever remember what was said few minutes ago. They may forget that they have taken meals. Remote events may be remembered. They may be able to recall their youth and childhood vividly. As the disease progresses, remote memory also gets involved.

Thinking and speech — Thought process is also effected. They may not be able to undertake complex task. Their speech becomes slow and they may be able to respond to simple questions only. If the patient has developed aphasias, then all the symptoms of aphasia may be present. Power of abstraction is reduced.

General behaviour — It starts showing gradual deterioration. Their dress may be improper and dirty. They may become naked in front of other people. They may show urinary and faecal incontinence. Their social and occupational behaviour deteriorates. They may show catastrophic reaction (Goldstein). Whenever they are faced with a difficult or novel problem which they may find difficult to handle, they react with acute anxiety and perplexity.

The patient should be thoroughly examined physically and one should specifically look for conditions mentioned under etiology.

The mental examination of the patient will reveal the following :

General Appearance and Behaviour — The patient is usually unkempt and improperly dressed. Their behaviour may range from being quiet and withdrawn to hilarious and over friendly. But the behaviour is generally not in accordance with social norms.

Consciousness — The patient is usually fully conscious, unless dementia is complicated with delirium or some other disease.

Attention and Concentration — Attention is arousable but concentration is poor.

Thought Process — Thinking is impaired. They may only speak few simple sentences. Other signs of aphasia may be present.

Some patients may exhibit delusions. Patients can have delusions of persecution or of grandiosity or of bizarre nature.

Perceptual Disorders — Normally patients of dementia do not exhibit hallucinations.

Mood — Demented patients often develop depression early in the course of illness. When they become aware of their failing abilities, they exhibit depressive symptoms. Some patients may show anxiety. Some patients will exhibit emotional lability. Mood swings from happiness to crying in momemts. Once dementia has advanced the affect becomes silly, flat and incongruous.

Memory — Memory for recent events is lost early. When the disease advances remote memory is also effected.

Intelligence — Intelligence deteriorates. The patients are unable to undertake complex tasks. Later, simple tasks also become difficult.

Insight and Judgement — Early in the disease insight and judgement may be intact, but as the disorder progresses these are lost. The patient does not consider that he is ill. He cannot take proper decisions regarding himself and others.

Diagnosis

The following are essential for diagnosis : (I.C.D.-X)

Decline in both memory and thinking, sufficient to impair activities of daily living.

Memory disturbances affect the registration, storage and retrieval of new information (recent memory), but previously learnt material may also be lost (recent and past memory).

Thinking is impaired and the patients find it increasingly difficult to communicate properly.

Consciousness is clear. If delirium is superimposed, then consciousness can be impaired.

Duration of at least six months is required for a definite diagnosis.

Differential Diagnosis

1. **Depressive Pseudodementia** — Some depressives may present as dementia. (detailed differential diagnosis under mood disorders).

2. **Subnormal Cognitive Functioning** — People living in severly impoverished states (slums) may not develop their cognitive abilities fully. These poor cognitive abilities may be confused with dementia.

Differentiation between various subtypes of dementia can be done on the basis of the following :

Type of onset — If the onset is acute (within days or weeks), then the following conditions could be expected : massive cerebrovascular accident, trauma, CO poisoning, meningitis, encephalitis. All the other conditions run a subacute or chronic course.

Investigations

Blood — Haemoglobin, TLC, DLC.

The evidence of anaemia may indicate deficiency state. Further examination should be done for Niacin and B_{12} deficiency.

Blood Sugar	—	for Diabetes
Blood Urea	—	for Renal disease
Serum Creatinine	—	
Liver function tests	—	Liver diseases
Thyroid functions	—	Hypothyroidism
Serum Calcium	—	Parathyroidism
V.D.R.L.	—	Neurosyphilis
Serum copper	—	Wilson's disease
K.F. Ring	—	Wilson's disease
H.I.V. Infection	—	A.I.D.S.
Fundus examination	—	Space occupying lesions
	—	Evidence of atherosclerosis
E.E.G.	—	May show slowing (non-specific) focal signs may also be present.
C.T. Scan	—	May reveal decrease in brain mass with dilated ventricles. It may also reveal any other brain pathology.

Sometimes, inspite of all investigations, it may not be possible to pinpoint the etiological diagnosis of dementia. It is important to rule out treatable causes of dementia, all of which can be identified from the above mentioned investigations. The common treatable causes are hypothyroidism, normal pressure hydrocephalus, subdural hematoma, deficiency diseases and some infective disorders.

Course and Prognosis

The majority of dementias usually run a progressive deteriorating course. Only 10% of the dementias are reversible if identified and treated early. The majority of dementias are due to primary degenerative disorder (Alzheimer's disease), which pursues a progressive course. The disease usually lasts for five to ten years. In later stages, the patients will need nursing care for their feeding, cleaning and toilet functions also.

Management

The patients are to be provided supportive care.

Psychological Support — These patients are unable to deal with novel situations due to deteriorating intelligence and memory. Such situations may induce intense anxiety in some of them. The aim of the psychological management is to avoid such situation and to help the patient to remain self-sufficient for as long as possible.

The environment of the patient should be structured. All their things should be kept at fixed places and within easy reach of the patient. It is better to give him meals at fixed time. These measures will help the patient to manage his day to day needs independently. These patients usually develop deterioration of behaviour whenever, they are shifted to a new place.

Everyone who comes to see them should be introduced instead of asking the patient to identify the person.

Nutrition should be maintained. Vitamin supplement should be added, if needed.

If the patient is depressed, antidepressants can be tried. Antidepressants having low anticholinergic side effects should be given. Fluoxetine can be a good drug, E.C.T. can be given if depression is severe.

If the patient shows restlessness or psychotic symptoms then Haloperidol 1.5mg once or twice a day may be given.

There are no specific drugs which can improve dementia, though many drugs are being marketed as helpful in dementia none of them had been found effective unequivocally in dementia.

SPECIFIC DEMENTIAS

Though there are large number of specific dementias their incidence is quite low. Moreover, the majority of them are difficult to diagnose clinically. The description of two commonest types is given below :

Alzheimer's Dementia (Primary degenerative Dementia of Alzheimer type). This is the commonest type of dementia seen in the elderly. It constitutes 60-70% of all cases of dementia in the west. Indian figures for its prevalence are not available. It usually starts after 65 years of age but, it can also start early. Then it is called presenile dementia. It is slightly more common in women.

Etiology and Pathology

There is some evidence to indicate that this disease may have hereditary basis.

A large number of patients exhibit positive family history for similar disorders. Some may have positive family history of Down's Syndrome. The abnormal proteins seen in both these conditions are identical. Some patients show high levels of Aluminium. Recently, this disorder has been found to be associated with degeneration of cholinergic neurons.

Typical neuropathological changes include, senile plaques, neurofibrillary tangles and granulovacuolar degeneration of neurons. These changes are generalized.

Clinical Picture

This illness starts insidiously. The earliest presenting features are memory impairment, inability to cope with work or social life. All the other symptoms described under dementia could be present. Many patients may exhibit, anxiety, depression and suspiciousness. As the disease advances, these symptoms may give way to inappropriate and flat affect. The course is progressive.

Case History

Mr. S a 62 year old man was brought to the clinic. His illness had started two years back. He had become slow in all his activities. He had started demanding food repeatedly (even when he has taken his food short time earlier). He forgets who had come to see him. Once or twice, he could not find his way home. The family thought that all these problems were due to old age. But from the last few months, he has become very unstable and suspicious. He has started suspecting that his sons are taking money out of his bank account. He has become irritable and stubborn. He occasionally passes urine at improper place. On examination, his memory and intelligence were impaired. He had delusions of suspiciousness.

Comment

This patient is exhibiting symptoms of a deteriorating illness. Investigations did not reveal evidence of systemic or brain pathology, except the C.T. scan of head, which showed generalized cortical atrophy. His memory and intelligence are impaired. He has lately developed delusions of suspicion. He was provisionally diagnosed as Alzheimer's dementia.

Management

Same as described under dementia. There is no specific treatment.

MULTIINFARCT DEMENTIA

This is the second commonest type of dementia. It accounts for nearly 10-15% patients of dementia. This disorder arises earlier than Alzheimer's disease usually between 50-60 years of age. It is slightly more common in males than females.

Etiology

This is associated with various vascular diseases. These patients generally have hypertension with hypercholesteremia. Pathologically lacunar infarcts are seen.

Clinical Picture

This disease shows a step ladder pattern. The patient develops multiple episodes of cerebral ischaemia which may or may not be apparent. The patient exhibits a worsening of mental activities after each episode, which stabilises for a short time and then worsens again.

Clinically, these patients show memory disturbances, intellectual deficits, along with focal neurological signs. They may have aphasias. These patients often show emotional incontinence (start weeping on trifles) and emotional lability. They may retain insight into their problems for quite some time, due to which they become severely depressed. The illness exhibits gradual deterioration.

Management

The basic factors behind the dementia should be properly treated. Hypertension should be effectively treated, Lipidaemia should be controlled both by diet and drugs. If the patient is a smoker, then cessation of smoking may also be helpful.

The general management of dementia should be followed. The role of various drugs which effect the blood supply of brain is debatable.

ORGANIC AMNESIC SYNDROMES NOT INDUCED BY ALCOHOL AND OTHER PSYCHOACTIVE SUBSTANCES

This syndrome is characterized by prominent impairment of recent and remote memory while immediate recall is preserved. The patient is unable to learn new material (antero-grade amnesia). The syndrome usually develops acutely.

The epidemiology is not well known.

Etiology and Pathology

It is commonly caused by bilateral involvement of mamillary bodies, hippocampus and fornix. In some patients, the frontal lobes may also be involved. The commonest cause is thiamine deficiency due to alcoholism. It can also occur due to neoplasm, trauma, cerebrovascular accidents involving this region. It can be seen in carbon monoxide poisoning and may be induced by drugs such as benzodiazepines and by E.C.T.

Clinical Features

The syndrome develops acutely. In alcoholics, it may follow Wernicke's encephalopathy (confusion ataxia, Nystagmus, Opthalmoplegia). The prominent clinical features are :

Loss of recent memory. Patient does not remember where he is, what he has taken even few minutes earlier. They cannot register, store and recall new information.

Immediate recall is intact. They may be able to repeat 6-7 digit forward.

Memories of recent past are also effected.

The patient may show confabulation. They fill up the period of memory gap with false material.

Other mental functions are normal.

The patient has no insight into his illness. He may deny it or may minimize it by confabulation.

Course and Prognosis

The course of the condition depends on its etiology. The onset is always acute . The course is benign when the syndrome is precipitated by vascular insufficiency, E.C.T., drugs and cardiac arrest. The outcome is poor in traumatic, CO poisoning, herpes simplex encephalitis.

Diagnosis (I.C.D.-X)

The main symptoms are the following :

a) Recent and past memory loss

b) Intact immediate recall

c) Evidence of disease of brain involving diencephalic and medial temporal structures.

d) Consciousness is clear.

The syndrome should be differentiated from delirium, dementia and depression.

Management

If the condition is induced by thiamine deficiency, then thiamine should be administered by injectable route. Other B complex factors should also be given. In all other conditions, the etiological factor has to be treated.

If the syndrome has become permanent then rehabilitative measures are needed.

DELIRIUM

This is an acute confusional state which occurs due to generalized brain dysfunction. The syndrome is characterized by confusion, disturbances in consciousness, hallucinations and delusions.

Epidemiology

The syndrome is quite common in medical and surgical wards. It is more common in children and the elderly people. Those who have had an episode of delirium are likely to have it again.

Etiology

Delirium occurs due to generalized disturbance in brain functioning. It may also occur due to poor sensory inputs as seen during cataract surgery (Black patch delirium). Psychological factors also play a part in the development of delirium. Patients who are fearful of surgery or patients kept in intensive care units, where normal perceptual inputs are diminished, are more likely to develop delirium. The etiological factors are given in accompanying table.

Etiology of Delirium

Traumatic	Head injury
Infection	
	Any systemic infection with high fever
	Meningitis

Encephalitis

Cerebrovascular Vascular insufficiency
Haemhorrage

Epilepsy

Systemic diseases

Pituitary dysfunction
Pancreas (Diabetes)
Adrenal disorders
Parathyroid disorders
Thyroid disorders
Liver failure
Renal failure
Carbon-dioxide narcosis
Cardiovascular
Arrythmias
Cardiac failure
Deficiency disease
Thiamine
Niacin

Drugs and Poisons

Sedatives and hypnotics
Tranquilizers
Anticholinergic
Anticonvulsants
Antihypertensives
Cimetidine
Disulfiram
Insulin
Salicylate
Steroids

Psychoactive substances Alcohol
Opium and its derivatives
Marijuana
L.S.D.

Post-operative states

Electrolyte imbalance

Clinical Picture

The condition usually starts acutely but some prodromal symptoms may be apparent for a few days before the acute illness becomes apparent. These prodromal symptoms could be irritability, memory lapses, occasional irrelevant replies, sleep disturbances and diminished appetite.

Some salient clinical symptoms are :

General Behaviour

The patient's activity may vary from stupor and lethargy to acute excitement. These behaviour changes occurs suddenly and without any provocation. The patient may show motor restlessness. They are usually not concerned about their dress. Their relatedness with people may vary from moment to moment.

Consciousness — Level of consciousness is variable. They may be fully conscious for few moments or hours and then may lapse into a semiconscious state. They are usually disoriented for time and may be for place and person.

Attention and concentration also vary from time to time. They are not able to focus on any topic for a sufficient period of time.

Speech — They may speak excessively or may not speak at all.

Thought Process and Content — Thinking is often disturbed. They may talk irreleventyly and incoherently. They may exhibit transitory delusions. Delusions are generally of persecution or grandiosity.

Mood — These patients often exhibit affect of anxiety, fear or perplexity. A few may show depressive affect with weeping spells. The mood is typically changing and variable.

Perceptual Disturbances — These usually dominate the clinical picture. The patients will have multiple hallucinations generally in the visual field, but the auditory and tactile hallucination are also common. They may see frightening figures, usually of animals. They may feel as if insects are crawling on their body or may hear music. Illusions are frequently present. They may misinterpret stimuli.

Memory — Immediate and recent recall may be impaired.

Intelligence — Usually cannot be tested.

Insight and judgement is lost.

Delirium usually shows worsening at night. Sleep is often disturbed. The patient may sleep in day and may remain awake at night.

Course and Prognosis

Delirium has an acute onset and usually resolves completely within a few weeks. It may last sometime up to six months, specially in chronic hepatic failure. If the delirium has developed in the terminal phase of a fatal disease, then it may terminate by death.

Diagnosis (I.C.D.-X)

For a definite diagnosis symptoms, mild or severe,

should be present in each one of the following areas : (I.C.D.-X)

a) Impairment of consciousness and attention (on a continuum from clouding to coma, reduced ability to direct, focus, sustain and shift attention) ;

b) Global disturbance of cognition (perceptual distortions, illusions and hallucinations most often visual, impairment of abstract thinking and comprehension, with or without transient delusions, but typically with some degree of incoherence ; impairment of immediate recall and recent memory but with relatively intact remote memory; disorientation of time, as well as in more severe cases, for place and person) ;

c) Psychomotor disturbances (hypo- or hyperactivity) and unpredictable shifts from one to another; increased reaction time; increased or decreased flow of speech; enhanced startle reaction);

d) Disturbance of the sleep - wake cycle, total sleep loss or reversal of sleep-wake cycle; daytime drowsiness, nocturnal worsening of symptoms, disturbing dreams or nightmares which, may continue as hallucinations after awakening ;

e) Emotional disturbances, e.g. anxiety or fear, irritability, euphoria, apathy or worsening perplexity.

The presence of the above mentioned symptoms with evidence of one or the other etiological factors will help in diagnosis.

Differential Diagnosis

It should be differentiated from the following :

1. Dementia — Dementia may precede or follow delirium. The clinical picture of dementia is characterized by stable memory and intellectual loss, while delirium may show both these symptoms but they vary from time to time. The onset is acute in delirium and insidious in dementia. Consciousness is clear in dementia while it is altered in delirium.

Acute psychosis, schizophrenia and acute mania may show confusional symptoms for a short time. But they should exhibit the classical features of these disorders and differentiation should not be difficult.

Etiological Diagnosis

Patients should be carefully examined for finding out the etiology of delirium. The following investigation may help to identify the specific cause.

1. Fundus examination - Evidence of papilloedema
2. Lumbar puncture (if indicated)
   Blood
   Hb, TLC, DLC
3. Blood urea
4. Blood sugar
5. Urine examination
7. Liver function tests
8. Serum electrolytes
9. X-ray chest — If indicated of other parts
10. Any other relevant investigation.

Management

Basically the management should be of etiological condition, if it is treatable. General measures include the following :

Maintain nutrition by IV drip or through nasal tube (Ryle's tube).

Maintain electrolyte and fluid balance.

The patient's back and pressure points should be attended to avoid bed sores.

The patient should be nursed in a quiet reasonably illuminated room.

A close relative (if available) should stay with the patient.

The number of visitors should be restricted.

Whenever, the patient is in clear consciousness, one should try to convey to him the exact clinical state and provide emotional support.

Symptoms of agitation and hallucination can be treated with small dosages of phenthiazines, e.g. Haloperidal 1.5 mg twice or thrice a day.

If the patient has sleeplessness, hypnotics, e.g. Nitrazepam 5-10 mg at bed time can be given.

The majority of the patients will improve, a few may pass into dementia or Amnesic syndrome and fewer will die when delirium is associated with fatal disease.

OTHER MENTAL DISORDERS DUE TO BRAIN DAMAGE AND DYSFUNCTION AND TO PHYSICAL DISEASES

This group includes miscellaneous symptoms, detailed under nonorganic mental syndromes like anxiety, depression, delusions, etc. Whenever these clinical states occur in the course of some organic brain disease or due to intake of certain substances (drugs and intoxicants), they are included under this category.

The decision to classify a clinical syndrome here should be supported by the following : (I.C.D.-X)

a) Evidence of cerebral disease, damage or dysfunction or of systemic physical disease known to be associated with one of the listed syndromes.

b) A temporal relationship (weeks or few months) between the development of the underlying disease and the onset of the mental syndrome.

c) Recovery from the mental disorder following removal or improvement of the underlying presumed cause.

d) Absence of evidence to suggest an alternative cause of the mental syndrome (such as strong family history or precipitating stress).

If (a and b) are present then a provisional diagnosis can be made but if all the four conditions are fulfilled then a firm diagnosis can be made.

The following conditions are associated with these mental symptoms :

1. **Intracranial**	**Drug**
Trauma	Propranalol
Infections : Tuberculosis,	Levodopa
Encephalitis and other	Methyldopa
infections of C.N.S.	Steriods
Extracranial neoplasm with	Antihypertensives
remote C.N.S. effects	Antimalarials
Cerebrovascular disease	Ranitidine
Cerebral Malformations	Anticholinergics
2. **Systemic disease**	**Psychoactive Substances**
Endocrinal	Amphetamines
hypothyroidism	
hyperthyroidism	
Cushing's syndrome	Alcohol
	Opiates
Metabolic disorders -	Marijuana
Hypoglycaemia, porphyria,	L.S.D.
hypoxia	

ORGANIC HALLUCINOSIS

It is characterized by prominent hallucinations in any sense modality in a state of clear conciousness and these hallucinations are presumed to be induced by an organic condition.

Epidemiology of this condition is not clearly known.

Etiology

It is commonly seen in association with use of various drugs like cocaine, alcohol, marijuana and L.S.D. Conditions producing perceptual disturbances like cataract, deafness, etc. can be associated with hallucinations in that sense modality.

Clinical Picture

Hallucinations in clear conciousness are prominent features. Alcoholics usually show visual and auditory hallucinations, while cocaine is associated with tactile hallucinations like bug crawling.

Course and Prognosis

When the syndrome is due to drugs then the chances of recovery are good. But in some other cases it may become chronic.

Diagnosis

This condition is diagnosed on the basis of following : (I.C.D.-X)

Prominent hallucinations
No clouding of consciousness
No evidence of delirium or dementia
No predominent disturbances of mood
No predominance of delusions
Fulfils general criteria (a-d) described earlier.

Management

If etiological factor is known (like drug or alcohol intake) then treatment should be of that disorder. For symptomatic relief, antipsychotic drugs like haloperidol and chlorpromazine can be used.

ORGANIC CATATONIC DISORDER

Some patients may exhibit stupor or acute excitement (details in chapter VII) which might be due to organic cause.

Often the history may be indistinguishable from schizophrenia. Careful evaluation will reveal certain organic symptoms which can distinguish this condition.

The epidemiology is not known. Etiologicaly common causes are encephalitis and carbon monoxide poisoning.

Clinical picture will reveal symptoms of stupor or excitement. The consciouness may be clear or may be clouded. The patient may exhibit other catatonic features.

The course of the disorder will depend on the

cause. If cause is treatable then the patient will improve.

Case History

A 32 year old male was admitted with history of not speaking, not replying to questions asked and only turning his head when called out to, by name, since one month prior to admission. On a longitudinal review of past history, it was revealed that the patient had had two manic episodes, 2 and 1 years ago. Eight months prior to present admission, the patient began to show head nodding without any reason, increased talkativeness which was relevant and coherent and devoid of any grandiosity. He exhibited marked suspiciousness against the family members, especially the wife. There was marked neglect of personal grooming and hygiene. By two months of antipsychotic (CPZ 600 mg/day) treatment both the talkativeness and head nodding decreased, sleep increased and suspicious behaviour decreased but was not abolished. After the initial improvement there was no further response even when CPZ was increased to 1000 mg/day. Since 4 months prior to admission patient, though ambulatory, began to show occasional unexpected incontinence of urine, and after a month developed faecal incontinence of which the patient remained unaware. At this time, he also developed a slight stuttering in speech, which assumed a childlike property and was progressive. One month prior to admission, the patient began to show marked decrease in appetite, episodic teeth clenching and replied to questions in monosyllables.

On examination, the patient remained mute and immobile, following objects with eyes but not responding to questions. A neurological examination failed to reveal significant findings. 3 DECT's were given, which caused no improvement in the pt's condition. 600 mg of CPZ likewise failed and, as intake further worsened. IV fluids were started. A GBP failed to reveal any significant abnormality. EEG showed generalized runs of slows waves, lasting for 1-2 secs. but no other significant findings. MRI revealed multiple areas of demyelination. A diagnosis of post viral demyelination was considered.

The patient revealed a past history of manic illness which may point towards the diagnosis of bipolar affective disorder. The present episode started with head nodding, and he developed incontinuance of urine and faeces which developed before he became fully mute. These symptoms should strongly arouse suspicion of organic brain disorder which was confirmed on M.R.I. This patient was diagnosed organic catatonia.

Diagnosis

For firm diagnosis following condition should be fulfilled : (I.C.D.-X)

a) Conditions (a to d) for this group should be fulfilled.

b) The patient may have stupor, excitement or both may shift from one to another

c) Other catatonic features will improve the reliability of diagnosis.

Management

The treatment of basic etiology should be done. Excitement or catatonia can be controlled by antipsychotic drugs or electroconvulsive therapy.

ORGANIC DELUSIONAL (SCHIZOPHRENIA LIKE) DISORDERS

These patients present with delusions, hallucinations and other symptoms seen in schizophrenia and delusional disorder. They are diagnosed here if an organic cause could be identified.

Epidemiology is not known.

Etiology

The majority of these disorders are induced by drugs like amphetamines or alcohol. Many other drugs can also be responsible. This disorder can also be seen in temporal lobe epilepsy and in conditions involving temporal and parietal lobes specially on right side.

Clinical Picture

This is similar to schizophrenia. These patients may not show flattening of affect and typical thought disorders seen in schizophrenia. Some evidence of other organic symptoms may be present.

Course and Prognosis

It is dependant on the underlying etiology. Drug induced disorders and epileptic psychosis usually respond to treatment.

Diagnosis (I.C.D.-X)

1. The general criteria for the group (a-d) should be met.

2. Symptoms characteristic for schizophrenia or delusional disorders like delusions, hallucinations, thought disorder or isolated catatonic symptoms should

be present.

Differential diagnosis from schizophrenia is described in chapter ( ).

Management

The underlying disorder should be treated. Otherwise the management is same as for schizophrenia.

ORGANIC MOOD (AFFECTIVE) DISORDERS

These disorders are characterized by mood of depression or mania which is a result of brain pathology or drug intake. If depression is a psychological reaction to a physical disease that will not be included here.

Epidemiology is not well known. Nearly 10% of the patients taking antihypertensive drugs develop this disorder. It is also frequently associated with cerebral strokes.

Etiology

Mood disorders could be induced by any of the conditions mentioned in chapter on mood disorders.

Clinical Picture

It is similar to depression and mania.

Course and Prognosis

The course is dependant on the underlying cause. The majority of the underlying symptoms will improve by medication and psychological help.

Management

If the condition is caused by some drugs it is better to discontinue it and use some other which does not effect mood. Otherwise symptomatic treatment as described in mood disorders can be done. Dosage required may be lower.

ORGANIC ANXIETY DISORDER

Many patients develop symptoms of anxiety or panic or both due to various systemic diseases or due to drug intake. Epidemiology is not clearly known.

Etiology

A large number of systemic disease and drugs can induce this syndrome. The common conditions are mentioned below :

COMMON PHYSICAL CONDITIONS ASSOCIATIED WITH ANXIETY

1. **Drugs and Toxins**
   Amphetamine
   Sympathomimetic agents like ephedrine
   Alcohol
   Caffeine
   Nicotine
   Withdrawal from any habit forming drug
2. **Endocrinal Disorders**
   Hypoglycaemia
   Pheochromocytoma
   Hyperthyroidism
3. **Mitral Valve Prolapse**
4. **Many other Neurological and Systemic disease can be associated with anxiety.**

Course and Prognosis

The course and prognosis is dependant on underlying cause.

Clinical Picture

This is similar to as described under generalized anxiety disorder and panic disorder. These patients should show evidence of underlying physical disorder which should be able to explain the anxiety symptoms.

Diagnosis

Diagnosis is made on the basis of following : (I.C.D.X)

1. Evidence of general factors (a-d) described for presence of this group.
2. Clinical picture of anxiety or panic disorder.

Management

Treat the underlying cause and anxiety can be symptomatically managed as described in chapter ( ).

ORGANIC DISSSOCIATIVE DISORDER

This disorder presents with symptoms of dissociative disorders but fulfil the criteria for this group of disorders. It has not been studied in detail so far.

ORGANIC EMOTIONALLY LABILE (ASTHENIC) DISORDER

This disorder is characterized by marked and persistent emotional incontinence or lability, fatiguability or variety of unpleasant physical sensations, (e.g. dizziness) and pains regarded as being due to the presence of organic disorder. This is thought to occur more with cerebrovascular disease or hypertension than with other causes. It should be differentiated from somatoform disorders.

MILD COGNITIVE DISORDER

Few patients may exhibit mild memory impairment and learning or concentration difficulties. These are not severe enough for the diagnosis of dementia or amnesic syndrome. These may accompany wide variety of infection and physical disorder. This condition should be differentiated from post-encephalitic and post-concussional syndrome by its different etiology.

PERSONALITY AND BEHAVIOUR DISORDER DUE TO BRAIN DISEASE, DAMAGE AND DYSFUNCTION

Some patients develop alterations in their personality and behaviour either concomitantly with a brain disease or in the residual state. The symptom may refer to a particular brain area but this should not be overemphasized because symptoms referring to a particular brain area may occur due to lesion elsewhere.

ORGANIC PERSONALITY DISORDER

This syndrome is characterized by significant and persistent changes in behaviour after or during the course of a disorder affecting brain functions. Present behaviour is apparently different from premorbid behaviour.

Epidemilogy is not clearly known.

Etiology

Common etiological factors are enumerated in the accompanying table :

Conditions Associated with Organic Personality Disorder

1. Head injury
2. Epilepsy
3. Cerebrovascular accidents
4. Brain tumours
5. Neurosyphilis
6. Manganese poisoning
7. Steroids (Anabolic)

Clinical Picture

Clinical picture is characterized by an abrupt change from premorbid behaviour. Some patients may show accentuation of pre-existing behaviour traits The patients may exhibit antisocial behaviour like stealing and lying, etc. Many patients are not able to stick to their jobs and they may show mild deficits in memory and intelligence. Mood is often sad or anxious. A few patients may also show emotional lability, other may have mild euphoria.

Course and Prognosis

If the illness is the result of structural changes in the brain, then the condition is likely to persist. In some instances when the cause is reversible like drug intoxication the personality change may be reversed.

Diagnosis (I.C.D.-X)

The definite diagnosis require evidence of brain disease or dysfunction. The diagnosis also require two or more of the following features :

a) Consistently reduced ability to persevere with goal directed activities, especially those involving a longer period of time and postponed gratifications;

b) Altered emotional behaviour characteized by emotional lability, shallow and unwarranted cheerfulness (euphoria, inappropriate jocularity and easy change to irritability, or short lived outburst of anger and aggression), in some instances apathy may be a more prominent feature;

c) Expression of needs and impulses without consideration of consequences or social convention (patient may engage in dissocial acts such as stealing, inappropriate sexual advances or voracious eating or may exhibit disregard for personal hygiene) ;

d) Cognitive disturbances in the form of suspiciousness or paranoid ideation and/or excessive preoccupation with a single or usually abstract theme, (e.g. religion, right and wrong);

e) Marked alteration of the rate of flow of language production with features such as circumstantiality, over inclusiveness viscosity and hypergraphia,

f) Altered sexual behaviour.

It has to be differentiated from post concussional syndrome and post encephalitic syndrome by their etiology. Differentiation from other personality change disorders, is by demonstrating different etiological factors and by absence of organic factors.

POST-ENCEPHALITIC SYNDROME

This syndrome is quite common in our country where viral and infectious encephalitis are common. This syndrome is quite similar to organic personality disorder and the differentiation is based mainly on history of encephalitis prior to the onset of this syndrome.

This syndrome is characterized by the following : General malaise, apathy or irritabilty, learning difficulties, altered sleep and eating patterns, change in sexuality and in social judgement. The patient may also have a variety of residual neurological dysfunctions such as, paralysis, deafness, aphasia, constructional aparaxia and echolalia.

The condition can some time be reversible.

POST-CONCUSSIONAL SYNDROME

This condition follows head injury. The head injury is usually sufficient to cause in unconsciousness. The main symptoms are headache, dizziness (usually lacking the features of true vertigo), fatigue, irritability, difficulty in performing mental tasks, impairment of memory, insomnia and reduced tolerance to stress, emotional excitement or alcohol abuse.

The patient is often concerned with the fear of brain damage. They are often depressed. Previously, such patients were considered neurotic because they wanted to obtain compensation. Now this syndrome is considered to be due to non-specific neurophysiological alterations. This syndrome is quite common. It is not necessarily associated with compensation motive.

The exact management of this syndorme is not known. The patient's problem should be accepted and he should be helped psychologically to overcome these symptoms. Drugs may be used for symptomatic relief.

EPILEPSY

This is a common neurological disorder. It's prevalence is estimated to be around 1% in general popultion.

Seizures is a transient paraoxysmal, pathophysiological disturbance of cerebral function caused by a spontaneous, excessive discharge of cortical neurones.

The clinical symptoms of epilepsy will depend on the location and spread of discharge.

Epileptic seizures are broadly classified into the following :

1. **Partial Seizures**
   a. With elementary symptoms
   b. With complex symptoms
   c. Partial with secondary generalization.
2. **Generalized Seizures**
   a. Petit mal seizures
   b. Myoclonus
   c. Tonic clonic seizures.

Patients with seizure disorders can have a multiple type of psychiatric disturbances. These can be divided into the following :

1. Psychological reaction to the diagnosis of epilepsy
2. Psychotic states
3. Personality disorders.

PSYCHOLOGICAL REACTION TO DIAGNOSIS OF EPILEPSY

Epilepsy is generally considered to be a chronic illness which may impair the patient's educational activities, and may hamper his vocational and social life. As soon as the patient learns that he has epilepsy, he becomes anxious or depressed. It may lead to behavioural changes because the patient may feel that there is no further purpose in his life and he may stop constructive activities and may become careless.

All these symptoms could be avoided, if the patient is explained that epilepsy can generally be controlled and if will not interfere in his education, vocation and personal life. The patient should not be advised to lead a resticted life. If restrictions are necessary (no swimming or driving), it should be explained that these are temporary and would be lifted as soon as the siezures are controlled.

PSYCHOTIC STATE

Psychotic behaviour in seizure disorder can be divided into the following :

1. Pre ictal
2. Ictal
3. Post ictal
4. Inter ictal.

PREICTAL PSYCHOTIC STATE

These are very infrequent. They are characterized by changes in mood, irratibility, mild cognitive deficit (repeating same sentence or difficulty in concentrating on a task), delusions and hallucinations. This conditions may last for few hours or days and is terminated by a seizure.

ICTAL PSYCHOTIC STATE

In these patients the ictal phase is represented by psychotic behaviour. It can be seen in Petitmal status or in complex partial seizures. The psychotic state is characterized by disturbances in conciousness inability to concentrate and certain phrases or behaviour may be repeated. There could also be acute excitement. This seldom lasts for more than a few hours to a weeks.

POST-ICTAL PSYCHOTIC STATE

These are most common. They may last from a few minutes to a few weeks. The patients are generally confused (disoriented to time, place or person). They may exhibit various kinds of thought disorders. The speech may be incoherent. There could be feelings of euphoria or perplexity. Delusions and hallucinations may be present. The patients are usually sleepless in this state. The condition usually terminates automatically.

INTER-ICTAL PSYCHOTIC STATE

These are quite common and can occur in quite a substantial number of patients of seizure disorders.

SCHIZOPHRENIA LIKE PSYCHOIS

This is the most clearly described psychotic state in epileptics. These patients exhibit paranoid delusions, thought disorders, may have hallucinations.The thought disorders in these patients are more of an organic kind, like difficulty in conceptualization. Other symptoms like sleep disturbances, poor personal hygiene, excitement, etc. are often present. The affect is often preserved. They do not show the flattening of affect seen in schizophrenia.

Management

Adequate control of epilepsy usually helps to control preictal, ictal and postictal psychotic states. Interictal psychosis often respond to antipsychotic drugs. The dosage required is similar to schizophrenia (see chapter 7). They should be given with antiepileptic drugs because antipsychotic drugs can lower the seizure threshold. The dosage of antiepileptics may have to be increased. Sometimes the psychosis worsens, when seizure control is better and development of seizure may terminate the psychosis.

Personality Changes

The subject of personality changes in epilepsy is quiet controvertial. Many investigators describe epileptic personality while others deny any evidence of typical epileptic personality.

Personality changes are seen in few epileptics. These changes are more commonly seen in temporal lobe epilepsy.

The common changes seen are : excessive religiosity, changes in sexual behaviour, viscosity and heightened experience of emotions. A few persons develop religious conversion after epilepsy. They become excessively precoccupied with religion, right or wrong and may even develop a religion of their own. In viscosity the person hovers around the same topic again and again, they may give many and unnecessary details. They find it difficult to shift from a topic. Their writing will often show similar disturbances. They often show hyperemotionality and may show a quick change of emotions and may at time appear unconcerned.

The management of this condition rests primarily on good control of seizures. Drugs like Carbamazepine may be more effective.

CHAPTER 6

MENTAL AND BEHAVIOURAL DISORDERS DUE TO PSYCHOACTIVE SUBSTANCE USE

This section deals with behavioural problems caused by the use of psychoactive substances. Psychoactive substances include all those agents which produce stimulant or depressive action on the brain and prolonged use of these substances can cause dependence.

These substances can lead to many different kinds of mental or behavioural problems. ICD-10 delineates psychoactive substance related disorders into the following subtypes.

Acute Intoxication

This is a transient condition which can be caused by any psychoactive substance use. This is characterized by the following.

a) Disturbances in Levels of Consciousness

There is usually an altered level of consciousness. The patient appears dazed and may not be able to recognize time, place or person.

b) Disturbances in Thinking, Intelligence and Memory

These persons will not be able to think clearly. They may give inappropriate or wrong replies. Their memory and intelligence is usually disturbed .

Perception — Such patients may experience hallucinations in any sense modality (usually visual and auditory).

Affect — The mood may vary from uninhibited hilarity to anger, sadness or fear. There may be changes from moment to moment.

Behaviour — These persons may show hyperactivity or motor-slowness. They may not take proper care of their dress or appearance. Such patients can behave obscenely and may become naked in public.

The symptoms of intoxication are usually dose dependent. They also can vary from one situation to another. A person may become hilarious in a party but may appear withdrawn when alone. The symptoms of intoxication can also be altered by the coexistence of other diseases or by interaction with other substances. A patient with organic damage of the brain may become intoxicated easily.

The symptoms of intoxication also depends on the nature of substance, eg. alcohol, opioid, cannabinoids, etc. Intoxication usually remits with time. It is further subdivided into the following :

Uncomplicated — When intoxication is dose related and settles as the time passes by.

With Trauma or Other Bodily Injury — When intoxication leads to head or other bodily injuries.

With Other Medical Complications — When intoxicated state shows other medical complications like fever, haematemesis, etc.

With Delirium — Some intoxicated patients may pass into delirium. They will show signs and symptoms of delirium.

With Perceptual Distortion — When patient with intoxication exhibits hallucinations and illusions.

With Coma — When intoxication leads to coma.

With Convulsions — When patient develops seizure during intoxication.

Pathological Intoxication — This term is only used for alcoholics. These persons may show signs of intoxication with very small amount of alcohol.

Harmful Use

When the intoxicating substance is causing bodily or mental problems even without dependence. This term is only used when definite disorders are present, e.g. development of heptitis due to I.V. drug use, or drug use may lead to psychological symptoms like depression.

The harmful use is not diagnosed if dependence is present.

Dependence Syndrome

Some individuals exhibit a need for continued intake of psychoactive substance and usually develops a withdrawal symptom if the drug is not taken. A definite diagnosis of dependence is made if three of the following are present simultaneously during the last one year : (ICD-X)

a) A strong desire or sense of compulsion to take the substance ;

b) Difficulties in controlling substance taking behaviour in terms of its onset, termination or levels of use ;

c) A physiological withdrawal state when substance use has ceased or been reduced as evidenced by:

the characteristic withdrawal syndrome for the substance; or use of the same (or a closely related) substance with the intention of relieving or avoiding withdrawal symptoms ;

d) Evidence of tolerance, such that increased doses of the psychoactive substance are required in order to achieve effects originally produced by lower doses. (clear examples of this are found in alcohol and opiate dependant individuals who may take daily dose sufficient to incapacitate or kill non-tolerant users) ;

e) Progressive neglect of alternative pleasures or interest because of psychoactive substance use, increased amount of time necessary to obtain or to take the substance or to recover from its effects ;

f) Persisting with substance use despite clear evidence of overtly harmful consequences, such as harm to the liver through excessive drinking, depressive mood states consequent to periods of heavy substance use, or drug-related impairment of cognitive functioning ; efforts should be made to determine that the user was actually or could be expected to be, aware of the nature and extent of the harm.

Dependence syndrome is further specified by :

Currently abstinent now, but in a protected environment (in a hospital or prison).

Currently on a clinically supervised maintenance or replacement regime (controlled dependence), (e.g. with methadone, nicotine gum, etc.).

Currently abstinent, but receiving treatment with aversive or blocking drugs (e.g. naltrexone or disulfiram).

Currently using the substance

Continuous use

Episodic use.

Withdrawal State

This is characterized by a group of symptoms which are specific for each substance, whenever the use of that substance is markedly reduced or stopped. The patient will have both psychological and physical symptoms. These symptoms are temporally related to withdrawal of the substance and they are relieved by intake of the substance.

Withdrawal State With Delirium

Some patients can develop symptoms of delirium during withdrawal phase. This is more commonly seen in alcoholics and leads to delirium tremens.

Psychotic Disorder

If symptoms of psychosis, e.g. thought disturbances, hallucinations, delusions and behavioural disturbances develop within 4 hours of substance use, then drug induced psychotic disorder could be diagnosed. These symptoms should resolve partially within one month and finally within six months.

Amnesic Syndrome

Some substance can cause an amnesic syndrome which is characterized by recent memory impairment. This is generally seen with alcoholics.

Residual or Late Onset Psychotic Disorder

Some patients may exhibit psychotic, cognitive or personality changes, much beyond the period during which a direct psychoactive substance related effect might reasonably be assumed to be operating.

Flash Backs

The patient reexperiences previous drug related experiences.

Personality or Behaviour Disorder

Meeting the criteria for organic personality disorder.

Residual Affective Disorder

Meeting the criteria of organic mood disorder

Dementia

Meeting the criteria of dementia

Other Persistent Cognitive Impairment

This is a residual category which includes patients with cognitive deficit who do not fulfil criteria for amnesic syndrome or dementia.

Late Onset Psychotic Disorder

Other Mental and Behavioural Disorders

Unspecified Mental and Behavioural Disorders

ALCOHOL USE DISORDERS

Alcohol is the most widely used intoxicant all over the world. It has been used in different forms since antiquity. Alcohol is a part of everyday food in some countries and cultures, while it is completely prohibited in others. Many cultures permit its use on certain occasions. Thus any use of alcohol should not be considered as abnormal. If alcohol intake fulfils the diagnostic requirement of any of the condition described under the classification of psychoactive substance use disorders, only then it should be considered abnormal.

Chemistry, Absorption and Metabolism of Alcohol

Alcohol is chemically called Ethanol (C_2H_5OH). It is rapidly absorbed by the stomach, and the large and small intestines. However the stomach can control the rate of absorption by secretion of mucus which coats the stomach wall and thus reduces the rate of absorption. The pyloric sphincter is closed and the alcohol cannot pass into the small intestines where the rate of absorption cannot be controlled. The closure of the pyloric sphincter can give rise to vomitting by which excess alcohol is vomited. Alcohol can be accumulated in the stomach over long periods which may be absorbed a few hours later and may give rise to delayed effects.

Metabolism

Alcohol is excreted unchanged by the lungs and the kidney. The remaining alcohol is oxidised mainly by the liver. It is oxidised by ADH (alcohol dehydrogenase) which converts alcohol into acetaldehyde. Aldehyde dehydrogenase (AldDH) converts acetyldehyde into acetic acid which is not toxic. Disulfiram inhibits conversion of acetyldehyde to acetic acid and this produces its toxic effects.

Rate of Metabolism

The rate of metabolism is fairly constant and approximately 10 to 15ml of absolute alcohol is metabolised in an hour. If a person consumes 1 peg of alcohol, i.e. 50 ml of 40% proof alcohol per hour he is not likely to get intoxicated as the same can be metabolised in that period.

Two types of alcoholic drinks are available in India which are classified as country made liquor (locally distilled alcohol) and Indian made foreign liquor. Both these types have similar content of alcohol.

Effect of Alcohol On Various Body Parts

Brain — Alcohol is a depressant of the brain. Euphoria or hyperactivity experienced after alcohol intake is due to suppression of critical control and the person may become disinhibited.

Effects on the brain are dependant on the blood level of alcohol. At 0.5% level the critical faculties become lax and the person may become euphoric, may show poor judgement and thought process may become disrupted. At 1% level motor action becomes clumsy and the person may show slurring of speech and unsteadiness of gait. At still higher level the person may become confused and disoriented. If still more alcohol is consumed the person may pass into a coma and death may ensue. Death usually occurs due to direct respiratory depression or due to regurgitation of vomits into lungs.

Liver — Chronic alcohol ingestion induces fatty infiltration of liver and later may lead to cirrhosis.

Stomach — Chronic ingestion of alcohol can lead to gastritis and ulceration of the stomach.

Pancreas — Alcohol use may lead to pancreatitis.

High Density Cholesterol — This is increased by alcohol intake. Small quantities of alcohol may prove preventive in heart attacks.

Sex — People usually take alcohol to improve sexual desire and performance. Alcohol may reduce inhibition and thus the person may be able to express his sexual desires without inhibition. It may be useful for anxious individuals.

It usually depresses the performance, the erection may not occur or may be lost. The non drinking partner may find the behaviour of the partner disgusting. Long term use of alcohol leads to poor sexual desire and impotence in man. The females will also have reduced desire and may have difficulty in obtaining orgasm.

Epidemiology

Alcohol use differs from culture to culture. It is a part of the diet in some of the western countries like the United Kingdom, U.S.A. and some European countries. The use of alcohol is much less in India. However its use is increasing rapidly in this country while in the United States the total consumption of alcohol has shown a decrease.

Alcohol is used all over this country. The state of Punjab seems to have much higher consumption of alcohol than other parts. It is more commonly used by the poor, slum dwellers and by people with semskilled jobs. Its rate of use is increasing in the upper middle classes and rich class. Use of alcohol is also increasing amongst students.

However, not everyone who takes alcohol can be

considered sick. Nearly 15% of the people who are exposed to alcohol develop alcohol related problems. Alcohol use is much more common in men, in India. Similarly, alcohol related problems are also commonly seen in men. There are no large scale studies on epidemiology of alcoholism in this country.

Etiology

Etiology of alcohol related disorders has to be considered on two parameters.

a) Factors leading to exposure to alcohol,

b) Factors leading to alcohol related disorders.

Exposure to alcohol is dependant on the following

a) **Religion** — Many religious rituals of the christians are associated with alcohol consumption and christianity in general does not prohibit alcohol use.

The Muslim religion prohibits the use of alcohol. Hinduism is a way of life with multiple approaches to life. In general, alcohol use is discouraged in the Hindu way of life. But certain subcultures are allowed alcohol use. There is no prohibition to alcohol use.

b) **Socioeconomic Groupings** — Certain groups and occupation lead to alcohol use, e.g. industrial workers, workers in marketing trade and business, daily wage earners, students, and upper income groups with westernised approach.

c) **Climatic Condition** — People living in colder parts of the country tend to use alcohol more frequently.

d) **Easy Availability** — Country made liquor is quite cheap and is easily available in most parts of the country, thus encouraging alcohol use.

Factors Leading to Dependence and Other Alcohol Related Disorders

Biological Factor — There is good evidence to indicate that dependence has a genetic basis. Many studies in the west have shown that, father's of alcoholic the also show a greater frequency of alcoholism. Monozygotic twins show a high conçordance for alcoholism.

It has been observed that alcohol may have specific effects on the GABA system. This also explains the additive effect of alcohol with minor tranquilisers (benzodiazepines) which also acts through the GABA system.

Psychiatric Disorders

Alcohol dependence is often associated with certain psychiatric illnesses like, depression, schizophrenia, anxiety states and dissocial personality disorders.

Psychosocial Factors

Social Factors — Social approval of alcohol, advertisments and movies showing alcohol use by idealised figures may lead to increased alcohol use.

Peer pressure and use of alcohol by friends often leads to the initiation of this habit.

Psychological Factors — Individuals in psychological distress due to any cause like failures, broken marriage or dissatisfaction with life, may find solace in the use of alcohol.

Alcohol Related Problems

1. **Alcohol intoxication** — Intoxication occurs after excessive intake of alcohol. The main symptoms are :

Person may exhibit irrelevant and incoherent talks. He may become querulous or indecent. Some may become quiet or stupurose.

Other symptoms include slurring of speech, staggering gait, and flushing of face. Symptoms subside with time.

Pathological Intoxication

A few persons may show signs of acute intoxication after the ingestion of a very small amount of alcohol. This is known as pathological intoxication. It usually occurs in older persons suffering from organic diseases of the brain, in persons taking hypnotics or sedatives or in persons who are very anxious. The symptoms are similar to acute intoxication.

Harmful Use

This condition is diagnosed when the person continues using alcohol even after it has been definitely established that he has developed an alcohol related physical disorder, like the liver disease. These persons need not be dependant on alcohol.

Alcohol Dependence

An alcohol dependant person uses alcohol compulsively and fulfils the conditions required for drug dependence described earlier.

The clinical picture can be variable. Such persons may use alcohol excessively. Their jobs, family relationship and economic status is usually compromised. They may develop various alcohol related disorders. A few persons may take alcohol in bouts. Each bout lasts for a few days with complete sobriety during the interval. It is also known as binge drinking.

Case History

M was a 36 years old male belonging to an economically affluent family. Alcohol use was common among the male members of the family. His father was also an alcoholic. M started drinking when he was 13 or 14 years of age. His drinking has continuously increased. Later he started the mornings with a bottle of alcohol. He hardly ate anything. His daily consumption was nearly one to one and half bottle of rum. He stopped looking after his business. He had strained family relationships. This patient later developed cirrhosis of the liver, gastric haemhorrage and then died.

Comment — This patient had a strong genetic loading of alcoholism and his affluence allowed him unrestricted availability of alcohol. The family could neither control his alcohol intake nor could motivate him for treatment.

Alcohol Withdrawal

This syndrome develops when a chronic alcohol user gives up alcohol suddenly.

The characteristic features are :

Anxiety, restlessness, irritability

General malaise or weakness

Excessive sweating, tachycardia, raised blood pressure

Insomnia

Headache

Few patients may develop seizures.

Management

Acute withdrawal states are generally managed by the following :

a) Benzodiazepines — Chlordiazepoxide is usually used. 40-80mg/day may be required.

b) Clonidine and propranalol have also been used.

c) Nutrition should be maintained.

d) Psychological support should be provided.

The patient will require help and understanding both from family and the treatment team. These patients are often blamed for their drinking due to which they feel disheartened and their self-esteem is lowered. This should be avoided and the patient is to be helped to work through his personal, family and job difficulties.

Alcohol Withdrawal Delirium (Delirium Tremens)

Some patients may develop delirium after stoppage of heavy drinking. The syndrome is characterized by :

a) The person is usually disoriented and his level of consciousness is fluctuating ;

The patient may have hallucinations which are usually visual and tactile ;

They may have tachycardia, sweating and high blood pressure ;

The patient usually has coarse tremors ;

They may also develop seizures.

Management

The patient should be nursed in a quiet single room.

He should be given chlordiazepoxide 40-80 mg per day orally or by injection if the patient cannot take it orally.

Maintain nutrition by intravenous drip.

Vitamin B complex should be given by injectable routes.

High calorie, high carbohydrate diet should be given.

Mortality rate is around 20% in fully developed delirium tremens.

Alcoholic Hallucinosis

Some patients may develop hallucinations after cessation of alcohol intake. This hallucinosis is not a part of delirium. These patients usually have auditory or visual hallucinations. They must be differentiated from schizophrenia by the absence of other schizophrenic symptoms.

The condition is usually short lasting. It should be managed by proper nutrition, vitamins and phenothiazines.

Alcohol Induced Amnestic Syndrome

Alcohol use can induce vitamin B1 (thiamin) deficiency. It may lead to Wernicke's encephalopathy, which is characterized by ataxia, opthalmoplegia, nystagmus and confusion. This state may later lead to amnesia or Korsakoff's Psychosis.

Alcohol Induced Dementia

Alcohol dependence can lead to dementia in some cases. Dementia usually occurs after prolonged heavy drinking. The person may have associated cirrhosis of liver; there could also be history of Wernicke's encephalopathy. Signs and symptoms will be the same as described under dementia ( ).

Management — The patient should be managed symptomatically :

If there are nutritional or vitamin deficiencies they should be treated.

If there is evidence of cirrhosis, proper management should be done.

Alcohol use should be stopped.

If substantial brain damage has occurred, recovery will not take place but further damage can be prevented.

Manangement of Alcohol Dependence

The aim of treatment of alcoholism is to help the patient to abstain from taking alcohol permanently. Some people do advocate reduction in alcohol consumption as an alternative. Quite often when reduction of dosage is attempted the patient generally reverts back to the earlier pattern.

Assessment of the Patient

Personality of the patient.

The patient with dissocial traits, (E.g. repetitive antisocial acts, lying, stealing, precocious sexuality) are likely to do poorly. Patients with stable well adjusted personality do better.

Psychosocial Support System

Patients who have a caring family are likely to do better. Patients with a stable job are also likely to do better. Availability of community support or groups like Alcoholic Anonymous can also be helpful.

Associated Illness

The patient should be carefully evaluated for evidence of physical or mental illness.

These patients should be screened for :

Physical Disorders

a) Liver cirrhosis

b) Diabetes

c) Peripheral neuropathy

d) Subdural haematoma

e) Brain pathology

Mental disorders :

a) Depression

b) Schizophrenia

c) Other minor mental disorders

d) Personality disorder.

If any one of the above are present, appropriate treatment should be done.

Motivation

Patients usually come for treatment because of pressure from their employers, or doctors or families. They may not be motivated by themselves. The treating doctor has to help the patient to develop motivation. It is done by the following :

a) The patient should be repetitively told about harmful consequences of alcohol the e.g. cirrhosis, dementia, loss of sexual potency amd other complications of alcohol use.

b) The patient has to be clearly demonstrated that the reasons for which he used alcohol are not being fulfilled.

e.g. instead of being a good company alcoholics are avoided by others ;

People usually make fun of them

Their social credibility is lost

It leads to family and occupational problems

Sexual performance deteriorates.

Repetitive emphasis on the above may help to maintain motivation.

Psychotherapy

The doctor should be active during the psychotherapy of the alcoholic. He should discuss the patient's problems sympathetically and help them to face these situations.

The family should always be involved in treatment. They should not consider alcoholism as an inherent moral depravity or wickedness. The alcoholic suffers much more himself than others can imagine. The family should learn to accept him and to help him overcome his habit. At the same time the family has to be warned that they should not allow themselves to be manipulated by the patient in providing him alcohol.

Medication

These patients would require drugs to overcome the withdrawal symptoms. This phase is characterized by restlessness, anxiety, craving for alcohol and sleeplessness. All these symptoms can be controlled by benzodiazepines.

The patient can be given chlordiazepoxide 20-60mg/day depending on the severity of the symptoms.

Patient should feel comfortable with the help of the drugs. Usually 40mg is enough. Other benzodiazepines can also be used. This drug should be gradually withdrawn once the withdrawal symptoms have abated.

Disulfiram — This drug competitively inhibits aldehyde dehydrogenase due to which metabolism of alcohol is stopped, when it is converted into acetyldehyde. Acetyldehyde is a toxic substance and produces the following symptoms :

a) Flushing of face and body
b) Nausea and vomitting
c) Palpitation and difficulty in breathing
d) Hypotension may lead to sudden death.

This response can occur even if the patient ingests alcohol in the form of tonics or vinegar. Disulfiram is used to help the patient to develop internal control on his craving. Disulfiram does not reduce craving but helps the patient in controlling his desire because of the fear of toxic reactions.

The patient should have the following explained :

a) This drug does not reduce craving or produce aversion for alcohol.

b) If he takes even small quantity of alcohol he may develop severe reaction which can at times lead to death.

c) This drug helps the person by helping him to remain abstinent because of fear of toxic reaction. It acts as an internal police man. The person can thus avoid those moments when his resolve of abstinence might become weak.

d) This drug should be given only to those patients who have understood the above and are voluntarily willing to take the drug. They may be asked to write an agreement.

Dosage

250 mg to 500 mg Disulfiram is given daily. The drug should be discontinued after six months.

Side effects of Disulfiram are :

Toxic psychosis
Liver damage
Diarrhoea.

Group therapy is also helpful. Voluntary organisation like Alcoholic Anonymous are also helpful in maintaining abstinence.

MENTAL AND BEHAVIOURAL DISORDERS DUE TO USE OF OPIOIDS

Opioid stands for all substances which are similar to opium. Opium is derived from the juice of the opium the poppy, known as Papaver-Somniferum. There are around 20 alkaloids of opium, out of them the morphine is most potent. Semi-synthetic opioids are made by minor alteration in the parent substance, e.g. Heroin, and hydromorphine (Dilaudid). Purely synthetic substances are propoxyphene, mepridine, methadone and diphenoxylate (lomotil).

There are some relatively new products like pentazocine, butorphenol, and buprenorphine having mixed characteristics of agonist and antagonist actions of opioids. Buprenorphine is getting more attention nowadays due to its potent abuse potential.

Epidemiology

India has a special place in opioid related trafficking. It is situated in the middle of the golden triangle (Thailand, Mynamar) and golden crescent countries (Pakistan, Afghanistan and Iran). Hence, India is on the transit route for the opiod trafficking from these countries. Besides, India itself produces opium by cultivating opium poppy as a cash crop. Opium has been used in certain areas and certain occupational groups commonly. Opium was used frequently by the farmers of Punjab. It is also being used in certain areas of Uttar Pradesh. It is commonly used in a crude form. Lately, heroin is being smuggled into our country. The last few decades have seen marked increase in the use of Heroin (Brown Sugar) in various parts of the country, much more so in the metropolitan towns. Some poor quality heroin is also being locally produced. The groups effected are the students, skilled workers and generally younger people. It is much used more by men than by women.

Many people also use other related compounds like Pethidine, pentazocine and buprenorphine which are manufactured for medicinal purposes.

The exact incidence or prevalence of opium abuse is not known.

Pharmacology

Opioids are metabolised rapidly by the liver and almost 90% of the metabolites are excreted through the urine and bile within 24 hours of intake (except very long acting substances like Methadone). Though some metabolites can be detected in the body up to 48 hours. That is why clinical tests to determine fresh intake are administered only after 48 hours of stoppage of drugs.

Most of the drugs are taken orally. However, morphine and heroin are hardly absorbed from gastrointestinal tract. Heroin is diacetyl morphine and it is rapidly converted into morphine in the body. Heroin is twice as potent as morphine. 3-4mg of morphine is equal to 1-2mg of heroin ; 15-20 mg of Mepridine and 25-30 mg of codeine.

Opioids act by binding to the specific receptor sites in brain called "opioid receptors". The finding of opioid receptor in the central nervous system in the early 70's led to the discovery of substances having opiates like characteristics such as encephalins and endorphines. These are endogenous polypeptides and are involved in the regulation of pain perception. These substances are also supposed to have some role in regulation of normal mood, neural transmission and possibly in mediation of some action of other drugs of abuse. The opioid receptors have many subtypes like : Mu receptor, Kapa receptor, Sigma receptor and Delta receptor. Mu receptors are mainly involved in causing euphoria, analgesia and development of dependence. They seem to be mainly responsible for opioid's reinforcing behaviour. Other receptor subtypes have different actions. Opioid antagonists are synthetic compounds which displace and block the opioid receptors thus reversing or blocking the action of opioids. The main antagonists are naloxone, naltrexone (Trexan), nalorphine, and apomorphine. These are important in the management of opiod overdoses and rehabilitation of opioid dependant subjects. Heroin is more lipid soluble than morphine. Hence, it reaches the brain early and induces more rapid action specially, euphoria.

Tolerance and Dependence

Tolerance is rapid with most of the opioids. However, tolerance is variable for different actions. Tolerance quickly develops for sedation, depression, analgesia and mood elevation. Pupillary constriction (Miosis) and tendency of constipation are resistant to this tolerance effect. It is clinically important as many a times chronic drug dependant subjects try to dodge the physician about their drug taking behaviour. In such cases, there is no visible sign of drug intake except that the pupil is constricted which gives clue to their surreptitious opioid intake. Some people can use very high amount of heroin per day. Cross tolerance is also commonly seen among the opioids.

Opioids have very high capacity of inducing dependence. It is both early as well as severe in nature, even after short term use of opioids for medicinal purpose. The degree of dependence is related to the potency of opioids, duration of intake and amount taken. Dependence is both-psychological and physical. In fact, opioids induces mild tolerance even when used in therapeutic doses for even a week. However, clinically the significant withdrawal reaction occurs only after the chronic use of opioid as continuous binding of receptors by opioids is required for it.

There are reports that due to long exposure to opioids, changes in number or sensitivity of receptors takes place, leading to phenomenon of dependence. At intracellular level alteration in levels of calcium and cyclic adenosine monophosphate (CAMP) occurs by chronic intake. The withdrawal symptoms are induced by stoppage of chronic drug intake and are more severe and rapid, if opioid antagonists are administered.

The development of supersensitivity of various neurotransmitter systems like dopamine, serotonin and cholinergic by prolonged intake of opioids is thought to be important in causing rebound over activity leading to withdrawal syndrome when chronic use is discontinued.

Etiology

The personality profile of drug abusers often indicate lack of resources to confront challenges of day to day life, inconsistent behaviour and feelings, antiauthoritarain attitude and poor regard for social norms. They usually exhibit poor social achievement, conduct and behaviour problems bordering to antisocial traits or actual delinquency. Some demonstrate acute feelings of anxiety and depression and take drugs to ward off the unpleasant emotions and later get hooked to it. Often, there is no history of drug abuse or alcoholism in the family. Usually family ties are not strong and relationships are chaotic.

Clinical Characteristics

All the opioids give rise to analgesia, sedation, alteration in mood, which is usually of euphoria and clouding of mental activites. However, depending upon the nature and potency of opioids there is considerable variation in the effects on various systems of body. Morphine is more effective analgesic while heroin produces more euphoric action. Besides there is a feeling of warmth, heaviness in extremities and dryness of mouth. There may be flushing and itching of face, particularily nose due to release of histamine. The mood gets elevated leading to euphoria in most of the persons, lasting for about half an hour. A naive person may experience the use of opioid as unpleasant due to associated feelings of nausea, vomiting and dysphoria. Respiratory depression caused by opioid is a clinically important phenomenon as many deaths due to overdoses occur on account of arrest of respiration. Effect on other systems like cardiovascular and cerebral circulation are not significant. Associated intake of phenothiazines, monoamines oxidase inhibitors (MAOI's) Barbiturates, etc. may augment the respiratory depressant effect and could lead to serious consequences. All opioids cause pupillary constriction (Miosis) except mepridine, contraction of smooth muscles and decrease in peristaltic activities of intestine leading to constipation. Analgesia, induced by opioids is of the central type. There is basically alteration of pain perception, leading to indifferent attitude towards pain. Opioids analgesia is quite potent hence is clinically used for amelioration for the severest of pain like myocardial infarction, traumatic injuries and other severe visceral pains. Lately use of opioids for relieving severe pain of advanced cancer patients has increased .

Pattern of Opioid Use And Dependence

Opioid trafficking and sale is a very profitable business. Hence, the underworld and the antisocial elements play a large role in illicit trade of opioids specially heroin. They have vested interst in recruiting new customers and once hooked, they maintain the drug taking behaviour due to opioid's high dependence potential and continuing pressure by the drug culture subgroup. Hence, opioid dependence is very readily established in users. A personality profile of an average heroin users is — a young male from a poor background with poor schooling and performance. Usually, there has been initial use of cannabis/tobacco called the gateway drugs at an early age of 13-14 yrs and soon followed by heroin/smack abuse. The person having antisocial traits has a poor prognosis as compared to an average street user.

The life span of an addict is short and many casualties occur due to drug related problems like infection, accidents and drug-overdoses. The prognosis for intravenous users is specially poor. The I.V. users are at a special risk of hepatits B, bacterial infections and AIDS.

Relapse is common and risk is maximum in the first six months of abstinence. Mainly, it is because of strong craving for opioids, depression and exposure to old milieu of drug subculture. However, gradually the rate of relapse declines. Good prognostic indicators are stable job and family atmosphere, marriage, few delinquent acts unrelated to drugs and lack of any psychopathology or psychiatric illness.

Acute Intoxication

Opiate overdose is usually an acute, life threatening condition and it is generally accidental. There is marked unresponsiveness, coma, respiratory depression, hypothermia, hypotension and collapse. The body is pale with blue lips, pupils are pinpointed and there may be pulmonary oedema and shock. There are usually needle marks on the body. In very severe cases cardiac arrythimia and convulsions may develop and death may occur due to respiratory arrest and pulmonary oedema.

Management

Rule out other causes of coma, e.g. head injury, hypo or hyperglycemia or electrolyte abnormalities. Clear airway should be establised and heart function should be aided and monitored. Hypotension is managed by plasma expanders and pressure drugs. Pulmonary oedema is managed with positive pressure oxygen. Administration of narcotic antagonist could be life saving.

1) Naloxone is drug of choice. Dose is 0.01mg/kg by I.V. route and repeated within 10 minutes if no response is seen. The patient should be monitored for at least 24 hours due to its short half life.

2) If naloxone is not available, nalorphine 3-5mg I.V. can be given, repeat if needed.

Dependence Syndrome

Withdrawal State — Acute withdrawal state result from abrupt stoppage of opiods or precipitated by antagonists. It usually begins within 5-8 hrs of last dose of morphine and heroin. Methadone withdrawal state begin after 24-72 hrs due to long half life. In general the drugs with short half lives produce more rapid and severe withdrawal symptoms in comparison to long acting drug which produce less pronounced and long-lasting symptoms. The intensity of withdrawal symptom is related to dose, the duration of use and physical health of an individual. For heroin and morphine, the withdrawal symptoms peak in 36-48 hrs and then subside. It is usually over by 7-10 days. The main withdrawal symptoms are : running nose, lacrimation, sweating, yawning and intense craving for drug, severe insomnia, morbid restlessness and anxiety, pain in muscles and joints dilatation of pupil, anorexia and goose flesh (piloerection). At the peak of symptoms the patient is in great distress, have severe aches in bone, marked abdominal cramps and flu like syndrome consisting of weakness, G.I.T. upsets, chills and muscle spasm develops. There is also tachycardia, tremors, increased blood pressure, fever and temperature dysregulation.

The withdrawal symptoms are rarely life threatening unless there is underlying physical illness of severe nature.

Protracted Abstinence

The acute withdrawal state is followed by a more protracted abstinence. It is characterised by autonomic disturbances, e.g. change in pulse, blood pressure, body temperature, insomnia and craving for opioids. It persists for many months or a year. Possibly due to this residual withdrawal state, there is a vague discomfort and dysphoria which leads to an increased tendency for relapse. All acute or protracted abstinence symptoms can be readily removed by intake of opioids.

Treatment of Withdrawal

Usually, the withdrawal is planned and it is a first step in management of opioid addicts. This is technically called detoxification. It is mainly symptomatic in nature. The patient is generally hospitalized and properly examined, to find out any associated physical problem.

Clonidine, an antihypertensive drug blocks alpha-2-receptors specially in the locus coeruleus area of brain (adrenergic neuron system) and thus reduces sympathetic overactivity seen prominently in withdrawal state. The usual dose regime is as under :

Day 1	3 tabs/day
Day 2	6 tabs/day in divided doses
Day 3	to 8/9 tabs/day in divided doses
Day 9	6 tabs/day
Day 10	3 tabs/day
Day 11	NIL

(Each tablet of Clonidine is of .1 ugm)

Drowsiness and hypotension are main side-effects of clonidine. Hence, a close monitoring of blood pressure is required. Clonidine does not affect insomnia and craving. Hence, a hypnotic/anxiolytic is usually administered. For other problems like pain and aches, analgesic may be given. In management of diarrhoea, Diphenoxylate is preferred.

Methadone Maintenance

Methadone is a long acting synthetic opioid and is used mainly for substitution of heroin/other opioids. It is an effective treatment for those opioid addicts who find it difficult to live without drugs. It tends to prevent and suppress withdrawal symptoms to a tolerable level and this helps the patient to remain abstinent. It is convenient to use by oral route. Titration of methadone doses depends upon the amount of opioids taken. Usually 20 to 80 mg per day dose is sufficient for most patients. The duration of action is more than 24 hrs. Methadone maintenence is widely prevalent in the western countries. Unfortunately it is not available in India. There is inherent risk of methadone addiction, hence, it needs to be used with caution in vulnerable subjects. However, detoxification of methadone is usually a simple affair as compared to heroin and morphine.

Levo-alpha-acetylmethadol (LAMM) is a longer acting synthetic opioid then methadone. It is used in opioid addicts in a manner similar to methadone maintenance. However, it has an advantage over methadone as it can be given thrice a week. Dose is 30 to 80 mg.

Apart from pharmacological treatment of opioid dependence psychological support and family involvement in treatment plan is quite important. The patient needs to be reassured and any life crisis shoud be managed to prevent relapse. Many patients need change of place and job to remain away from the clutches of drug sub-culture of old acquaintances and friends. This may not be easy and require concerted effort of government agencies and voluntary organisations.

Role of Opioid Antagonist in Mangement

Opioid antagonists tend to block the effects of opioids, specially euphoriant action. Naltrexone, long acting (72 hrs) opioid antagonist, is used for this purpose. The dose is usually 350 mg per week. It can be given 100 mg on alternate days and 150 mg on last day. It is not addictive and it is devoid of any major side-effects.

Therapeutic Community — The emphasis is on self-reliance. Role taking confrontation and group discussion are encouraged. Usually the patient has to stay for long (from 6 months to 1-2 yrs). He has to adopt a new life-style and values. There has been conflicting reports of success of such programmes. They have high drop-outs. However, it has been seen that if a patient continues for more than six months he is likely to be benefited by this modality of self-help-programme. In India, most of the metropolitan cities have such therapeutic community centre.

CANNABIS

Cannabis is a well known intoxicant-euphoriant and it is widely used in Northern India. Cannabis is the generic name for various preparation of Cannabis Sativa or India hemp plant, which has been quite popular among the Chinese, Indian and some of the middle East countries. Its use spread in Europe and U.S.A after the 17th century, when the soldiers returned to Europe from the Indian subcontinent. By the 19th century, it had gained popularity as an analgesic, anticonvulsant and hypnotic. However, in the 1960's and 1970's, it attracted the attention of the youths in the UK and USA and it was quite popular in persons below 30 years of age. Though the trend has declined, it is still a common drug of abuse all over the world.

Sources and Preparation

Cannabis Sativa has many varieties which differ in the concentration of active ingredient - delta-9-tetra hydro cannabinol (THC). The plant grows well in the warm climate. The active ingredient (THC) is in higher concentration in flowering tops and nearby leaves. The female flowering top is known to be more potent than the male plant.

Bhang and Marijuana is the mildest of all preparations. It is prepared from dried leaves and stems of a hemp plant. Usually, it is smoked but may be mixed in sweets or sweetened drinks. This drink is more popular in Uttar Pradesh.

Charas or Hashish — It is dried resin of flowering tops and nearby leaves. It is supposed to be about ten times more powerful than Bhang or Marijuana.

Ganja — It is quite popular in India and is used widely by hermits for smoking. It is of intermediate potency and is prepared from the leaves near the flowering top and stem. It can also be used in drinks and sweets.

General Characteristics

The predominant effects of marijuana in usual doses are euphoria and alteration in the level of consciousness. The average cigarette contains 2.5-5 mg of Delta 9 THC. However, usually half of this amount is used through this route of administration. The peak plasma level are achieved in 10 mins. but it takes about half an hour for its main physiological and subjective effects to develop. The intoxication usually persists for 2-3 hours when the drug is smoked. When the drug is taken by an oral route, the larger amount of drug are absorbed, resulting in longer intoxication. Peak blood levels are obtained in 2-3 hrs and the effect lasts for as long as 8 hrs. Delta 9 THC is rapidly metabolised and tends to disappear from the plasma rapidly and gets absorbed in body tissues with special affinity for fatty tissues, e.g. brain and testes. The plasma half life is about 7 days mainly due to its accumulation in tissues. Some metabolites can be seen in urine and faeces even upto 8 days or more. However, the plasma half-life is greater in individual taking cannabis for the first time than the experienced ones. It indicates that cannabis induces its own metabolism. The chief metabolites of Delta 9 THC is 11 Hydroxy Delta 9 THC which is active and about 20% more potent then Delta 9 THC.

Acute Effects of Cannabis

There is a disturbance of short-term memory and impairment in the capability of carrying on multi step tasks. However, changes in mood not only depend upon the amount of cannabis taken but also the setting in which it is consumed. When a naive person takes cannabis in a new or strange environment, he harbours some anxiety about its intake and he is likely to experience marked anxiety and apprehension. He may feel suspicious of people and if consumed in higher amounts, may even develop hallucinations which are usually visual and may be at times accompained by paranoid delusions. There may be associated disorientation and feeling of panic. There are usually fine tremors, dry mouth, 'blood-shot eyes' and poor muscular coordination. Some persons experience nausea, headache, nystagmus and hypotension. THC may also induce seizures in epileptic. In general intoxication by cannabis is rated as mild to moderate in comparison to other substances of abuse like LSD, Phenylclidine, etc. To some extent effects of cannabis can be modulated by conscious control. In fact, many people who take cannabis regularly in mild to moderate quantity emphasize its positive aspect — it helps them to work better, for more hours and with more concentration.

Flashback

An abstinent cannabis user may experience spontaneous recurrence of the drug effect, specially when feeling exhausted. There is usually an interval of few days or weeks, rarely of months between cannabis use and flashback phenomenon. However, the flashback phenomenon is more characteristic of psychedelic drugs other than cannabis.

Acute Physical Effects of Cannabis

The main effects in a healthy individual are dryness of mouth, conjuctival injection (red conjunctiva due to dilatation of blood vessels) tachycardia and tachypnoea. Initially, there is bronchial constriction but later bronchial dilatation occurs. This effect of cannabis is utilised in treatment of asthma. The other significant effect is lowering of intra-ocular pressure, this is being employed for treatment of glaucoma. There is no effect on blood sugar level implying that the effect on hunger induction is unmediated through the mechanism of hypoglycemia. There is reduction of plasma testostrone level to a significant level 2-3 hours after cannabis intake.

Tolerance and Dependence

Though still controversial however, there is an increasing agreement about the phenomenon of mild dependence and tolerance after the continued use of cannabis. Some of the effects of cannabis like bronchial dilatation, decrease in intraocular pressure and tachycardia tend to diminish over a period of time. Likewise, abrupt stoppage of drug leads to tremor, increase salivary flow, increase body temperature and intro-ocular pressure along with psychological symptoms like anxiety, insomnia, anorexia, restlessness and sweating, etc. The effects could be reversed immediately by intake of cannabis suggesting development of some physical dependence. However, the intensity of withdrawal symptoms is overall mild and can be managed easily. Further, there is no drug seeking behaviour or craving after stoppage of cannabis use, indicating mild degree of psychological dependence.

Immediate Adverse Psychological Effects

The ratio of lethal to effective dose is thought to be in the range of 20,000 to 1 to 40,000 to 1. Hence, the drug is very safe. However, drug sensitive person may experience depression, marked anxiety, persecutory ideation, dizziness and visual impairment or distorted perception. There may be poor control of behaviour and clouding of consciousness, and feeling of heaviness in head and gastro-intestinal upset, etc. Severe cases of intoxication may exhibit frank hallucination, marked excitement, depersonalization, and delirium.

Long Term Effects of Cannabis Use

There are many reports indicating the development of apathy, inertia, poor drive, poor social judgement and withdrawal from activities needing long hours of work or persistence. This syndrome is known as a motivational syndrome and is seen in chronic heavy users of cannabis. It is now believed that this syndrome is more likely due to earlier personality traits of the patients and cannabis may have no role in its development.

Psychosis

It is a transitory psychotic state characterised by paranoid behaviour and hallucination occurring in setting of clear sensorium. It usually develops following heavy use of cannabis. However, recent research work does not support the existence of prolonged psychosis after cannabis use.

Medical Problems of Long Term Cannabis Use

General cannabis intake is not associated with complications. Medical problems associated with cannbis intake are of mild and temporary nature. Some important systems affected by cannabis are :

1) Respiratory System — Cannabis, when smoked can cause irritation of lung mucosa resulting in Bronchitis. It clears with stoppage of drug use. It also leads to destruction of lung parenchyma. There is tendency for development of asthama like syndrome. Initially cannabis causes bronchial dilatation but long term use eventually leads to constriction. There are some reports of carcinogenic changes in lungs produced by chronic cannabis intake. Cannabis is supposed to have 50% higher levels of carcinogenic hydrocarbons than tobacco.

2) Nose and Throat — Chronic sinusutis, pharyingitis are seen in chronic heavy cannabis smokers.

3) Cardiovascular System — Cannabis induces tachycardia and reduced strength of cardiac contraction. This could be important for a cannabis user with

a underlying cardiovascular disease. However, the underlying clinical implications are not clear.

4) Immune System — There are some reports suggesting sensitivity of lymphocytes to THC, which may impair the immune system. This may lead to lowered resistance to infections. However, hardcore evidence of this effect is lacking.

Reproductive System

Heavy cannabis use may lead to chromosomal destruction and decreased spermatozoa production. There are reports of decrease in prostrate and testicular size in men and disturbances in menstruation and ovulation in females. There is a lowering of testosterone in the males.

Brain

Cannabis use may induce EEG changes and there are few reports of some brain damage in heavy chronic cannabis users. These reports of cerebral atrophy seen in chronic cannabis users have not been confirmed.

Treatment

Cannabis intake is common in Northern India. It is a mild and cheap agent leading to relaxation and enjoyment. Many such people do not have any complaints ; neither is there any adverse effect on their work and social relationship. Such people do not require any treatment. When there are physical problems or psychological effects, then cannabis use has to be stopped. However, the tendency of using cannabis in younger population should be curbed heavily as a preventive strategy. The use of any mind altering drug may lead to loss of productivity in immature young persons. It may provide a substitute for more healthy recreational activities like sports. Hence education, social awareness of illconsequences and other harmful effect should be highlighted to dissuade potential or occasional drug users before they seriously embark upon regular or heavy drug using behaviour. The main emphasis in management is on psychological approach. There are no serious withdrawal symptoms on sudden cessation of cannabis use. For acute anxiety and panic reaction minor tranquilizers and reassuarance is required.

MENTAL AND BEHAVIOURAL DISORDERS DUE TO USE OF SEDATIVES AND HYPNOTICS

Sedatives and tranquilizers are being prescribed extensively in our country. Most of these drugs produce dependence on prolonged use. The following group of compounds are included :

Benzodiazepines —Diazepam, Lorazepam, Alprazolam, Chlordiazepoxide, Flurazepam, Nitrazepam.

Hypnotics — Pentobarbital, Secobarbital, Phenobarbitone, Methaqultone, Glutithemide.

Epidemiology

Most of these drugs are medically prescribed and often the dependence is a result of repititive intake without medical prescription. Individuals are able to purchase these drugs from dispensings chemists without prescription, though the Indian law does not allow this sale.

The exact extent of misuse of these drugs is not really known, but it is certain that these drugs are being misused at a large scale. Medical profession should take special care that these drugs are not unnecessarily precribed and the prescription is only for a limited period.

BARBITURATES

The manufacture and sale of Barbiturates is restricted in this country. Phenobarbitone is the only barbiturate whose sale is allowed on duplicate prescription. The phenobarb is used for seizure disorders and it is not generally misused. However, phenobarb is often used for suicidal attempts.

Management of Phenobarbitone Overdosage

The patient should be treated in an intensive care unit. The patient should be kept awake if he is not already comatose. He should be put on I.V. drip. Airway should be kept patient either by endotracheal intubation or if needed by tracheostomy. The patient should be given gastric lavage with activated charcoal. Vital signs should be monitored.

BENZODIAZEPINES

Benzodiazepines are the most commonly prescribed drugs and are often misused. These drugs are generally used by people to suppress anxiety or to obtain sleep. The drug often lead to tolerance so that a larger dosage is required to achieve the same effect. Many patients increase the dosage as time passes by. Often the drug use remains limited and does not produce much harm. These drugs also do not lead to lethal consequences because there is large difference between therapeutic and lethal dosage.

The drug use may continue for years because whenever the individual tries to reduce the drugs insomnia, anxiety reappears.

Management

These drugs can be gradually withdrawn if there is no preexisting psychiatric or physical disorder which warrants their use. The limited use in certain chronic conditions does not produce any perceivable harm.

MENTAL AND BEHAVIOURAL DISORDERS DUE TO COCAINE USE

Cocaine is a psychic stimulant and leads to euphoria, increased energy and increased activities. The effect of drug may last for few hours and is followed by dysphoria, feeling of being let down and agitation. This can be relieved by another dose of cocaine. Cocaine is often used as an aphrodisiac for delaying ejaculation. However, the repetitive use of cocaine leads to impotency.

Fortunately this drug has so far not become a drug of common use in our country. Cocaine use can lead to delirium, which is characterized by perception of bugs crawling on or below the skin. These persons may develop persecutory delusions (people are trying to harm them). They may also show excitement, sexual disinhibtion and disorientation.

MENTAL AND BEHAVIOURAL DISORDERS DUE TO USE OF OTHER STIMULANTS INCLUDING CAFFEINE

This group includes drugs like amphetamines, and ephedrine. The manufacture and sale of these substances has been banned in our country, due to which their use is very limited.

However, the banning of drugs like amphetamine has affected proper management of conditions like hyperactive attention deficit disorder of children, narcolepsy and obesity.

CAFFEINE

Caffeine is part of daily diet for most Indians in form of tea or coffee. Tea or coffee produce an alerting effect on the individual, their concentration increases and tiredness decreases. The psychomotor performance improves. The effect may last for 3-10 hours. Non-availability of caffeine to a habituated individual may lead to headache and fatigue. Most persons do not require intervention. If a person develops anxiety and tremulousness due to excessive intake, then withdrawal may be attempted.

BEHAVIOURAL AND MENTAL DISORDERS DUE TO USE OF HALLUCINOGENS

This group contains those drugs which induce hallucinations. Common drug in this category are LSD, phencyclidine, Fortunately, the use of these drugs is quite rare in this country.

MENTAL AND BEHAVIOURAL DISORDERS DUE TO USE OF TOBACCO

Tobacco (Nicotine) has been in extensive use throughout the world. It has been so popular among all sections of the society, that nobody apprehensive that it may lead to health hazards. Contrary to general belief, tobacco causes serious dependency which is generally realised when one wishes to stop its use on medical advice or otherwise. There is severe craving in an abstinent person along with irritability uneasiness and sleep disturbances, which may persist in protracted form for many months to years after cessation of tobacco use. Psychiatric patients tend to use tobacco excessively. In one study in USA, 88% of schizophrenic outpatients and 70% of bipolar affective disorder outpatients were found smoking cigarettes.

Epidemiology

In the west, the use of Tobacco gained momentum after the World War I and reached its peak in 1960. During this time a study reported that 52% American males and 32% American females were taking Tobacco. However, in recent years, there has been a drastic decline in use of Tobacco in Western world specially in America for adult population, possibly due to the world wide campaign against smoking. In India, the exact figures of tobacco use are not available. Tobacco is also used for sniffing and chewing (Zarda and Khaini). Tobacco is quite popular in northern India. Tobacco in Paan (Beetal) is in popular use and is socially approved. Due to this route of tobacco intake, oropharyngeal carcinoma is on the increase. The number of youth and student population consuming tobacco is increasing. The children of smoking parents are at a special risk. Many reports suggest that there is a genetic predisposition. Smoking usually starts in adolescents and it is more in youths having adjustment problem, poor scholastic achievement and tendency to take risk.

Pharmacology

Nicotine, the active ingredient of Tobacco is consumed mainly by smoking or chewing Tobacco leaves, and at some places it is sniffed in nasal cavity. Smokers inhale large number of substances, e.g. Nitrogen oxide, Ammonia and aldehydes depending on the temperature of burning. There are 3 major compounds of tobacco 1) Tar 2) Carbon-monoxide (CO) 3) Nicotine. The Tar contains aromatic amines which possibly are carcinogenic. The carbon monoxide decreases oxygen carrying capacity of blood which gives rise to an increased number of RBC, and it ultimately may result in increased incidences of cardiovascular problems, due to enhanced arteriosclerotic process.

Nicotine was first isolated in 1828. It is rapidly absorbed through GIT and lungs. One puff of smoke produces appreciable amount of Nicotine within seconds. The average cigarette contains 1.5 to 2.5 mg Nicotine. A filter cigarette may have slightly lower levels of Nicotine but may give rise to more CO (carbon monoxide). When taken through oral route peak plasma levels are in the range of 25-50 mg/ml and half life is 30-120 minutes. Nicotine is oxidised mainly by liver and it has enzyme-induction property. Hence, metabolism of some drugs, like theophylline, phenacetin, caffeine, propranolol and imipramine is increased. Nicotine thus, increases the need of higher doses of benzodiazepines and decrease the antianginal activity of Nifedipine, atenolol and propranolol. Nowadays, smokeless tobacco is more popular in some parts of the world specially in India, Pakistan, Bangaldesh. The smokeless tobacco (chewing tobacco and sniff) has its own hazards of nasopharyngeal irritation and is implicated in the increased incidence of oropharyngeal malignancies in these countries. Nicotine affects many systems of body through the nicotine receptor, a subclass of acetylcholine receptors. CNS has more pronounced effect where it induces alertness and arousal, followed by calmness. Many smokers believe that tobacco increases clear thinking and concentration and there is some truth in it. Some studies do actually demonstrate enhanced recall and rapid information processing. Nicotine leads to suppression of appetite. The respiratory system is more adversely affected. There is chronic irritation of bronchial mucosa leading to irritating cough. A smoker's cough is due to the development of chronic bronchitis. There is an increased incidence of lung carcinoma due to smoking, 2-4 times more than general population. It induces tachycardia, increased cutaneous vasoconstriction high blood-pressure and possibly enhanced platelet stickiness.

The endocrine system reacts to Nicotine by release of epinephrine and catecholamines. Nicotine effects the sleep pattern, specially REM sleep is disturbed. It also leads to development of fine tremors. Nicotine is otherwise very toxic and 60 mg may be a fatal dose for many. Nicotine poisoning may exhibit increased salivation, pain in abdomen, nausea and vomiting, increased heart rate and blood-pressure, confusion and dizziness, headache, jitteriness, ataxia with tremulousness, which may ultimately lead to fainting, hypotension, decreased respiration, convulsion and death may occur due to respiratory failure.

Dependence

Tolerance and dependence on Nicotine is rapid. Usually people have a feeling that dependence of nicotine is of mild nature and they can stop smoking as and when they want. This however, is a wrong notion as persons tend to increase their quota of daily smoking in a short time. In general, people tend to smoke 20 to 30 cigarettes everyday. Behavioural, metabolic and pharmacological factors are involved in the development of dependency. Most of the persons, specially youth, smokes for psychological gain, they feel themselves to be more stylish, forward looking and get "status" in their peer group. In adults, smoking is usually associated with pleasurable activities like cocktails, dinner, celebration and club activities. Catchy advertisement also contributes in maintaining tobacco consumption. Tolerance to unpleasant effects of tobacco like nausea, vomiting, dizziness and irritation of bronchial mucosa occurs rather early.

The Withdrawal Syndrome

The withdrawal syndrome starts within hours of stopping intake of nicotine and peaks within 24 hours. The most characteristic is intense craving for nicotine. There are irritability, anxiety and restlessness. The person tend to become nervous, has poor concentration and bad temper. There is a disturbed sleep pattern and the patient feels dull and drowsy and performance is impaired. There is a positive correlation between level of tolerance and intensity of withdrawal symptoms. Usually, there is appreciable weight gain due to increased appetite. The symptoms wane after a month or so, however, craving and some discomfort may last for a long time, at times as long as 10 to 20 years. The withdrawal symptoms in general are of mild intensity. Unlike other drugs of dependence, nicotine is reported to have more intense symptoms when withdrawal is gradual, i.e. tapering off. Hence, abrupt stoppage of nicotine is recommended to cut short the duration of withdrawal symptoms.

Long-Term Complications of Chronic Nicotine Use

Apart from lung cancer and malignancies of oropharynx, vascular and cardiovascular complications like strokes, heart-attacks and angina are quite common in chronic tobacco users. With the increase in number of smoking mothers specially in the western culture, problems in neonates are on the rise. Low birth weight of the child is common in such women. There is also an increased risk of abortion, premature delivery and congenital anomalies. Children tend to be unstable and overactive which may persist for long time.

Nowadays, there is a growing concern for health hazards of passive smoking. The problems of eye irritation, heaviness in head, choking sensation as well as tendency for more serious hazards faced by non-smokers is getting more attention. Spouse and children of chronic smokers are at a special risk. In view of the above many restrictions are being imposed to curb smoking in public places. The "Non-smokers Zone" concept is catching on.

Treatment and Prevention

The management of tobacco dependence involves education and counselling to increase motivation and maintain abstinence. Most people can control this habit by stopping smoking suddenly, but quite often their motivation fluctuates and they may restart smoking.

Behavioural Approaches

Since many patients find it difficult to remain abstinent inspite of well meaning efforts to do so. Behavioural modification techniques are being increasingly applied for such cases. These strategies do show good results but need refresher/reinforcement sessions for long term benefits. Behavioural approaches require detailed analysis of tobacco consuming patterns. Thereafter, behavioural modification is attempted according to individual requirements.

One technique is "self control" strategy. This involves repeatedly reminding the patient about cessation of smoking and he is allowed to smoke only at times which are least pleasurable. He is asked not to smoke after food or in parties.

Other behavioural techniques are based on aversive conditioning, like administration of mild electric shock while smoking. Many other techniques are based on "flooding", i.e. forced intake of a heavy quantity of tobacco in short times or rapid chain smoking. Others use coupling of unpleasant images, like serious medical complications associated with tobacco intake with the act of smoking. All these techniques produce aversion towards smoking.

Pharmacological Treatment

On the line of substitution therapy like methadone, the maintenance in severe opioid dependants, nicotine gum have been promoted to take care of withdrawal symptoms in heavy tobacco users. Nicotine gum contains 2 mg of nicotine bound to an ion-exchange resin in each piece, when chewed slowly, nicotine is released in circulation at a relatively low level and is usually enough to curb withdrawal symptoms. Thus after abrupt cessation of heavy smoking, the nicotine gum is used for 3-4 months and is then gradually tapered off. It is an effective regime but has its own drawbacks like a tendency for addiction to nicotine-gum itself ; and GIT ulcers/inflammation and toxic reaction, if used excessively. Nonetheless, when coupled with good therapeutic supervision and education about its use, nicotine-gum has a promising role to play in heavy smokers. Recently people have used clonidine (alpha-2-adrenergic receptors agonist for amelioration of withdrawal symptoms like restlessness, anxiety, irritability and craving, etc.).

In the conclusion, it can be said that in view of high morbidity and mortality associated with chronic tobacco consumption, every effort should be made to stop its use.

THE NARCOTIC DRUGS AND PSYCHOTROPIC SUBSTANCES ACT 1985

The Government of India has enacted the above mentioned act to effectively curb the illegal manufacture, sale and use of substances notified under the act. The substances included are

Barbiturates, Tranquilizers, Opioids, Cannabis, Cocaine and other psychoactive substances.

The act provides stringent penalities of imprisonment for minimum of 10 years and penalty of Rs. 10 lacs or more for drug pedlars. A subsequent offence may lead to enhanced penalty including death penalty. The act also identifies drug addicts and forbids their prosecution, if they agree to take the treatment provided they are not involved in any other serious offences under the act.

The main purpose of this act is to provide deterrent punishment so that drug trafficking could be stopped.

(For details consult the original Act.)

CHAPTER 7
SCHIZOPHRENIA, SCHIZOTYPAL AND DELUSIONAL DISORDERS

These group of disorders are characterised by symptoms which were previously called psychotic symptoms. These symptoms are delusions, hallucinations and thought disturbances. It is not necessary that all these symptoms should be present in each category. This grouping is provisional and has been done on the similarity of clinical picture. These disorders are further classified as under :

Schizophrenia

Paranoid schizophrenia
Hebephrenic schizophrenia
Catatonic schizophrenia
Undifferentiated schizophrenia
Post-schizophrenic depression
Residual schizophrenia
Simple schizophrenia
Other schizophrenia
Schizophrenia unspecified.

The course of these disorders may be classified as —

Continuous
Episodic with progressive deficit
Episodic with stable deficit
Episodic remittent
Incomplete remission
Complete remission
Others
Course uncertain / period of observation less than one year.

Schizotypal Disorder

Persistent Delusional Disorder

Delusional disorder
Other persistent delusional disorders
Persistent delusional disorder, unspecified.

Acute and Transient Psychotic Disorders

Acute polymorphic psychotic disorder without symptoms of schizophrenia

Acute polymorphic psychotic disorder with symptoms of schizophrenia

Acute schizophrenia like psychotic disorder

Other acute predominantly delusional psychotic disorder

Other acute and transient psychotic disorders

Acute and transient psychotic disorder, unspecified.

Presence or absence of associated acute stress may be identified

Without associated acute stress
With associated acute stress

Induced Delusional Disorders

Schizoaffective Disorders

Schizoaffective disorder, manic type
Schizoaffective disorder, depressive type
Schizoaffective disorder mixed type
Other schizoaffective disorders
Schizoaffective disorder, unspecified.

Other Non-Organic Psychotic Disorders

SCHIZOPHRENIA

Schizophrenia is a common mental disorder. It is mainly characterised by disturbances in thinking, feeling and behaviour. The thinking of these patients becomes so disturbed that often, it is difficult to identify the logic in their expressed ideas. Their emotional state is also quite abnormal. While some may exhibit a totally unwarranted anxiety, perplexity or unaccountable fear, others may exhibit poor emotional response which is known as flatness of emotion. As a result of these disturbances, their overall behaviour becomes inappropriate, e.g. they may become quiet and non-responsive, and may show purposeless excitement or repetitive activity. Their work and social relationship are usually disturbed seriously.

Most of the researchers in this field, believe that schizophrenia is not a single disorder, but it may be subdivided in future into different subtypes depending on genetic and biochemical differentiation.

Epidemiology

Prevalence of the disease is almost similar in all parts of the world except in the few areas where the rates are unusually high. The point prevalnce of this illness is roughly between 1 to 2 per thousand. The rates will vary according to the age structure of the population.

The illness generally starts between 15 and 25 years, but can occur at any age. There is no difference in prevalence between the two sexes.

Till recently the reproduction rate of schizophrenics was quite low as majority of these patients developed the illness during adolescence before they could produce. In recent times, many of these patients can be treated and thus are able to marry and reproduce. Possibly, this may increase the prevalence of this disorder.

The socio-economic factors were earlier implicated in the genesis of schizophrenia, as the illness was found more often in lower socio-economic strata of society. However, current researchers have not affirmed these findings.

Epidemiology of Schizophrenia

Incidence	.05 - .25%
Prevalence	.2 - 1%
Life prevalence	1.5%
Sex	Equal
Age	15 - 25 years (could be any age)
Socio-economic status	No difference

Etiology

Exact etiology of this disorder is still not known. However, a large number of investigators have identified many neurophysiological and biochemical abnormalities, but none of these could be consistently demonstrated. It appears that this category may be etiologically heterogenous.

Following are some of the main observations concerning etiology of schizophrenia.

A) **Genetics** — It is now generally accepted that genetics plays an essential role in the development of schizophrenia. The illness tends to develops in only those who are genetically vulnerable for this disorder. The evidences in favour of genetic hypothesis are :

(i) Close relatives of schizophrenic probands show much higher risk of schizophrenia compared to general population.

(ii) Monozygotic twins have a high concordance rate for schizophrenia.

(iii) The biological parents of a schizophrenic show higher prevalence of this disorder then the adopted parents.

Currently, linkage studies are being undertaken to identify the exact mechanism of genetic transmission.

B) **Biogenic Amines** — Most of the antipsychotics act by blocking the dopaminergic neurons. It is postulated that these neurons are hyperactive in schizophrenia. Indirect evidence for this hypothesis is also provided by worsening of psychosis when dopamine agonists like amphetamine are administered to these patients.

Other neurotransmitters have also been implicated and studied in schizophrenia and inconsistent findings have emerged.

C) **Neuropathology** — Recent investigative techniques have demonstrated some changes in structure and functions of the brain of these patients. Common findings are :

Increased size of lateral and third ventricles.

Decrease in brain mass

Hypoactivity of frontal lobes

Minor abnormalities in basal ganglion, limbic and frontal lobes.

The exact nature of the lesion or its site has so far not been identified.

Many investigators have also demonstrated changes in immunoglobin level and endocrinal abnormalities.

D) **Psychosocial Theories**

i) **Socioeconomic Status** — Earlier observers had reported schizophrenia to be more prevalent in lower socioeconomic class. But later researchers could not substantiate this observation.

Family Psychopathology — Many researchers have observed that inappropriate communication amongst the family members is common in schizophrenic families. Unhealthy parent-child interaction has been heavily emphasised by several workers. Although none of these observations could be consistently demonstrated, it is however postulated, that the family interaction may be partially responsible for precipitating this disorder.

ii) **Stress** — Schizophrenia commonly develops during adolescence or in post-partum phase and both these periods are of intense endocrinal disturbances as well as psychological stress. It is possible that some biological or psychological stress may be associated with the precipitation of the disorders in the vulnerable individual. It has now been quite consistently shown that relapse of schizophrenia is more common in those families where family members show over-emotionality and critical attitudes towards the patient.

Conclusion : Although the exact nature of etiopathology is not known, the evidence is quite robust that this illness occurs in those who have a genetic vulnerability. Such individuals may however develop this illness when they experience a stress which could be of a biological or psychological nature, (e.g. endocrinal changes, stress of marriage or examinations, etc.).

TABLE

Summary of Etiological Theories of Schizophrenia

1. **Genetic** — The evidence is robust but some precipitating factors have to be presumed.

2. **Biochemical**	
a. Dopamine hypothesis	Etiological role still hypothetical
b. Nor-epinephrine	
c. Gamma-Aminobutyric acid	
d. Other neurotransmitters	

3. **Brain Pathology**
a. Dilatation of lateral and third ventricles
b. Decreased brain mass
c. Changes in basal and ganglion limbic lobes
d. Brain imaging techniques indicating hypoactivity of frontal lobes

4. **Endocrinal and immunological abnormalities**

5. **Psychosocial** — Family pathology, stresses

CLINICAL PICTURE

Scizophrenics present with such a varied clinical picture that an untrained observer may not find any similarity amongst them. A closer scrutiny will however, exhibit disturbances in thoughts, emotions and overall behaviour in all of them.

Premorbid Personality

Premorbidly these patients are usually quiet and obedient. They are often described as ideal children, many of them may do very well in studies and may also score high marks. Their social interaction are very limited. They prefer to participate in lonely pursuits e.g. watching television, listening to radio, body building, etc. Nevertheless, depending upon the genetic loading and other factors, the illness may also develop in individuals having other types of personality make up and the clinical presentation is largely coloured by the basic personality attributes and it is responsible for so may differences in the symptomatology of schizophrenia.

Prodromal Symptoms —

Many patients can show mild behaviour abnormalities for few days or few weeks prior to the onset of florid symptoms. These may include irritability, withdrawal, sleep difficulties, lack of interest in studies or work.

Symptomatology — For the purpose of clinical examination symptomology of schizophrenia is given here under the following sub-heads :

A) **General Behaviour**

i) Overt behaviour may appear fully normal so that a casual observer may consider them normal, although a closer scrutiny for an appreciable period would enable the examiner to detect several abnormalities in the behaviour.

ii) **Withdrawal** — Such patients may appear unconcerned with surroundings. This may also reflect in their dress which may be unkempt or untidy, their hair may be overgrown and poorly cared. They might start keeping a beard. The nails may be dirty and long. In short, they do not take care of their appearance.

iii) Other patients may show marked overactivity, excessive talkativeness, abusiveness or destructiveness.

Most patients avoid eye to eye contact with the examiner.

iv) Some patients may exihibit symptoms of catatonia. These symptoms are —

a) **Catatonic Stupor** — The patient is almost mute. He lies in bed motionless. The bladder and bowels are full and there could be urinary or faecal incontinence. However, the patient is otherwise fully conscious and responds to painful stimuli. Though the patient is mute and unresponsive he may register everything that is going on around him. The attending personnel should be therefore, careful about their behaviour towards the patient because he is likely to recall it later.

b) **Waxy Flexibility** — When the patient's body parts, limbs or head are put in uncomfortable posture the patient may not revert that body part for a long time to a comfortable position.

c) **Posturing** — The patients may show bizarre postures, e.g. standing on one feet for long time, standing in hot sun or gazing at the sun, etc.

d) **Negativism** — Some patients may show oppositional behaviour, e.g. if the examiner asks them to open the mouth, they might close it tightly.

e) **Automatic Obedience** — Certain patients may exhibit complete obedience to every command. If the examiner asks the patient to protrude the tongue and tells him that he will prick it with a pin, the patient will let him do so, while ordinarily in such a situation a normal person will withdraw the tongue.

f) **Echolalia** — Some patients tend to repeat the words spoken by the other person, if examiner asks to open the mouth, he may instead repeat the spoken words "open your mouth".

g) **Echopraxia** — Some patients may repeat the acts done by the examiner, e.g. if the examiner scratches his face during the interview, the patient also does the same.

h) **Catatonic Excitement** — Such patients exhibit purposeless intense activity and may appear destructive, quarrelsome or hostile.

Speech — Some patients may be mute (not speaking) or may speak in monosyllables (yes/no or I don't know, etc.) Whereas, other's may speak excessively. Often the modulation of speech may be lost.

Disorders of Thinking — Although disorders of thinking are the corner stone of schizophrenic illness, in some patients thought disorder is quiet a prominent feature while in others it may be more or less minimal. Thought disorder is usually inferred from speech, although writing or other activities of the person, may also provide a reliable account of the individuals thought process.

Thought disorder can be categorised as disturbance in thought process or thought content and types of presentation in each of these two are given below.

a) **Disturbances of Thought Process**

i) **Irrelevant Speech** — The patient does not answer questions appropriately. The speech is not easily understandable. For instance, if the examiner asks the patient to tell his name he may reply "The moon is going down into the river. All men are worthless".

ii) **Incoherent Speech** — The answer of the patient starts relevantly but the latter sentences do not have any relation with each others. The example quoted above also shows incoherence.

iii) **Loosening of association** — This means that the normal association process is disturbed and this leads to irrelevance, or incoherence or both.

iv) **Circumstantiality** — The disturbance is characterized by the inclusion of unnecessary details in the answer although the answer is relevant to the question to a great extent.

A patient was asked how he came to the hospital. He replied "It was a nice day. I got up early in the morning. There was no water. I asked my uncle to accompany me to the hospital. We took a cycle rickshaw for coming to the hospital."

v) **Tangentiality** — The patient's answer may just touch the point but later, deviate to related but not required details.

vi) **Neologism** — Some patients develop a morbid habit of coining new words by condensing two or more words, which may not appear meaningful to others.

vii) **Verbigeration** — The patient repeats one or two meaningless phrases repetitively.

viii) **Word Salad** — Incomprehensible mixture of words.

ix) **Poverty of thought** — These patients present with impoverishment of thoughts and as such they are found to be frequently repeating one or two ideas or sentences.

x) **Thought block** — The patient may stop abruptly while talking and after a few seconds, he may be able to complete the answer. On being asked why he stopped, the patient will say that all of a sudden his mind went blank.

xi) **Perseveration** — The phenomenon is characterised by patient's repeatation of the answer to a previous question. For instance the examiner asks the patient to tell his name and he tells his name but later on being asked where he lives he may again repeat his name.

xii) **Poor Abstraction** — Abstraction is the ability to identify commonness as well as differences in various things, objects or concepts. The schizophrenics often lack this ability. To assess it, the patient may be asked to tell the similarities between orange and banana (both are fruits), bird and aeroplane (both can fly) or differences between chair and table. Similarly, they may not be able to give abstract meaning of simple common proverbs.

xiii) **Thought being read** — These patients complain that other people mysteriously come to know, whatsoever they are thinking, without the former disclosing the same. Some may compain that their thoughts are being broadcasted on radio or television.

xiv) **Thought control** — The patient feels that his thoughts are being controlled by some external power, e.g. Radio, T.V., C.B.I., etc. A patient used to complain that his former Guru is controlling his thoughts so that he should marry his daughter.

xv) **Thought Withdrawl** — Some patients may complain that their thoughts have been withdrawn or stolen by some external agency.

b) **Disorder of Thought Content**

i) **Delusion** — This is a firm false belief which can not be corrected by reason and it is not normally accepted by the patient's sociocultural group. Common delusions is that people are trying to harm or are conspiring against him. In delusions of grandiosity, the patient feels that he has too much power or money. There could be delusions of love. There could also be other bizarre delusions, such as the patient believes that he can cause the destruction of the earth or he is the chosen one to save the mankind from disaster.

Delusion of control — The patient is convinced that some external power is controlling his thoughts and actions. It is also called passivity phenomenon. "A patient felt that a transmitter has been fitted into his brain by some evil person and his actions are being controlled through this transmitter."

ii) **Ideas of reference** — Some patients may feel that people are talking about them or they are making signals to them. One patient used to complain that whenever he walked on road, people made faces at him. When these ideas are not firmly held and there is an element of doubt, they are called ideas of reference but if the patient is fully convinced about them, then these are called delusions of reference.

D) **Disorders of Perception** — It is another commonly observed phenomena during which the patient experiences a perception without a stimuli (hallucination). This disorder of perception or hallucination can occur in any sense modality, e.g. hearing (auditory), seeing (visual), smelling, (olfactory) taste (gustatory) or touch (tactile). In cases of schizophrenia, hallucinations are usually auditory (E.g. voices accusing, threatening or commenting on the patients behaviour). Typical hallucinations seen in schizophrenics are :

Running commentary on patients behaviour : These voices will repeat what the patient is doing or thinking ; they may also advise or reprimand the patient.

Two voices may discuss about the patient and comment on him. The patient may complain that the hallucinating voices are coming from his chest or stomach.

Visual hallucinations are rare. Though there can be hallucinations in other modalities, if hallucinations of touch and smell are present, one should strongly suspect an organic illness.

E) **Mood and Affect**

Most patients of schizophrenia have flattening of affect. These patients appear emotionally indifferent to most of the situation or circumstance. Some may, however, show an affect of extreme fear, or perplexity or depression. These affective states are usually not appropriate to their thoughts and often the patient is unable to explain as to what is making him fearful, anxious or depressed. There could be silly, purposeless laughter or giggling in some cases.

Since schizophrenic patients are unable to relate emotionally to other people, the examiner cannot feel with the patient. This is known as lack of rapport or empathy.

F) **Attention and Concentration**

It is often difficult to arouse the attention of the patient. They may not respond to questions. Concentration is generally poor. They cannot pursue a given task for sometime (E.g. task of serial substraction of sevens from hundred).

G) **Impulse Control**

Impulse control of these patients is usually poor. They may all of sudden become hostile and destructive. Their behaviour is often unpredictable.

H) **Orientation and Consciousness**

These patients are fully conscious and their orientation to time, place and person is intact.

I) **Intelligence and Memory**

Intelligence and memory is usually not affected

but due to poor attention and concentration, it may be difficult to evaluate it in a substantial percentage.

J) **Insight and Judgement**

These patients generally do not consider them to be ill and so the insight is often poor or lost. They cannot make proper judgement.

K) **Other Symptoms**

a) **Sleep** — Sleep is invariably disturbed. Total sleep is reduced. Further, there could be frightening dreams.

b) **Somatic Symptoms** — Many patients may complain of various aches and pains in different parts of the body but there are no specific somatic symptoms. Many patients may show rise in systolic blood pressure with dilated pupils and moist palms. These symptoms are due to sympathetic hyperactivity. Constipation is usually present.

In a large number of patients, the appetite may be poor or almost lost, but in some patients it may be increased.

Diagnosis

Diagnosis of schizophrenia is based both on history and examination. History will reveal an episodic illness characterised by disturbances in social and occupational functioning. The patient's behaviour would show a distinict change from premorbid functioning.

According to ICD 10, the following symptoms are required for diagnosis :

a) Thought echo, thought insertion or withdrawal and thought broadcasting.

b) Delusions of control, influence or passivity, clearly referred to body or limb movements or specific thoughts, actions or sensations and delusional perception.

c) Hallucinatory voices giving a running commentary on the patient's behaviour, or discussing him between themselves, or other types of hallucinatory voices coming from some part of the body.

d) Persistent delusions of other kinds that are culturally inappropriate and completely impossible, such as religious or political identity or superhuman powers and abilities (E.g, being able to control the weather or being in communication with aliens from other world).

e) Persistent hallucinations in any modality, when accompanied either by fleeting or half formed delusions without clear affective content or by persistent over-valued ideas or when occurring every day for weeks or months on end.

f) Breaks or interpolations in the trains of thought resulting in incoherence or irrelevant speech or neologism.

g) Catatonic behaviour, such as excitement, posturing or waxy flexibility, negativism, mutism and stupor.

h) "Negative" symptoms such as marked apathy, paucity of speech and blunting or incongruity of emotional responses usually resulting in social withdrawal and lowering of social performance. It must be clear that these are not due to depression or to neuroleptic medication.

i) A significant and consistent change in the overall quality of some aspects of personal behaviour, manifest as loss of interest, aimlessness, idleness, and self absorbed attitude and social withdrawal.

According to ICD-10, for the diagnosis of schizophrenia the minimum of one very clear symptom (and usually, two or more if less clear cut) belonging to any of the groups listed a to d above or atleast two of the groups referred to as (e) to (h) the should have been present for most of the time in the past one month. Prodromal symptoms are not considered in this time frame of one month. If the duration is less than one month than the diagnosis of acute schizophrenia like psychosis is made. The group (i) in the above list applies only to the diagnosis of simple schizophrenia and duration of at least one year is required.

Differential Diagnosis

For a firm diagnosis of schizophrenia following conditions are to be excluded :

a) Symptoms of depression or mania should not be prominent. If schizophrenic symptoms occur only during a stage of elation or depression, then the diagnosis of depression or mania should be made. If affective symptoms occur after development of schizophrenic symptoms then the diagnosis of schizophrenia is made. If symptoms of both the conditions are clearly present in the same episode then the diagnosis of schizo affective disorder is made.

Schizophrenia	Mania and Depression
1. Premorbid personality is often schizoid.	1. Premorbidly the patient is usually extroverted or cyclothymic.
2. The symptoms often develop insiduously but may be acute in some cases.	2. Onset is often acute (within a week) in mania. Depression may however start insidiously.
3. Classical symptoms of schizophrenia (thought disorders, hallucinations or affective incongruity) are often present	3. The patient will usually show basic mood of depression or elation. Their thinking and action are appropriate to the presenting mood.
4. Depression or elation may be present, but the mood state is not appropriate to behaviour, e.g. a schizophrenic may say that he is the King of India but he will not mind sweeping the floor.	4. Manic acts according to his mood. If he has a delusion that he is a king, he will like to order people around.
5. A schizophrenic usually does not relate to the interviewer.	5. Manic or depressive, generally relates to the interviewer.
6. Interval period between the two episodes are usually not fully normal.	6. Interval period is generally normal.
7. The family history of schizophrenia.	7. Family history of Mania or Depression (M.D.P.)

b) History of intake of psychoactive substances like amphetamines, alcohol, cannabis, opium should be elicited. If the history of intake of these substances clearly precedes the psychotic symptoms then the possibility of drug induced psychosis should be considered. Quite often the persons start using various intoxicants to calm down their anxiety due to psychosis. Further, drug induced psychosis will have symptoms specific to the substance used ; Evidence of confusion and disturbed orientation to time, place and person.

Thought disorders as seen in schizophrenia are often not present.

Other signs of intoxication will be present.

c) **Organic brain disease** — The evidence of organic brain diseases which can produce symptoms similar to schizophrenia should be elicited, e.g. diseases of frontal, parietal, temporal and limbic lobes or deeper structures. Careful neurological examination may reveal various lobe signs. History of epilepsy should be carefully asked because sometimes, epileptics can develop a psychosis which is similar to schizophrenia. This usually develops after 10-15 years of epileptic fits. The picture resembles paranoid schizophrenia but these patients do not show thought disorder as seen in schizophrenia. The affect is also not as impoverished.

SUBTYPES OF SCHIZOPHRENIA

Schizophrenia has been subdivided into subtypes on the basis of symptomatology. These subtypes sometimes merge into each other and a large number of patients often do not fulfil the diagnostic requirements of any one subtype. Some investigators have tried to subtype schizophrenia on the basis of presumed etiopathology but these attempts have so far not yielded a satisfactory system of classification.

Subtypes

Paranoid Schizophrenia
Hebephrenic Schizophrenia
Catatonic Schizophrenia
Undifferentiated Schizophrenia
Post-schizophrenic Depression

Residual Schizophrenia
Simple Schizophrenia
Other Schizophrenia
Schizophrenia Unspecified

PARANOID SCHIZOPHRENIA

This is the commonest type of schizophrenia. The following symptoms are prominent :

a) Delusions of persecution (''people are trying to harm or poison''), delusions of love or infidelity, or any other type of delusions. These delusions are fairly clear cut and stable.

b) Hallucinations — Usually auditory, voices commanding, threatening or any other type of hallucination may be present.

c) Thought disturbances though present are not prominent.

d) Affect is usually of hostility, anger or suspiciousness.

e) Negative symptoms like flat affect, poverty of speech and poor activity level are not prominent. The onset is in late twenties and the illness may have episodic pattern or chronic course.

Case History

Mrs M, a 32 year old married house wife developed the illness nearly 5 years back when she started suspecting her husband of an illicit relationship. She used to get outbursts of rage whenever her husband tried to talk to her. She would check his pockets, handkerchief, etc. She improved spontaneously three months later. A couple of years later she again became suspicious. Now in addition to infidelity, she also started suspecting that her husband is trying to poison her and their two chidren. She would not eat anything purchased by her husband or kept in the refrigerator. She used to insist that her children have become weak because of slow-poisoning. Her sleep was reduced. She did not like to go out of the house and also did not take care of her dress. She could do her household work, though slowly. Mental status examination revealed poor abstraction ability, flatness of affect, loss of insight and judgement and systematic delusions.

Comments

This patient's illness is primarily characterised by delusions of persecution which started with delusions of infidelity and progressed to the delusion of being poisoned. She showed inappropriateness of affect and poor abstraction ability. Illness started in the episodic from and later became chronic.

HEBEPHRENIC SCHIZOPHRENIA

This type is characterized by :

a) Flattening of affect or senseless giggling . The affect is grossly inappropriate.

b) Thought disturbances are prominent. The patient is usually incoherent and irrelevant. They show poverty of ideas.

c) Delusions and hallucinations can occur but they are fragmentary and changing. They are not prominent.

d) The patient's behaviour is remarkably aimless and their occupational and social acitivities deteriorate.

e) Illness usually starts during early adolescence and becomes chronic.

Case History

Mr M, 18 years old, was brought for consultation after he has failed in high school twice. He would not talk to anyone. He was confined to his room where he did not allow anyone to come. He had collected many useless articles in his room. He did not allow anyone to clean his room. He would get angry on trifles. He had grown a beard and his dress was shabby and unclean. During a clinical interview, he was muttering to himself and answered to the questions in monosyllables. On being asked what is wrong with him he replied ''stars and moon are all going to end. Nobody will survive''. He showed complete lack of concern with surroundings, His affect was flat ; at times he showed silly laughter without any stimuli. Hallucinations could not be demonstrated. His attention was difficult to arouse. Memory and intelligence could not be tested due to poor cooperation. He lacked insight and judgement.

Comments

Illness in this young boy started at the age of fifteen or sixteen. The failure in examination was due to illness. He showed prominent thought disturbances and flatness of affect. Collection of rubbish is quite common in this subtype. The illness usually become more or less chronic.

CATATONIC SCHIZOPHRENIA

Catatonic schizophrenia is becoming uncommon in the western countries. Even in India, the number of catatonic patients are decreasing. The reason for this observation is not clearly understood.

Characteristic symptoms of this disorder are :

a. Acute purposeless excitement which may include abusive and destructive behaviour.

b. Stupor — The patient may become immobile, may stop oral intake of food, may develop urinary and faecal retention. Such patients are generally fully conscious.

c. They may show any of the symptoms described under catatonia.

These catatonic symptoms alone are not sufficient for diagnosis. The patient should exhibit other characteristic symptoms of schizophrenia, either before they become mute or stuporose or afterward. Catatonia can be seen in organic illnesses also.

Case History

Mr J, a 18 years old, developed the illness six weeks back. He was an agricultural worker. One afternoon after having returned from the fields he said he was not feeling well. For a couple of days he became moody. He would get angry on trifles. His sleep became disturbed and his appetite was sluggish. One night at around 1 a.m. he got up from his bed and tried to run away. He was held back by his family members. Soon he started abusing them. After few hours of excited behaviour he slept for sometime. Next day he started shouting and abusing again. He was restless most of the time. He did not eat anything except liquids and became fearful whenever anybody approached him. He felt that some voices were telling him that he would die. These voices also told him that he should save himself from other people around. The content of these voices was fluctuating. He was taken to some Ojha for faith healing where he became quiet for sometime but after coming back home he started showing similar behaviour. His sleep and appetite were decreased. M.S.E. revealed acute excitement, irrelevant talks, auditory hallucinations, fearful and inappropriate affect and loss of insight and judgement.

Comments

The patient showed an acute onset of illness which was characterized by acute excitement, thought disturbances, auditory hallucinations and affect of fearfulness which was inappropriate.

UNDIFFERENTIATED SCHIZOPHRENIA

Patients who fulfil the diagnostic criteria of schizophrenia but do not satisfy the criteria of any other subtype of schizophrenia are included in this group.

TABLE

Clinical Characteristics of Subtypes of Schizophrenia

	Paranoid	Hebephrenic	Catatonic	Undifferentiated
Age of Onset	Late 20's to early 30's	15-25 yr.	15-25 yr.	?
Thought disturbance	mild	Prominent Irrelevent Incoherent	Prominent Irrelevent Incoherent	+
Delusions	Prominent Delusions are systematised and clearly expressed	Delusions are not prominent	Delusional are not prominent	+
Affect	According to delusions but	Flat affect purposeless giggling	Flat and inappropriate	+

	inappropriateness could be demonstrated	inappropriate		
Hallucinations	+	+	+	+
General Behaviour	Nearly normal hostile and argumentative	Shabby unkempt Poor social contact	Stupor Excitement	±
Negative Symptoms	Very few	Prominent	+ -	+

POST SCHIZOPHRENIC DEPRESSION

Many schizophrenics develop depressive symptoms during the recovery phase. This condition is thought to be caused by the following :

a) Depressive symptoms : Negative symptoms of schizophrenia may be wrongly diagnosed as depression.

b) Depressive symptoms may appear due to development of insight in the patient. He may be acutely conscious of his problem. He may be unable to work and he may he feel that he is a burden on others. He might understand that the illness can be recurrent and disabling. These may induce depression in him.

c) It could be the result of antipsychotic drugs which are likely to induce depression. The other side affects like restlessness are also responsible for producing depression.

d) The depressive illness may be independent and may be coexisting with schizophrenia.

The exact pathogenesis of post-psychotic depression is not clearly understood. Many patients in this phase may attempt suicide.

The diagnostic features are :

1. The patient has had a schizophrenic illness meeting the criteria of schizophrenia in past twelve months ;

2. Some schizophrenic symptoms are still present;

3. The depressive symptoms are prominent and distressing fulfilling the criteria of depressive episode and have been present for at least two weeks.

If no schizophrenic symptoms are present, then diagnosis of a depressive episode should be made.

RESIDUAL SCHIZOPHRENIA

This state devlops after one or more episodes of schizophrenic illness. This is usually a chronic stage though not necessarily irreversible, which has prominent negative symptoms.

Diagnostic Guidelines — (ICD-X)

1. Prominent 'negative' schizophrenic symptoms, i.e. psychomotor slowing, underactivity, blunting of affect, passivity and lack of initiative, poverty of quantity and content of speech, poor non-verbal communication by facial expression, eye contact, voice modulation and posture, poor self care and social performance.

2. Evidence in the past of at least one clearcut psychotic episode meeting the diagnostic criteria of schizophrenia.

3. The period of at least one year during which the intensity and frequency of the florid symptoms such as delusions and hallucinations have been minimal or substantially reduced and the negative schizophrenic syndrome has been present.

4. Absence of dementia or other organic brain diseases or disorder and of chronic depression or instituionalism sufficient to explain the negative symptoms.

SIMPLE SCHIZOPHRENIA

This is a rare and difficult diagnosis to be made. Some workers believe that this category should be given up. The illness is characterized by insiduous onset of oddities of behaviour, withdrawal, and increasing evidence of negative symptoms described above. The differentiation from residual schizophrenia is made by absence of a clearcut episode of schizophrenic illness.

This disorder usually runs a chronic course and the patients become vagabond or drifters. This disorder can be confused with schizotypal disorder. The later disorder may run a fluctuating course with similar symptoms but usually will not lead to deterioration. Many authors do not differentiate between these two conditions.

POSITIVE AND NEGATIVE SCHIZOPHRENIA

Mr. Crow divided schizophrenia into two types as positive and negative.

Positive Schizophrenia

This type has predominently positive symptoms like hallucination, delusions gross thought disorders. These patients do not show much abnormality on CT scan of brain and respond well to treatment.

Negative Schizophrenia

This is characterized by negative or deficit symptoms which include the following :

1. **Affective flattening** — The patient does not express emotions of any kind. They appear to be lost in their own world. The face appears emotionless. The eye contact is poor.

2. **Poverty of speech** — They talk in monosyllables or short sentences. They have a very few ideas and may often repeat them.

3. **Apathy** — They do not take any initiative. They are often careless about their hygiene and dressing. Patients usually avoid taking bath or cleaning their teeth. They may not shave and usually grow a beard.

4. **Poor sociability** — They do not establish human relationships and usually avoid social contact. Whenever visitors come to their home they will try to avoid them.

5. **Initiative and planning** — They lack initiative. They will not start anything new and they may also give up the work, already started.

These negative schizophrenics tends to show dilated lateral ventricles on CT scan and respond poorly to the treatment. Most of the recent researches have however, failed to confirm the independence of these two syndromes. Most patients tend to have a mixture of both type of symptoms. Very few remain purely negative or positive.

Course and Prognosis

Schizophrenia is generally considered to be a chronic illness. It starts with an episodic course and may later become persistent and chronic. Initially, it was thought that all the patients of schizophrenia show a deteriorating course but now it has been clearly established that nearly a quarter of patient may have complete recovery and one quarter may have chronic down hill course while remaining fifty percent show intermediate prognosis.

The prognosis in schizophrenia can be divided into the following :

a) Risk of death
b) Deterioration in mental symptoms
c) Deterioration in work performance
d) Deterioration in social relationships.

a) **Risk of Death**

Schizophrenics have higher then normal risk of death by malnutrition, infections and suicide. Risk of suicide in schizophrenia is 10-15%.

b) **Mental Symptoms**

Clinical symptoms of schizophrenia tend to diminish with the passage of time. Many recent studies show that even in chronic schizophrenics, some improvement in symptomatology appears with the passage of time. Paranoid and catatonic schizophrenia show much better symptom resolution then other subtypes. Patients having prominent negative symptoms tend to do poorly.

c) **Work Performance**

Most schizophrenics show deterioration in their work ability. This deterioration will be dependant on the type of work they had been involved prior to their illness. People in executive jobs, sales jobs or jobs that require quick decision making or social interaction may not have the same efficiency. On the other hand, labourers, artisans and people working in mechanical professions may be able to work unimpaired. Housewives may be able to continue their household chores reasonably. Work deterioration is much more in hebephrenic schizophrenics while it may be very little in paranoid schizophrenics.

d) **Social Relationships**

Social relationships generally tend to deteriorate.

Most patients withdraw and do not establish new relationships. Paranoid schizophrenics may maintain more or less normal relationship with people who are not part of their delusional system.

It has been observed that the course of schizophrenia is much better in developing countries. In course and outcome study of schizophrenia (ICMR) it was found that nearly 68% patient showed a good prognosis. The factors relating to good prognosis were :

1. Good drug compliance
2. Short duration of illness
3. Absence of dangerous behaviour
4. Acute onset
5. Absence of economic difficulties
6. Rise in socio-economic level
7. Rural background
8. Lower education
9. Absence of schizoid traits
10. Lower socio-economic status
11. Nuclear type of household
12. Absence of negative symptoms
13. Younger age of onset
14. Regular occupational history.

Many of these were earlier considered poor prognostic factors. It appears that social and familial acceptance of deviant behaviour, poor demands on the patient and good family ties have bearing on the prognosis of schizophrenia. Most of the homeless in the west are found to be mentally ill. It is largely because the families in the West abandon the deviant relatives and they become drifters.

TABLE

Outcome of Five Year Follow up

	Best	Intermediate	Worse
ICMR	23.7	71.8	4.5

ICMR FACOS Study 1988

Management of Schizophrenia

The management of schizophrenia can be divided into the following :

A) Management of acute episode
B) Maintenance treatment
C) Rehabilitation
D) Prevention.

A and B) **Management of Acute Episode and Maintenance Treatment**

The patient in acute episode present with excitement, suspiciousness, socially disruptive behaviour, with problems of food intake and sleeping difficulties. Initially, the clinician has to decide whether the patient has to be treated as an out-patient or is to be hospitalized. In our country most of the patients are to be treated as outpatients because there are very few hospital beds available. Secondly, most of the families are quite willing to look after the patient at home.

The clinician should ensure the following :

a) Patient can be given medications.
b) His food intake is adequate or can be supervised.
c) He can be safeguarded against harming himself or others.

If these conditions cannot be fulfilled, then the patient will need hospitalisation.

Pharmacotherapy — The mainstay of treatment is antipsychotic drugs. These drugs effectively control delusions, hallucinations, thought disturbances, overactivity and normalize sleep. They do not cure the disease. They may not improve the negative symptoms substantially. The antipsychotic drugs are the following :

Phenothizines	**Dosage Equivalence**
Chlorpromazine	100mg
Thioridazine	100mg
Trifluperazine	3-5mg
Pimozide	1mg
Others	
Loxapine	10mg
Flupenthixol	
Clozapine (not available in India)	

Most of the drugs have equal antipsychotic properties but their side-effect profiles differ.

Dosage— Dosage of these drugs differ from each other. Dosage equivalence of these drugs have been given above. Dosage by oral and injectable routes also differ. Oral drug requirement is 1.5 to 3 times the injectable drugs because a part of the oral drugs are metabolised in the liver.

The commonly used dosage for schizophrenia is 200 to 400 mg of chlorpromazine orally per day in two divided dosages. Haloperidol is used in 5-10 mg/day in two divided dosages. However, when the patient does not respond to this dosages within four weeks then the dosage can be increased up to 1000 mg of chlorpromazine or to 30-40 mg of haloperidol. These higher dosages should not be given for more than one month, if there is no response. The dosage should not be escalated in the first four weeks as the therapeutic effect usually takes four weeks. The agitation and sleep improves first and other psychotic symptoms gradually disappears thereafter. The same dosage needs be continued for three to four months or till such time the improvement is occurring. When the patient stabilizes, then the dosage is reduced.

Duration of Treatment — When the patient has come in first attack, the effective dosage may be continued for 3 months. Thereafter the dosage is reduced to half for another 2-3 months. This quantity could be further halved and after another 2-3 months the treatment can be stopped. If there is a second attack than the same regiment may be used with slight prolongation of treatment. If a relapse has occurred within 3 to 4 months of stoppage of treatment, then the drug may be continued for a year or more. If more than three attacks have occured within last three to four years than the treatment may have to continue indefinitely. The maintenance dosage is around 100 to 200 mg of chlorpromazine or 2.5 to 5 mg of haloperidol.

Side-effects— All antipsychotic drugs have many annoying and a few severe side-effects.

Anticholinergic Effects — Common anticholinergic side-effects are dry mouth and nose, constipation, blurring of vision and urinary retention. Some may also develop nausea and vomiting . These side effects are more with low potency drugs like chlorpromazine and less with high potency drugs like haloperidol.

Postural Hypotension — There is a drop in blood pressure when the patient gets up from a lying position and the patient feels dizzy and may fall down. This side effect is also more common with low potency drugs.

Endocrine Effect — These drugs produce hypersecretion of prolactin which may decrease libido (sexual desire) and cause erectile difficulties. Females may also develop reduction in sexual desire. Many men develop gynaecomastia and the women may experience amenorrhea and milk discharge from the breast.

Skin Effect — Many patients show photosentivity reaction when exposed to the sun. This is more common in the West. Long term medication may result in pigmentation of the exposed parts of the skin.

Opthalmalogic Effect — Some patients may develop lenticular and corneal opacities. Patients on thioridazine, may develop pigmentation of the retina. These side-effects are quite uncommon and occur only on high dosage.

Weight Gain — Many patients gain weight which is often complained as the swelling of the body. These patient should be advised to restrict their diet and increase exercise.

Cardiac Effects — There are E.C.G. changes with phenothiazines. Common changes are prolongation of QT and PR interval, blunting of T waves and depression of ST segement. These changes are more common with chlorpromazine and thioridazine.

Haematological Changes — Some patients may develop leukopenia. Agranulocytosis is more common with clozapine.

Jaundice — It was a common complication of phenothiazines earlier but is seen much more rarely these days. Jaundice usually occurs within first four to six weeks of treatment and is of the obstructive type.

Sedation — Most of these drugs induce sedation. Generally the patient become accustomed to the sedative effect and after few a weeks of treatment they do not show day-time sedation, specially when on low dosage of drugs.

Central Anti-cholinergic Syndrome — This is characterized by confusion , delusion like symptoms, agitation and pupillary dilatation. Quite often, it is confused with worsening of psychosis, and drugs are increased. The phenothiazines should be stopped and physostigmine 2 mg may be given by slow I.V infusion. It can be repeated after one hour if necessary

Neurological Side-effects — These drugs have

many neurological side effects. Neurological side effects are more common with high potency phenothiazine and are lowest with thioridazine. Clozapine is not reported to have these side effects.

Dystonias — They are the most alarming side effects for the patient. The common symptoms are twisting of the body, protrusion of tongue, blepharospasm and opisthotonus. These symptoms occur within the first few days. They can be treated by injection of anticholinergic drugs like orphenadrine. They also respond to promethazine 50 mg (IMI). These dystonias disappear later. If dystonia is severe, then the drugs may be changed to low potency compounds, like thioridazine or chlorpromazine.

Parkinsonian Effects — A large number of patients receiving antipsychotic drugs develop parkinsonian symptoms. These symptoms occur due to dopamine blockade in nigrostriatal system. Some patients are able to compensate for the blockade and do not develop parkinsonian symptoms. Generally, 15-20% patients develop these side effects.

The common parkinsonian symptoms are :

1. Mask-like face. The patient does not show any emotion.

2. The body becomes like a statue. Upper limbs are flexed and usually do not show normal swing while walking.

3. Coarse tremors of hand and feet can be seen. These tremors are more apparent on rest.

4. Few patients may show rabbit syndrome, which is generally seen after a few months of medication. The patient shows perioral tremor which is similar to lip puckering seen in rabbits.

5. Slowness of movement in all the parts of the body may develop.

6. Speech becomes slow and monotonous.

7. Speech may be affected by oral tremors.

These symptoms are more frequent in elderly females. They are seen more often with high potency drugs like haloperidol and are less common with chlorpromazine and thioridazine.

Parkinsonian symptoms can be treated by adding anticholinergic like Trihexyphenydyl (Pacitane), Procyclidine (Kemadrine) or Orphenadrine (Disipal). These drugs will generally reduce such symptoms. Drugs like amantadine may be more effective in some cases. Levadopa is not effective in drug induced parkinsonism. If the symptoms are too troublesome, then one can change the antipsychotic drug to chlorpromazine or thioridazine. These anticholinergics should be reduced after three months. It is expected that the patient will become habitual to these symptoms by that time. But if these symptoms reappear after stoppage of anticholinergics, then these drugs should be continued.

In our country, antipsychotic-anticholinergic combinations are quite popular, eg. Trifluperazine and Trihexyphenydyl, Haloperidol and Trihexyphenydyl. The advantages of these combinations are :

1. The likelihood of developing dystonias and parkinsonian symptoms is reduced,

2. It is specially useful in our population where the majority of patients are illiterate and they often wish to reduce the number of tablets. If both the drugs are given separately, then it is likely that, they may reduce either one of them resulting in treatment failure or side effects.

However, this problem can be overcome if the different purpose of the two drugs can be explained to the patient and the relatives.

The main disadvantage of the combination is that if one wants to increase antipsychotic drugs, one automatically increases anticholinergics. This may increase the chance of developing anticholinergic syndrome.

Akathisia — This is a common side-effect of antipsychotics. These patients complain of motor restlessness. They cannot sit in a place even for a short time. They may feel like pacing up and down for hours. This is often misinterpreted as worsening of psychosis. However, the difference between the two are :

a) Patients with akathisia is distressed by this symptom and complains that he cannot sit still. Patients with motor hyperactivity will not complain of it.

b) Motor restlessness of akathisia is not associated with psychological abnormalities of psychosis.

Akathisia can be treated by adding Propranolol (40-120 mg/day) Benzodiazeipine (5-15 mg) or Clonidine (.1-.5 mg day).

Tardive Dyskinesia — This is by far the most serious side effects of antipsychotic drugs. This symptom can be disabling and may be irreversible, if not controlled in time. This is characterized by the following :

a) Choreoathetoid movements of the limbs, head and trunk.

b) Movement of facial and jaw muscle leading to lip smacking, chewing movements of the jaws and perioral tremors.

c) Movements of tongue : Generally to and fro movements.

d) Neck may be kept in any abnormal position (torticollis).

These movements may range from mild to severe. They may sometimes lead to difficulties in eating and walking.

Tardive dyskinesia is a delayed side effects and occurs after prolonged use of the drugs. The etiopathology of the symptoms is considered to be the hypersensitivity of the dopaminergic receptors in nigrostriatal system.

The incidence of this side-effect is more in females and elderly. It is associated with higher dosage of the drugs. It is advisable to treat the patient on the lowest possible dosage to reduce the incidence of this side effect. These drugs should be used with caution in females and in the patient who have pre-existing neurological diseases.

Management of tardive dyskinesia rests in reducing or stopping the drugs. This may lead to worsening of the symptoms. Gradually, the tardive dyskinesia will subside. If detected early 50 to 90% of the patients with T.D'S. can be controlled. Many drugs have been tried but none have been found effective so far. Such patients can be treated with Lithium/Carbamazepine or benzodiazipines for their psychotic symptoms.

Neuroleptic Malignant Syndrome — A very few patients develop hyperpyrexia, high blood pressure, muscular rigidity, confusion and agitation when they are receiving antipsychotic drugs. The laboratory findings are, increased white blood cell count and a massive increase in creatinine phosphokinase (C.P.K.) and liver enzymes. Myoglobin is increased which may result in renal shutdown.

These symptoms can occur at any time during treatment. Whenever, these patients develop hyperpyrexia one should get the serum level of C.P.K.. If there is manifold increase in its values then N.M.S. should be suspected.

The treatment lies in stopping the phenothiazines and treating the hyperthermia by cooling the patient. Nutrition should be maintained by I.V. drip. Many specific drugs have been tried but their superiority over life sustaining management has not been proved. Bromocriptine 1.25 mg can be given twice daily.

Atypical Anti-psychotic Drug

Clozapine — This drug does not induce extrapyramidal side effects as seen with other antipsychotic. This drug is not a dcpamine antagonist but its therapeutic effect is presumed to be due to its blockade of serotonin receptors. This drug is found to be effective in some drug-resistant schizophrenics. It is also claimed to be effective against negative symptoms of schizophrenia. Major drawback of this drug is that it produces agranulocytosis in 1-2 % of patients, which can be fatal. The drug has to be used cautiously and close monitoring of blood counts is needed. This drug is very costly.

Other Drugs

Other drugs may be required for two reasons :

1. For control of symptoms of anxiety, agitation and sleeplessness.

2. When the antipsychotics alone are not effective or they cannot be given due to side effects.

The drug used are :

a) **Lithium** — Lithium alone or in combination with antipsychotic drugs can be quite effective in controlling schizophrenic symptoms. Dosage required are 900 to 1500 mg/day. The details of lithium treatment are given in treatment of mood disorders.

b) **Carbamazepine** — Carbamazepine alone may not control schizophrenic symptoms but it can be useful in controlling violent behaviour. Dosage - 600 to 1200 mg/day.

c) **Benzodiazepines** — Drugs like Diazepam and Lorazepam can be used in addition to antipsychotics. They may decrease the quantity of antipsychotics. Some patients who cannot tolerate antipsychotics may be given these drugs alone.

E.C.T.

E.C.T was once used as a major treatment method for schizophrenia. It has now been shown that E.C.T is only indicated in following situations :

a) Acute catatonic excitement or stupor which is not responding to drugs.

b) Patients who either cannot take drugs due to

side effects or in whom drugs are not showing much response. Patients who develop T.D. may also be treated with E.C.T.

Psychosocial Management

Though the drugs are mainstay of treatment in schizophrenia, yet the psychosocial treatment plays a crucial role in the management. The following methods could be used.

1. **Family Education and Therapy**

The family members should be clearly explained the nature of the disease. They must be told that this illness tends to have relapses and after each relapse the patient may develop some personality defect. The patient usually becomes less social, i.e. they like to stay aloof. They do not like to mix with others. They do not bother about their future and their ability to plan becomes less. They become emotionally less responsive and may not show either happiness or sorrow. The patients find it difficult to adjust in social and occupational life.

The family members are often guilt-ridden because they feel that the illness in their child is because of their fault. Some may accuse other agencies like schools, employees or in laws for development of this illness. Their fears and guilts are to be allayed by explaining to them that this illness does not seem to have direct correlation with life stresses. Adverse life situations may at best trigger off the illness in a predisposed person. Usually the patient's pre-illness behaviour (prodormal period) may show such disturbances due to which they come in conflict with their friends and relatives.

It has now been shown that relapses in this illness are dependant on overemotionality and critical attitudes of the family memebers. The family members often become so exasperated by the behaviour that they criticise them for being lazy and lethargic. They have to be explained that this behaviour of the patient is a result of the disease process and it can be overcome with gentle persuasion. The patient should be encouraged to lead a structured life, i.e. to get up at a fixed time. The activities of whole day should be planned. This type of time-table living would help the patient.

These patients should be encouraged to work. The relatives often feel that the patient should rest, till such time he recovers. On the contrary, regular work will hasten recovery.

Individual Psychotherapy

The patient may be involved in a man to man relationship with the doctor. The aim of the relationship is to help the patient to understand the various difficulties he experiences in his day to day life and to help him to understand misinterpretations, which he might experience because of psychotic experiences. Psychoanalysis is not indicated in this illness.

Various types of group therapies may be undertaken to improve sociability and to reduce abnormal behaviour.

Rehabilitation

As this illness can produce long lasting changes in patients behaviour, it is essential to rehabilitate them.

Some patients may not be able to adjust with their family members or spouses and will require counselling to improve this relationship. If no relatives are available to look after the patient, then he or she may have to be placed in an after-care home.

Some patients will require job rehabilitation as the disease process may limit their job abilities. Most of these patients can do those jobs efficiently, where they do not need to interact excessively with other people. Professions like sales, law like, etc. may be difficult for them. They may be able to do clerical and simple technical jobs, etc. efficiently. Job rehabilitation has to be individualised. In our country, agriculture can provide work for a large number of patients from the rural area.

Prevention

Effective strategies are not known which may help the prevention of this illness. However, many of the workers feel that the number of schizophrenics seeking help in hospitals are decreasing. It may be the result of prompt outpatient treatment. Current treatment have reduced both morbidity and mortality in schizophrenia. It is advisable that the families having schizophrenic off-springs, should not intermarry.

Schizotypal Disorder

This disorder is usually seen in the first degree relatives of schizophrenic patients. Previously, it was also called pseudoneurotic or border-line schizophrenia. These patients show a continuous illness for two or more years. The illness is characterized by the following (I.C.D.-X) :

a) Inappropriate or constricted affect (the individual appears cold and aloof) ;

b) Behaviour or appearance that is odd eccentric or peculiar ;

c) Poor rapport with others and a tendency to social withdrawal ;

d) Odd belief or magical thinking, influencing behaviour and inconsistent with subcultural norms ;

e) Suspiciousness or paranoid ideas ;

f) Obssessive ruminations without inner resistance, often with dysmorphophobic sexual or agressive contents ;

g) Unusual perceptual experiences including somatosensory (bodily) or other illusions, depersonalisation or derealisation ;

h) Vague, circumstantial metaphorical, over elaborate or sterotyped thinking, manifested by odd speech or in other ways, without gross incoherence.

i) Occasional transient quasi-psychotic episodes with intense illusions, auditory or other hallucination and delusion like ideas, usually occurring without external provocation.

The patient should exhibit three or four of the above symptoms continuously for two years or more.

This disturbance is difficult to diffrentiate from simple schizophrenia and schizoid personality disorder.

Course and Prognosis

The disorder runs a chronic course, a few patients may develop overt schizophrenia.

Management

These patients should be treated with a low dosage of antipsychotic drugs (Haloperidol 3-5 mg/day)

PERSISTENT DELUSIONAL DISORDERS

This category includes all those disorders, where persistent delusions are the main clinical presentation.

Delusional Disorders (D.D.)

These group of disorders are characterized by well systemetized delusions. They may have hallucinations but these hallucinations are not prominent and are not of the type seen in schizophrenia. These patients do not show any other disturbances of thinking.

Epidemiology

The exact prevalence of these disorders is not known because many of these patients do not seek treatment. They may only be identified when they come in conflict with law or create social and familial problems. These disorders are said to be more common in the females. The usual age of onset is around forty years. Though they can occur earlier.

Etilogy

Their etilogy is not known. Some consider them to be incomplete manifestations of schizophrenia. However, the families of delusional disorder patient do not show excess of schizophrenia.

Psychoanalytic literature is replete with psychodynamic formulation leading to paranoid development. These hypothetical formulations are not very much favoured these days. However, certain psychological states are said to be conducive to paranoid development :

a) Social isolation

b) Poor achievement

c) Defective perception.

Clinical Feature

The illness may develop acutely. Usually, it starts with misinterpretations and anxiety. Later, symptoms crystallize into clear cut delusions. This condition may last from many months to many years. The patients may be functioning normally except in areas of delusion. The sleep may be disturbed. Appetite is normal. Delusion can be of any type.

Persecutory Delusions : These are very common. The patient feels that some people are conspiring against him or they are poisoning him. One fifty year old patient felt that he had been poisoned by his wife who has given him lead. This lead has been deposited in his body mainly in his skin. He used to scratch his skin Throughout the day, which has lead to marked thickening and discoloration of the skin. He was working as a clerk reasonably well. He did not show any other thought disorder.

Somatic delusions can be in any form of emitting faecal or bad odours. In our country, we commonly come across a condition in which the patient feels that his skin is infested with insects or worms. They feel that these worms are crawling all over their body. They are so convinced about, it that they may pick up some dead skin or dirt from their body and state that this is the worm. They often experience depression and may even attempt suicide.

Delusions can also be of erotomanic type where a person feels that he is in love with a person of high status. One of our patients believed that he is in love with Queen Elizabeth. He wrote a large number of letters to the queen and to the British high commission.

The clinical examination of these patients will reveal normal general behaviour. Their dress is appropriate and they communicate normally.

Consciousness is clear and attention can be easily aroused and concentration is well sustained. Their thought process is normal and they show systematized delusions. They may have transitory hallucination which do not dominate the clinical picture. They may have poor impulse control. They can commit suicide or homicide or other criminal act because of their delusional system. One should directly ask them about their plans of tackling delusional situation. The memory and intelligence are normal. The sence of judgement is impaired in the delusional area. Insight is always lost. They do not consider their delusions to be false.

Course and Outcome

The illness generally runs a chronic course. Though, nearly half of them may show recovery on long term follow up.

Diagnosis

For diagnosis of delusional disorder the following conditions should be fulfilled : (ICD-X)

a. Delusion constitutes the most conspicious or the only clinical finding. They must be related to the person only.

b. They must last at least for three months.

c. Hallucinations if present should be transitory.

d. There could be full blown depressive episode during the course of illness but the delusional symptoms should also be present in the absence of depression.

e. There should be no evidence for schizophrenia.

f. There should be no evidence for organic brain disease.

Differential Diagnosis

1. Schizophrenia — Delusional disorders have to be differentiated from schizophrenia. Schizophrenics may have similar delusions. The differences are :

a) Thought process disturbances seen in schizophrenia are absent in D.D. Schizophrenics may show incoherence, irrelevance and circumstantiality.

b) The mood is usually congruous to delusion. Inappropriate effect is not seen.

c) Hallucinations in schizophrenia could be commanding, commenting or discussing the patient as a third person. Hallucination in D.D. are usually transitory and not the main feature of the disease.

d) There is not much deterioration in personality and behaviour in D.D.

Organic Brain Disorder

These are differentiated by the presence of following :

Disturbances in level of consciousness,
Disturbances in attention and concentration,
Memory disturbances,
Any other neurological signs.

Management

These patients often harbour suspiciousness and may plan to take revenge or may try to kill themselves, if they are convinced that they can not alter the situation. One has to decide whether the patient can be treated as an outpatient or inpatient. If the risk of homicide or suicide is greater then the patient should be hospitalized. These patients usually do not agree to take drugs. If the drugs compliance is a problem, then the patient may either be hospitalized or given long acting drug by injections.

Pharmacotherapy

The drugs used are antipsychotics. (details already given under schizophrenia) The dosage required may be low. It is advisable to start Haloperidol 5 mg per day. Patients showing somatic delusions (insects crawling) tend to respond well to Pimozode 4-8 mg per day.

The result of drug treatment is uncertain.

Psychotherapy

Individual psychotherapy may help some patients. The psychotherapist has to attempt to build a trusting relationship. The aim of psychotherapy is to help the patient to understand the absurdity of delusions. The patients can often be helped to live their life comfortably inspite of the delusions.

OTHER PERSISTENT DELUSIONAL DISORDERS

This is a residual category and those persistent delusional disorders that do not fulfil the criteria of schizophrenia are included here.

Delusional Dysmorphophobia

Many patients may have the firm conviction that

some part of their body is misshapen or ugly. These patients usually contact a plastic surgeon for the removal of this defect. A young man of around 20 years felt that his ears are ugly and long. First he grew his hairs and started combing them over his ears. Later, this did not satisfy him and he consulted a plastic surgeon. The surgeon did not find anything wrong with his ears. So, he was referred to psychiatrist. He did not benefit with treatment and a few years later he comitted suicide.

ACUTE AND TRANSIENT PSYCHOTIC DISORDERS

A large number of clinicians felt that many patients suffer from acute psychotic illnesses which do not follow the course of schizophrenia. They remit within a few weeks or a maximum of few months. Such conditions were reported more often from India and other developing countries. I.C.D.-10 classificatory system has included this subgroup to fulfil the need of identifying these short lasting psychotic episodes. This group also includes those patients of schizophrenia, who consult within thirty days of the onset of the disease. Thus this category is a mixed descriptive group.

These disorders usually have an acute onset from 48 hours to about 2 weeks. The onset is often associated with stress. This stress should be acute and easily identified, e.g. bereavement, unexpected loss, trauma of terrorism and torture. A complete recovery should occur within 2-3 months.

These disorders should not satisfy the criteria of organic brain syndromes, drug intoxications, depression and mania.

These can be further subclassified into the following:

Without associated stress

With associated stress

Epidemiology and Etiology

The epidemiological and etiological data for these disorders is not available.

Classification

These disorders are classified into the following:

Acute polymorphic psychotic disorder without symptoms of schizophrenia. (APPD without S.).

Acute polymorphic psychotic disorders with symptoms of schizophrenia. (APPD with S.).

Acute schizophrenia like psychotic disorder. (ASLPD)

Other acute predominanatly delusional psychotic disorders.

ACUTE POLYMORPHIC PSYCHOTIC DISORDER WITHOUT SYMPTOMS OF SCHIZOPHRENIA

This is an acute psychotic disorder, which is characterized by changing symptomatology. The patient will exhibit delusions, hallucinations and other perceptual disturbances like illusions. They may show marked emotional turmoil which may range from ecstasy to fear and perplexity.

Diagnosis (I.C.D.X.)

For a definite diagnosis :

a) The onset must be acute (within 2 weeks or less);

b) There must be several types of hallucinations or delusions, changing in both type and intensity from day to day and within the same day ;

c) There should be a similarly varying emotional state ;

d) Inspite of the variety of symptoms, none should be persistent with sufficient consistency to fulfil the criteria of schizophrenia or mania or depressive episode.

Management

These patients are treated with antipsychotic drugs. Minor tranquilizers can be added to control severe anxiety. Drugs are required only for short periods. The dosage should be kept on lower side. Initially injections can be used (Haloperidol 5 mg or Choloropromazine 50 mg). When obvious stress is present psychological mangement is also required. As soon as the patient is able to communicate his/her reaction to stress should be inquired. Their fear and anxieties should be explored and they should be helped to reevaluate the situation realistically.

ACUTE POLYMORPHIC PSYCHOTIC DISORDER WITH SYMPTOMS OF SCHIZOPHRENIA

These patients exhibit symptoms of acute polymorphic psychotic disorder along with typical schizophrenic symptoms.

If the schizophrenic symptoms persisit for more than one month, then the diagnosis is changed to schizophrenia.

Management

The same as described for acute polymorphic psychotic disorder without symptoms of schizophrenia. If symptoms of schizophrenia persists beyond one month, then they should be treated as schizophrenia.

ACUTE SCHIZOPHRENIA — LIKE PSYCHOTIC DISORDER

This disorder is characterized by acute onset and stable schizophrenic symptoms. There may be mild variability of symptoms but this is not to the extent seen in acute polymorphic psychotic disorders.

Diagnosis (I.C.D.-X.)

For a definite diagnosis :

a) The onset of the psychotic symptoms must be acute (2 weeks or less).

b) Symptoms that fulfil the criteria for schizophrenia, must have been present for the majority of time since the establishment of an obvious psychotic clinical picture.

c) The criteria for acute polymorphic psychotic disorder are not fulfilled. When symptoms persist beyond one month, the diagnosis is changed to schizophrenia.

Management

The same as described under schizophrenia.

OTHER ACUTE PREDOMINANTLY DELUSIONAL PSYCHOTIC DISORDERS

These are acute psychotic disorders which are characterized by stable delusions and hallucinations. The patient may feel that people are conspiring against him because their misdeeds have become known to his. Many of the patients develop paranoid delusions after an act which is considered wrong or sinful. One patient had a sexual relation with a girl of different religion. From that day he felt that this has become known to the people of her community and they are planning to kill him. He could also hear voices.

Diagnosis (I.C.D.X.)

For a definite diagnosis :

a) The onset of psychotic symptoms must be acute (2 weeks or less).

b) Delusions and hallucinations must have been present for the majority of time, since the establishment of an obviously psychotic state ;

c) The criteria for neither schizophrenia nor acute polymorphic psychotic disorder are fulfilled.

If delusions persist for more than 3 months, than the diagnosis is changed to persistent delusional disorders; if hallucinations persist then other nonorganic psychotic diorders should be diagnosed.

A large number of patients where the illness is acute and their is a precipitating stress could be managed with psychotherapy and high dosages of benzodiazepines, e.g. Lorazepam 4-6 mg/day or Diazepam 20-30 mg/day. Psychotherapy is essential to dispel their paranoid doubts and to help them to accept reality.

INDUCED DELUSIONAL DISORDER

A rare delusional disorder where the delusions are shared by two or more persons. Only one person suffers from a genuine delusional disorder, but the other who has a dependant relationship with this person starts showing the same delusions.

The disorder can be managed by separating the dependant person and the patient with genuine delusions should be treated appropriately.

SCHIZO-AFFECTIVE DISORDERS

These disorders exhibit symptoms of schizophrenia and mood disorders in the same episode of illness. Symptoms of both disorders may be simultaneously present or may follow within interval of few days. These patients generally run an episodic course with more or less complete normality between the episodes. They do not show as much deterioration in personality as seen in schizophrenia but the course more deteriorating than affective disorders.

Epidemiology

The exact epidemiology of these disorders is not known as the concept of these disorders have been changing.

Etiology

Etiology is not clearly understood. At one time they were considered to be variants of schizophrenia at others of mood disorders. It was also thought that they may represent chance association of schizophrenia and affective disorder but their prevalence is much more then can be expected by chance.

Clinical picture

The illness usually run an episodic course. Some patient may show past history of schizophrenia or affective illness.

The clinical picture is characterized by schizophrenic symptoms like delusions, hallucinations, thought disturbances, and disturbances of behaviour and social relationships. They will simultaneously exhibit symptoms of depression, hopelessness, worthlessness, guilt, etc.

Some patients may have manic symptoms of elation, grandiosity and hyperactivity.

Course and Prognosis

This illness runs an episodic course. The illness may remain stable or in some patient deterioration can be seen. Prognosis is intermediate betwen schizophrenia and mood disorders.

Diagnosis

Diagnosis is confirmed on eliciting signs of both depression/mania and schizophrenia in the same episode.

Management

The management of these patients are done either on the line of mania or depression as the case may be. If the patient does not respond to this regime then a combination of Lithium/Carbamazine with antipsychotics can be used. The patients who are not responsive to drug treatment, can be given a trial of E.C.T.

For a long term management, Lithium and or Carbamazepine are used.

CHAPTER 8

MOOD (AFFECTIVE) DISORDERS

Human beings react to external or internal events by initiation of a series of thoughts, actions and feelings. Normally individuals exhibit a variety of feelings which may range from happiness to sadness, from irritability to anger and anxiety, depending upon the circumstances. These feelings are appropriate to the situation and can be terminated at will or with changed circumstances. When a particular feeling state persists for some time it is referred to as mood. A few individuals lose the normal reactivity of feelings and remain persistently in one mood state, of either happiness or sadness, and their thinking and behaviour is also consequently influenced by their mood. Such conditions are called MOOD DISORDERS. Conventionally mood disorders include only two affective states - of sadness (or depression) and happiness (or euphoria).

Mood disorders are characterised by the following :

a) Persistent mood of depression or elation most of the time, everyday for more than two weeks. There can be minor fluctuations of mood from day to day, or within the same day.

b) The thinking process is preoccupied either by depressive and negative thoughts or by grandiose and euphoric thoughts.

c) Psychomotor activity is decreased or increased. The patients in depression, will become slow and may appear withdrawn, while the patients with elation will be hyperactive.

CLASSIFICATION

Mood disorders are divided into :

Manic Episode

Hypomania
Mania withcut psychotic symptoms
Mania with psychotic symptoms
Other manic episode
Manic episode (unspecified)

Bipolar Affective Disorder

- Bipolar affective disorder, current episode hypo-manic
- Bipolar affective disorder — current episode manic without psychotic symptoms
- Bipolar affective disorder — current episode manic with psychotic symptoms
- Bipolar affective disorder — current episode mild or moderate depression
  Without somatic symptoms
  With somatic symptoms
- Bipolar affective disorder — current episode severe depression without psychotic symptoms
- Bipolar affective disorder, current episode severe depression with psychotic symptoms.
- Bipolar affective disorder, current episode mixed
- Bipolar affective disorder, currently in remission.
- Other bipolar affective disorders.
- Bipolar affective disorder, unspecified.

Depressive Episode

- Mild depressive episode
  Without somatic symptoms
  With somatic symptoms
- Moderate depressive episode
  Without somatic symptoms
  With somatic symptoms
- Severe depressive episode without psychotic symptoms
- Severe depressive episode with psychotic symptoms
- Other depressive episode
- Depressive episode, unspecified

Recurrent Depressive Disorder

- Recurrent depressive disorder, current episode mild
  Without somatic symptoms
  With somatic symptoms
- Recurrent depressive disorder, current episode moderate
  Without somatic symptoms
  With somatic symptoms
- Recurrent depressive disorder, current episode severe, without psychotic synptoms
- Recurrent depressive disorder, current episode severe, with psychotic symptoms.
- Recurrent depressive disorder, currently in remission.
- Other recurrent depressive disorders.
- Recurrent depressive disorder, unspecified

Persistent Mood (Affective) Disorders

Cyclothymia

Dysthymia

Other persistent mood disorders

Persistent mood (affective) disorder, unspecified

Other Mood (Affective) Disorders

- Other single mood (affective) disorders
  Mixed affective episode
- Other recurrent mood (affective) disorders
  Recurrent brief depressive disorder
- Other unspecified mood (affective) disorders

Unspecified Mood Disorders

The classification of mood disorder may appear daunting at first sight, basically the subdivisions are dependant upon the following :

Single episode/multiple episode

Only depressive episode

Both depressive and manic episodes

Further subdivision is based on severity

Mild, moderate and severe in depression and Hypomania and mania.

Symptomatology : Depression is subdivided with or without somatic syndrome (described later)

Both mania and depression are classified with or without psychotic symptoms

Basically mood disorders can be classified into the following :

A — Bipolar affective disorders

B — Major depressive disorders (unipolar)

C — Persistent affective disorders

A) BIPOLAR AFFECTIVE DISORDERS

This group of disorders are characterised by occurrence of attacks of depression and mania in the same patient. The episodes of mania and depression can occur in any sequence, e.g. mania - depression - mania, mania - mania - depression, depression - depression - mania, etc. The patient having recurrent manic episodes only are also included.

Bipolar disorders are further classified into Bipolar I and Bipolar II. Bipolar I patients have severe attacks of mania which necessitates treatment, while bipolar II patients only show mild hypomania which does not require treatment.

This differentiation is meant to identify disorders which may have different course, prognosis and management.

B) MAJOR DEPRESSIVE DISORDER (UNIPOLAR)

These patients may have a single episode of depression, or may have recurrent episodes. They do not show any symptoms of elation between attacks. However, some patients may have mild elation after the attack of depression which may occur as a result of antidepressants drug treatment or sometimes even without drugs. But this elation is mild and short-lasting. The depression is further subdivided into mild, moderate and severe, according to the severity.

C) PERSISTENT MOOD AFFECTIVE DISORDERS

These patient's have persistent mood symptions for two years or more, without any symptom-free period. They include dysthymia and cyclothymia.

Epidemiology

Most of the Western researchers estimate the life-time prevalence of bipolar disorders to be around 1%. Indian studies have not differentiated between unipolar and bipolar disorders, but the general feeling is that the life-time prevalence of bipolar disorders will be around the same as in the West. This illness does not show different rates in the two sexes. The age of onset can vary from childhood to old age but usually occurs in the third decade. Other socio-economic factors do not appear to be causally related.

Unipolar mood disorders are much more common than bipolar disorders. The life-time prevalence is around 5%-6%. The female to male ratio is around 2:1. Psychosocial factors seem to play a more important role in some patients. A large number of patients report negative life experiences at the time of onset as well as during the illness.

Etiology

Mood disorders show a familial tendency. Bipolar and unipolar disorders are considerd to be genetically different illnesses, but genetic studies in both disorders show prevalence of both types of illnesses in first degree relatives though the same kind of disorder is more often seen in their families. The reason for this observation could be that among bipolar relatives, some may not have so far experienced a manic episode. It appears understandable that unipolar depression is a mixed group, which may include some bipolar disorders, some psychogenic depressives and some true primary major depression.

Genetic Theory — There is good evidence that these disorders run in families. The points in favour are :

25% of the first degree relatives of bipolar disorders probands exhibit unipolar or similar disorders, while the percentage of affective illness in the first degree relatives of unipolar probands is slightly lower.

The risk of developing a bipolar illess is nearly 27% if one parent has had this illness while the risk doubles if both parents have similar illness.

a) **Lifetime Prevalence**

	Bipolar Disorders	Unipolar Disorders
General population	.2 to 1.8%.	.7 to 5.8%
Ist degree relative of bipolar probands	2.8 to 17.7%	.5 to 23%
Ist degree relatives of of unipolar probands	.3 to 5.4%	5.9 to 28.6%

b)	Monozygotic Twins	Dizygotic Twins
Concordance rates for affective disorders	33%- 75%	0% - 24%

In studies of adopted children, it has been observed that the risk of such illness is much more in biological parents than in adoptive parents indicating that the illness develops more due to biological factors than because of psychosocial factors.

The pattern of inheritance is not clear; it is thought to be multifactorial in nature. Recently linkage studies have been initiated which may be able to unravel the inheritance pattern more clearly.

Biological Factors

Neurotransmitter Abnormality — Most of the antidepressants drugs act by increasing the availability of Norepinephrine, or 5-Hydroxytryptamine or Dopamine, either by decreasing the re-uptake of these substances by the synaptic vesicles or by inhibiting the destruction of the monoamines by monoamine oxidising enzymes. Thus, the relative deficiency of these biogenic amines is proposed as factors associated to depression. Decrease or increase of these amines or their metabolites have not been consistently demonstrated in depressives or manics.

Moreover, most antidepressants take 2-3 weeks to act while the increase in bioavailability of these biogenic amines appears soon after the intake. So it is postulated, that the effectiveness of treatment is related to the down regulation of various receptors which takes nearly 3 weeks, rather than to increase in the availability of these amines. Recent evidence has also shown disturbances in other neurotransmitters like Gamma-aminobutyric acid and acetylecholine.

It is not clear whether these changes in biogenic amines and other neurotransmitters are the cause of depression or they are only an accompanying event.

Neuro Endocrine Abnormality — Changes have also been reported in the neuroendocrine axis. It has also been reported that the thyrotropin release response to Thyroid Release Hormone (TRH) is blunted. Dexamethasone is unable to suppress cortisol secretion in many patients. Both these tests are positive in some of the patients and are also positive in some other conditions.

Sleep — Sleep abnormalities are consistently seen in depression. Patients develop the first REM phase much earlier than usual (decrease REM latency) and exhibit increased density of REM sleep particularly in the first part of the night.

Brain Structure — Recently brain imaging techniques have shown decrease in blood flow and glucose metabolism in the frontal lobes, especially on the left side, though the evidence so far is not fully consistent.

There appears to be reasonable evidence of some neuroendocrine dysfunctions in these disorders, but the precise nature of the defect as well as its use as a diagnostic procedure is not yet established.

Psychosocial Factors

Though the association of various psychosocial stressors is often reported with the onset of the bipolar disorder, there is yet, no clear evidence that any such event is essential for the onset of an episode of the illness. Unipolar depressives frequently experience negative life experiences at the time of onset of the illness. Higher prevalence in females could also indirectly favour the stressor hypothesis. Females in almost all cultures undergo more stresses and strains than males. Some believe that the preponderance of females could be due to hormonal changes.

BIPOLAR AFFECTIVE DISORDERS (CLINICAL FEATURES)

The patient develops the disorder in their twenties. Most of the bipolar patients would have started their illness by 35 years of age. The bipolar disorder may begin with mania or depression. A few patients may have only recurrent episodes of mania.

MANIA

The illness starts acutely and may often develop within hours, the full severity being generally achieved within 7 days. The illness is characterised by excitement, elation and overactivity.

The history of the patients will reveal excessive activities, marked talkativeness and excessive spending. The patients start making wild plans to improve their work, or may even plan for the betterment of the country or the religion. Many of them may take part in current political issues. During the 1992 Ayodhya episode, many patients developed grandiose delusions of building the temple and some even went to Ayodhya.

Interpersonal Relationships — They often get involved in quarrels with family members and work mates. They are always in such a hurry that even a little delay makes them angry.

Sleep — Their sleep is reduced to a few hours. They sleep late at night and get up early in the morning, yet feel fresh in the morning.

Appetite — Appetite may be increased and they usually demand rich food.

Sex Drive — They may have excessive libido, demand sex frequently and may make obscene remarks.

Mental status examination will reveal the following :

General Appearance and Behaviour — The patient may be flashily dressed or dishelved. He is usually very excited, psychomotor activity being increased. He talks incessantly and is often quarrelsome and angry.

Consciousness is clear. Attention may be difficult to arouse and his concentration is difficult to sustain.

Speech — The patient talks rapidly and the speech often appears incoherent. He may show punning and rhyming.

Thought Process — Thought process may reveal excessive talking, irrelevance and incoherence.Few patients may exhibit the flight of ideas. In a flight of ideas, the thought are connected together, not by logic but by commonness of meaning, sounds or appearances. One patient, for example, said 'My name is Rama; God is most powerful ; Ravana should be killed'. This is an example of the flight of ideas, where the name Rama got associated with God, God to power and power to Ravana.

Thought Content — These patients usually have delusions of grandiosity. They may consider themselves to be the richest and the most powerful person. They may also have delusions of persecution. They may believe that some people are trying to kill them or steal their riches.

Mood — The mood is often of cheerfulness. It may range, however, from happiness, anger and irritability to hostility. The latter three affective states often develop when their wishes are being thwarted.

Impulse Control — They are generally implusive.

Perception — These patients generally do not show perceptual disturbances.

Memory and Intelligence are difficult to test but are generally not impaired.

Judgement and insight are impaired — The patients do not consider themselves to be ill.

Case Example

Mr R, a 38 year. old male, farmer by occupation

had stopped working 2 weeks ago. When he was questioned by his family members, he retorted that a man like him, who has been blessed by Lord Hanuman, need not do ordinary work. After a few days, the patient began to show a marked increase in psychomotor activity along with decreased sleep, which, however, did not impair his daily activity in anyway. The patient had two earlier episodes of similar grandiose behaviour, 3 yr. and 1 yr. prior to this illness, which had lasted about a month each, for which the family had consulted faith healers only. There was no known family history of psychiatric disorders.

On examination, the patient was found dressed shabbily in a torn vest and dhoti, and appeared not to have bathed since the past many days. When questioned about this, he replied in a loud voice that those blessed with the power of Lord Hanuman, need not bathe and wash daily. He further said that he could turn all he touched into silver and had a bank account worth millions of rupees. When challenged by family members who said that he never owned any bank account, he vaguely replied that he had donated everything to 'the needy'. On further probing upon this point, he became irritated and said that if this pointless interview was not stopped immediately, he would put 'a curse' on all the doctors.

The patient was admitted and started on Tab. Lithium 900 mg/day and Tab. Chlorpromazine 800 mg/day, to which he responded well. Within 2 weeks, no grandiose delusions could be demonstrated, the patient was sleeping well at night and was participating well in all the activities. Chlorpromazine was slowly tapered off and the patient was maintained only on lithium, with a serum level of 0.83 mmol/l. The patient was discharged on the same treatment after a month of hospitalization.

Comments — This patient exhibits typical manic symptoms. He had past history of manic attack, which lasted for a month or so and then he remained normal during the interval period. Present episode started with grandiose delusions. He felt he has special powers and he has been blessed by lord Hanuman. He also felt he could turn anything into gold and silver. He responded well to a combination of lithium and CPZ. He will require maintenance on lithium.

Diagnosis

A careful history from relatives and work-mates should be obtained. If the patient has had previous episodes of mania or depression, the diagnosis becomes easier. A family history of mood disorder should also be elicited. A history of suicide or attempted suicide can be a pointer towards affective disorder in the family.

Hypomania (Diagnostic Features) (ICD X)

This is a milder form of mania in which delusions and hallucinations are absent. The characteristic features include :

Mild elevation of mood for 1 week or more

Increased energy and activity.

Marked feeling of well being

Increased sociability and talkativeness, overfamiliarity, increased sexual energy.

A decreased need for sleep.

Some disruption in work and social activity.

For a diagnosis of hypomania, a patient should exhibit most of the above symptoms.

Mania (Diagnostic Features) : (ICD X)

Extremely jovial mood, which may lead to marked excitement

Increased energy and activity

Speech is excessive and under pressure

Flight of ideas and incoherence may be present

Attention may be difficult to sustain

Social inhibitions are lost

Grandiose and persecutory delusions may be present

Sleep is reduced

General behavior will exhibit excessive spending, making wild schemes

Tendency to pick quarrels, and inapproprite flashy dressing.

A diagnosis of mania can be made if most of the above are present for 1 week or longer.

Differential Diagnosis

Organic Brain Diseases

Manic symptoms can occur in some neurological diseases. Some of the common diseases needing differentiation from mania are : Epilepsy, HIV disease, diseases of the frontal lobe, head injury, strokes, systemic lupus erythematosus, vitamin deficiencies and General paralysis of Insane, etc. All these conditions exhibit symptoms of basic disease and should not be difficult to differentiate from mania. When needed, relevant investigations can also be done.

DRUGS — Drugs like amphetamine, cocaine, cannabis, INH, corticosteroids, levodopa and bromocriptine can produce symptoms resembling mania. Temporal correlation of the drug intake with symptoms and other symptoms specific to each drug will be helpful in the differential diagnosis.

Schizophrenia — Manic symptoms can be confused with schizophrenia. Both conditions can have delusions of grandiosity, hyperactivity, excitement and volubility. The differentiating features are :

Manic illness develops more rapidly.

Manics will show more interest in the environment and like to interact with others, while the schizophrenics behave more due to internal cues and do not relate to external events.

Manic thoughts are appropriate to the mood; while schizophrenics, for all their grandiose talks do not show grandiose behaviour.

Course and Outcome

The attack of mania usually lasts for 1-3 months. Those who tend to have longer episodes often develop schizophrenic symptoms. Approximately 7% of the patients have a single episode, only 45% have a recurrence and 40% have a chronic illness.

DEPRESSIVE EPISODES AND RECURRENT DEPRESSIVE DISORDERS (CLINICAL FEATURES)

Depression usually develops gradually but sometimes may develop acutely, when it is associated with severe loss (deaths, failures, financial loss, etc.). The clinical picture is characterized by :

Depressed mood — The patient generally feels sad most of the time, and everyday. He often complains, "I feel sad most of the time. The things which used to give me pleasure no longer do so. Even when my children or my wife want to talk to me, I wish to avoid them". This sadness varies in grade from mild to severe. Depression is usually experienced as painful and agonizing. The patient may start crying and at times the weeping becomes uncontrollable. The patients often lament their inability to laugh.

Anhedonia — This is said to be a characteristic feature of depression. The patients generally complain that they are not able to enjoy activities that were normally pleasurable. Thus, happy events like marriage, success in job or examination, etc. may not produce any pleasure in the patient. This incapacity to feel pleasure is often very painful to the patient.

Lack of energy or easy fatigability — These patients usually complain of tiredness and lack of energy. They find even normal day to day activities like bathing, dressing, eating, etc. to be too tiresome, and often like to avoid or postpone them.

Impaired concentration and memory — Many patients complain of difficulty in concentration due to which they give up too easily. They may also experience forgetfulness due to which, many elderly depressed patients may be wrongly diagnosed as dementia. Some may also complain of difficulty in thinking.

Reduced self esteem and self-confidence — Patients usually feel that they cannot achieve anything and complain of severe loss of confidence.

Ideas of guilt and unworthiness — Many depressive patients start blaming themselves for their own difficulties as well as for the difficulties of others. Patients may state that they have taken all the wrong decisions in their life, which are responsible for their current miseries. They feel that they are good for nothing and are a burden on others. In India, the guilt can be expressed in terms of sins committed in the previous birth.

Bleak and pessimistic view of the future — The future appears bleak and without any hope. Patients feel that they must not initiate any work because nothing will succeed. Negative thinking predominates. If any family member has gone out, the patients may believe that evil may befall him.

Ideas or acts of self harm and suicide — The patients may feel that life is not worth living, and many experience fleeting ideas of killing themselves while others plan to commit suicide or actually make attempts to kill themselves. Rarely patients may kill their near relatives, to save them from future misery and then kill themselves. Depressive mothers may at the same time kill their children and then attempt to kill themselves. Successful suicides are seen in about 10%-15% of the patients.

Disturbed sleep — Sleep is often disturbed. The patient generally goes to sleep as usual but wakes up early in the morning or in the middle of the night and then fails to go to sleep again. There may also be difficulty in falling asleep, and in severe cases, sleep may be completely lost. Few patients paradoxically complain of excessive sleep.

Diminished appetite — The appetite is generally

reduced, maybe more, so in the day and the patient may be a able to eat better in the evenings. There may be a significant weight loss (i.e. 5% or more of body weight per month). Few patients paradoxically have increased appetite.

Diurnal variation—Many patients feel that their depression is much worse in the morning, and they feel better in the evenings, while with others the opposite holds true.

Loss of libido — Sexual desire is usually diminished both in the males and the females.

Psychomotor agitation and retardation — The patient generally appears to be slow and retarded. They lie quietly, may not move their limbs and may even talk very little and slowly. A few patients develop a depressive stupor in which the patient is mute, does not respond to a stimuli and may not even pass stool and urine. Some patients may exhibit marked restlessness and may not be able to sit quietly, even for a short time. They may also talk excessively, but the content is generally depressive in nature.

Somatic symptoms — Patients often complain of pains and aches in various body parts. Poor digestion and constipation are common symptoms. Some patients may complain of an emptiness of body parts. Quite often, the somatic symptoms are the presenting complaints, the depression being identified only by direct enquiry. It is important to keep this in mind, when dealing with patients complaining of vague somatic symptoms.

Anxiety — Anxiety is often seen in patients with depression. The patients develop a feeling of unknown apprehension and may also exhibit symptoms like palpitation, dry mouth and sweating, etc. Some patients may also experience panic episodes, characterised by acute anxiety with a fear of dying.

Social behaviour — Depressive patients usually avoid meeting people. They like isolation and prefer a dark room. Their work performance deteriorates.

Psychotic symptoms — Some patients may develop delusions. They can be of the following types :

Nihilistic delusions : The patient may feel that his intestines have rotted or that there is nothing in his head.

Some patients may be totally convinced of their abject poverty, worthlessness, or may feel that the future holds no hope for them. All these ideas are held firmly and cannot be removed by any argument.

Paranoid delusions : Some patients may have delusions of suspicion that people are planning to kill them or are plotting against them.

Psychotic delusions : Rarely patients may have bizarre delusions as seen in schizophrenia.

Hallucinations : Very few patients of depression have hallucinations. They can have auditory, visual or olfactory hallucinations which are usually depressive in nature. Patients may hear voices condeming them for their misdeeds or voices may inform them of the possible misfortunes which are going to befall them. One patient, for example used to hear voices stating that her time of death had already passed, which prompted her to attempt suicide. The smell of burning flesh or bad odours emanating from the body have also sometimes been reported. Patients with psychotic features are always severely depressed.

Somatic (Melancholic) Symptoms of Depression

These symptoms were earlier considered essential for the diagnosis of endogenous (genetic) depression. These are now called somatic symptoms of depression. These include :

Loss of interest or pleasure in activities that are normally enjoyable ;

Lack of emotional reactivity to previous pleasurable surroundings and events ;

Waking up in the morning 2 hours or more before the usual time ;

Depression worsening in the morning ;

Objective evidence of definite psychomotor retardation or agitation (as reported by other people) ;

Marked loss of appetite

Weight loss (often defined as 5% or more loss of body weight in the previous month) ;

Marked loss of libido ;

Somatic symptoms are regarded as present, when four or more of the above symptoms are present.

Case Example

Mrs K, a 40 year old female patient, an uneducated housewife, could not date the exact onset of her symptoms. But her family members gave a history of approximately 2 months, when the patient began to show less interest in her work, would take hours to do kitchen chores, and would like to lie down much more often than before. She would complain of fatigue and loss of interest and headache most of the time of the day. Since past two weeks, she hardly left her room, would keep lying in her bed the whole day and when the questioned, would only say that no one can save her now. There was history of suicide in the patient's maternal uncle but the attendants were unable to give details of his psychiatric problem. The patient had never had such an episode earlier.

The patient walked slowly into the examination room, groaning and sat down only when repeatedly told to do so. She swayed to and fro and refused to answer questions, but suddenly began to cry loudly, she said "Please save me, doctor, I have two unmarried children, who will look after them selves after I am gone, you must save me," then lapsed into silence again.

The patient was admitted and started on Tab. Imipramine, 150 mg per day. After 3 weeks of above dosage the patient began to take some interest in her surroundings and after a month, began to ask about the welfare of family members, took interest in her grooming and hygiene and by 6 weeks no depressive symptoms could be demonstrated. The patient was discharged after 2 months of hospitalization on the same treatment.

Comments — This patient developed her first depressive episode around forty years of age. There were no precipitating factors. She showed slowing of activities, lack of interest, depressive mood and crying. The family history of suicide was present. The patient is a typical patient of depressive episode.

Diagnosis

A careful history should be obtained and one should specifically ask if the patient had similar episodes in the past or episodes of persistant elated bahaviour in which the patient was spending too much or making big plans, etc. The diagnosis becomes easier, if there is a history of past episodes of mania or depression.

If the presenting episode is the first ever, one has to carefully differentiate the illness from other psychiatric and physical disorders ;

Confirm whether the patient fulfils the following essential conditions for a diagnosis of depression (ICD-X).

1. Persistently sad mood continuously present for two weeks or more ;
2. Loss of interest and enjoyment ;
3. Reduced energy leading to increased fatiguability and diminished activity ;

a) Reduced concentration and attention ;
b) Reduced self-esteem and self-confidence ;
c) Ideas of guilt and unworthiness ;
d) Bleak and pessimistic view of the future ;
e) Ideas or acts of self-harm or suicide ;
f) Disturbed sleep ;
g) Poor appetite and weight loss ;

All the above may not necessarily be present but the first three and a few of the latter symptoms must be present for a diagnosis of depression. In general practice, many patients may present with only somatic symptoms, with mild depressive features. For the confirmation of the diagnosis of depression, one may need to directly elicit the symptoms in the above list. Once these symptoms are identified, a diagnosis of depression can be entertained.

Differential Diagnosis — When the clinical picture is suggestive of depression, the following need to be excluded :

Drugs

A history of drug or intoxicant intake which can result in depression. Some drugs which can cause depression are given below.

Drugs Inducing Depression

Antihypertensive drugs

Propanolol
Clonidine
Alpha-methyldopa
Digitalis
Reserpine

Analgesics

Ibuprofen
Indomethacin
Opiates
Phenacetin

Neuropharmacological drugs

Amantadine
Antipsychotics
Sedatives and Hypnotics
Bromocriptine
Carbamazepine

Steriods and Hormones

Corticosteroids
Oral contraceptives

Antibacterial and Antifungal

Ampicillin
Cycloserine
Metronidazole
Nalidixic acid
Nitrofurantoin
Streptomycin
Miscellaneous
Cemetidine
Disulfiram
Acetazolamide

Drug induced depression will not have all the characteristics of depression. There should be a temporal correlation between drug intake and depression. Stopping of drugs should result in improvement within a reasonable time-period.

Physical Disease— Evidence of a physical illness which may be associated with depression should be carefully looked for. Cerebral stroke, parkinsonism, dementia and chronic diseases are likely to be associated with depression.

Grief— If the depression has resulted from acute grief (death of loved ones), the diagnosis of depression is unwarranted since, the grief is likely to be overcome with the passage of time. Normal grief is worst in the first two weeks following the bereavement and usually resolves within 6 months.

Schizophrenia — Evidence of schizophrenia should be carefully looked for as schizophrenics often present as apparent depression. One should ask for all the positive symptoms of schizophrenia before discarding the diagnosis. Schizophrenics will generally complain of sadness but will not show the agony and pain experienced by the depressives. (discussed in detail in the chapter on schizophrenia).

Anxiety Disorders — Often anxiety disorder with depressive symptoms can be confused with depression because both may have symptoms of depression. Patients with anxiety, usually show anxiety symptoms to begin with and develop depression secondarily. The emphasis in these patients is on a baseless apprehension, while the depressive patients will show sadness and inability to cope with life.

Obsessive Compulsive Disorder— Patients with obsessive disorders often develop depression. They may hide their obsessive symptoms and complain only of depression. It is always a good practice to ask every depressive for obsessive compulsive symptoms, e.g. certain repetitive ideas which they consider absurd.

Dementia — Some elderly depressives may complain of memory loss and they may be confused with dementia. The differentiating features are :

Memory loss in depression is global while in dementia it is merely for recent events.

Depressive patients generally do not make the effort to answer questions while patients with dementia will try to give answers and may confabulate.

Dementia progresses more slowly than depression.

Myxoedema — Myxoedema can also mimic depression but a thorough clinical examination should normally exclude the diagnosis. When in doubt, thyroid function tests will confirm the diagnosis.

Course and Outcome

A) Unipolar Depression

Unipolar depression begins later than bipolar depression, though usually before 40 years. Some bipolar patients begin with depression and are usually labelled unipolar depressives, until they turn out to be bipolar disorders. Duration of the total depressive episode ranges between 6-9 months.

A majority of unipolar depressives show recurrence of the illness. The duration of episodes and frequency increases with time but tends to stabilize after 3-5 episodes. On long-term follow-up, approximately half of the patients show no impairment while 30% show some and 20% show significant impairment. Mortality is high and about 15% patients commit suicide.

B) Bipolar Diosrders

These patients show more frequent relapses amd more chronic course than unipolar disorders. Often, the management may be difficult due to switch from mania to depression. Mortality is nearly the same.

Management

Patients will be diagnosed in one of the following groups :

Depressive episode : The first episode of depression with no previous episodes of depression or mania.

Recurrent depressive disorder : These patients would have had one or more previous episodes of depression but none of mania.

Mania : Patients with only one episode of mania and no previous history of depression.

Bipolar disorder : The patients show depressive and manic episodes or only manic episodes.

A) Manic Episode

Manic patients usually do not consider themselves to be ill and often refuse treatment. Such patients have to be treated against their will. The consent of their close relatives must be obtained and often a legal procedure may be necessary for admission and treatment for some of such patients. In our country, a large number of relatives agree for the management of the patient at home. In such cases, the relatives have to ensure that the patient takes the drugs as prescribed and that he does not go out of the house and create problems for himself or others.

Pharmacotherapy

Lithium — Lithium is available as lithium carbonate. It is also available in sustained release form. The sustained release form does not offer any major advantage. Lithium is readily absorbed from gastrointestinal tract. The stable level of serum lithium are achieved within a week of regular administration.

The dosage of lithium required are 600 to 1500 mg/day. Lithium level in blood has to be monitored because lithium has a small therapeutic window. It is effective between .6 m mol/lit to 1.2 m mol/lit. It is ineffective below this level and toxic above this level.

Lithium is the drug of choice in mania. The therapeutic effects are evident in 2 to 3 weeks. The serum level for treatment of acute episode is maintained between .8 to 1.2 m mol/lit.

Carbamazepine — Carbamazepine in dosage of 600-1200 mg/day can also be used for control of acute mania. It is effective with in few days.

Antipsychotics—Haloperidol or Chlorpromazine can be used to control excitement in the first few weeks. Initially, Haloperidol 10-20 mg/day IMI or Chlorpromazine 50 mg-150 mg IMI is given. When the patients take drugs orally Haloperidol 10-30 mg/day or Chlorpromazine 600-1000/day in divided dosage should be given. Some patients can also be treated only by these drugs. The disadvantage of using antipsychotic drugs are :

a) Their side effects are more disturbing

b) They may induce depression.

Hypnotics

If the patient does not get sleep by above mentioned drugs hypnotics can be used :

Nitrazepam 10 mg h.s.; or
Lorazepam 2 mg h.s.

E.C.T.

It is indicated in mania in the following situations :

a) The patient is so excited that it is difficult to feed him or control him.

b) If the antimanic drugs are ineffective.

The majority of patients will respond to the treatment in one or two months. Few chronic patients may take longer.

If this is the first episode then the drug can be gradually tapered off in three to four months.

Bipolar Depression

Bipolar depressive episode should also be treated by lithium alone. If the patient does not respond within four weeks then antidepressants can be used. Antidepressants may cause switch to mania.

Indications of Prophylaxis of Bipolar Disorders

If the attacks of mania or depression occur at intervals of 2 or more years, prophylactic treatment may not be started. However, if the patient's job is such that an episode of illness can materially affect his life, (e.g. an Army or Police officer, railway driver, etc.), then prophylaxis may be required even without frequent episodes. Usually, if 2 or more attacks occur within 2 years, prophylactic treatment should be started.

Lithium is the drug of first choice for prophylaxis. Patients who cannot tolerate or fail to respond to lithium can be put on carbamazepine. Patients who do not respond to either alone may be put on a combination of both.

The following precautions are to be observed during prophylaxis :

Patients should be explained that that these drugs do not cure but only control the disease for as long as the treatment is continued.

The drugs may be required lifelong. However, if the patient has been symptom free for 3 years than one may taper the drugs gradually and stop. The patient should be carefully followed, and if there are symptoms of a relapse, prophylaxis should be reinstituted.

The patient may have minor relapses even while

on prophylactic therapy. These are termed as breakthrough episodes. They are usually controlled merely by minor adjustments of the dosage.

Serum lithium should be monitored once in two months or more frequently, specially during the summer months.

If the patient develops an illness where salt loss is excessive (e.g. diarrhoea, vomiting or even excessive diaphoresis), then lithium should be temporarily discontinued.

Kidney functions should be monitored 6-monthly.

Thyroid functions should be monitored annually.

Side Effects of Lithium — The side effects include nausea, loose stools, fatigue and muscle weakness, polydipsia and polyurea. Hand tremors may occur at the time of starting treatment. Weight gain and a mild memory impairment may also be noticed.

Lithium treatment reduces the T_3 and T_4 levels which is compensated by increase in the TSH levels. Mild increase in the TSH levels is common with lithium therapy. Clinical hypothyroidism develops in only about 5% of patients. Long term lithium therapy can, at times, induce tubulo-interstitial nephropathy. The clinical symptoms include polydipsia and polyurea.

Lithium Intoxication — If serum levels of lithium exceed 2 mmol/litre, the patient may develop symptoms of toxicity, including nausea, vomiting, diarrhoea and coarse tremors. Later, the patient develops confusion, muscular hypertonia, hyper-reflexia and epileptiform seizures. It is managed by monitoring of serum sodium and potassium levels. If hyponatremia is present, saline may be infused. Diuresis is induced by intravenous infusion of urea and mannitol, and the seizures are managed by intravenous diazepam or phenytoin. In severe cases, haemodialysis may be required.

Management of Major (Unipolar) Depressive Illness

Management of depression has to be individualized. The treatment should be tailored according to the severity of the disorder and the work status of the patient. One must assess the patient for the following :

Severity of depression — The patient may have mild depression where the illness is not interfering too much with his life. These patients may do well with psychological treatment. Mild depressives patients have few symptoms and are usually able to function reasonably well in their job as well as at home. Psychologically one has to focus on the current interpersonal and occupational difficulties. Quite often, the patient perceives the problem inappropriately ; he is then helped to revaluate the situation and support from the family members and colleagues may help him further to cope with depression.

If the anxiety symptoms are prominent then one of the following drugs could be used :

Alprazolam 0.25-0.5 mg twice or thrice a day as it has antidepressant properties as well.

Other minor tranquilizers may also be used.

If the severity of the illness ranges from moderate to severe, then antidepressant drugs are essential. These patients find it difficult to carry on their normal tasks. They usually stop working and the illness is quite disabiling.

Suicidal Risk — Suicidal risk should be evaluated in each patient. If the patient has suicidal thoughts, the risk will depend on the following :

Previous history of suicidal attempts.

Elderly, loners and widows/widowers have a higher suicidal risk.

Poor family support is also an important suicide risk

Patients having delusions of poverty, worthlessness and hopelessness have greater suicidal risk.

If suicidal risk is present, then the patient has to be hospitalized and guarded against the risk.

Before the treatment is started, the patient and the family members should be explained the nature of the disease, because many patients are convinced that (because of the negative expectations induced by the illness) there is no use taking any treatment, as they can never get well. They must be told that most patients of depression are likely to improve. Generally, depression is a self-limiting disease and chances of full recovery are very high. The symptoms of hopelessness and worthless which the patient is experiencing, are part of the illness and will improve with the treatment.

The patient should also be explained that most antidepressants, normally require 3 weeks for the antidepressant action and hence they should not expect immediate relief. Most antidepressants have annoying side affects including dryness of mouth, constipation, blurring of vision, giddiness due to postural hypotension and drowsiness. These side effects are often perceived to be the result of 'heat' caused by the medication. They must be explained that no permanent harm will ensue and that most of these side effects will disappear as time goes by. Sleep often improves first, followed by anxiety and appetite. Depressive thoughts are the last to disappear.

Pharmacotherapy

Antidepressant drugs are usually classified into the following :

Tricyclic Antidepressants : Amitryptyline, Imipramine, Clomipramine, Trimipramine, Nortryptiline, Doxeipin, Dothepin.

Atypical Antidepressants : Mianserin, Trazadone.

Monoamine Oxidase inhibitors : Not available in our country, which is rather unfortunate since they have been found to be quite useful in atypical and tricyclic resistant depression.

Most of the antidepressants have similar antidepressant properties but differ in thier side-effects profile. The main side-effects include :

Sedation : A large number of antidepressants induce sedation specially in the early part of treatment. This effect is therapeutically utilized by using more sedative drugs in anxious and insomnic patients. Patients who are working should preferably be given less sedative drugs.

Postural hypotension : The blood pressure does not rapidly change when the patient gets up from a lying posture. The systolic B.P. may fall more than 20 mm. Hg, though this fall is compensated in the next few minutes, the patient will feel giddy and may fall down. It is specially serious in elderly patients who may fall down and sustain fractures of the long bones. The patient should be advised to take support of some object while getting up, and should continue to take support until the giddiness passes off.

If the symptom is very severe, then the drug may need to be changed.

ECG : The drugs may cause prolongation of the PR interval and QRS complex.

Anticholinergic side effects : These include, dryness of the mouth, blurring of vision, constipation, difficulty in micturition and urinary retention in the elderly.

Weight changes : Some drugs may induce hyperphagia with resulting weight gain. Fluoxetine, however, is not known to cause this symptom.

Neurological and psychiatric side effects : The drugs may reduce seizure threshold. Some patients develop an anticholinergic confusional syndrome.

Haematological : Blood dyscrasias can rarely occur.

Some of these drugs can be fatal in overdose.

It is best to be totally conversant with two or three drugs. One must know their side effects, pharmacokinetics and drug interactions. Two commonly used drugs, imipramine and amitriptyline, are almost similar in their efficacy. Amitriptyline is slightly more sedative. The antidepressants dosages of these drugs ranges from 100-300 mg. The most common cause of treatment failure is inadequate dosage. It is essential to use the drugs upto their maximum permissible doses provided the patient can tolerate it. These drugs should be started in doses of 75 mg/day and gradually increased to the maximum tolerated dose in two weeks, upto a maximum of 300 mg/day. If, after six weeks of this dosage, the depression is not alleviated, other drugs or ECT should be considered.

Fluoxetine is a new drug with no sedative and very little anticholinergic side effects. This drug should be given in the morning, as it can interfere with sleep. The other common side-effects of this drug include headache, appetite loss, nausea and anxiety. The usual dosage is 20-40 mg/day. Night time sedatives can be given if the problem of sleep is not corrected by anti-depressants alone. This drug also needs three weeks to produce its effects.

The depressive symptoms will resolve in 4-6 weeks in most (60-70%) of the patients.

Drugs should be continued in the effective therapeutic doses for six months if this is the first episode, or longer, if the previous episode lasted longer than 6 months.

In recurrent depression (i.e. more than 2 attacks in the last two years), drugs should be continued upto three years in the same doses.

Patients who do not respond to one antidepressant within 6 weeks (30%) may require another drug with a different mode of action. Lack of antidepressant effect should be confirmed by giving the drug in full doses for six weeks.

If the patient does not respond to single drugs, ECT can be used. ECT is given biweekly and usually six sessions are sufficient. While another 20% of the patients respond to ECT, yet a small group remain who may not respond to single drug therapy and ECT. For the last group augmentation of antidepressants with other drugs can be tried. In drug resistant depression, the following drugs can be used to potentiate antidepressant action :

Lithium Carbonate : Can be added to the antidepressant in a dosage of 300 mg thrice daily for 3-4 weeks. The combination may relieve depression. However, this is effective only when given after baseline antidepressant treatment for 3-4 weeks.

Thyroxine : In doses of 0.25-0.5 ug/day may help to improve depression in some patients.

Monoamine oxidase (MAO) inhibitors : Some patients may respond to MAO inhibitors, especially those with atypical depression (i.e. increased appetite, hypersomnia and weight gain).

A combination of MAO inhibitors and tricyclics : This treatment can only be given in specialized clinics as severe side effects may result.

Psychological Treatment

A large number of patients with depression lose hope of the future, develops negative thinking and may harbour suicidal ideas. It is imperative that the therapist instill in them a ray of hope and explain to them that their negative thinking is a consequence of the disease and will improve with treatment.

Many patients have difficulties in their domestic life, in their occupations or on the financial front. These issues are discussed and the patient is helped to percieve the situation in its realistic perspective.

Some specialized treatment programmes have been devised for depressive patients. These require training and cannot be undertaken by persons not properly trained in these techniques. They include :

Cognitive Therapy — It is thought that the depressive patient develops a negative view of life and a negative evaluation of the self. Since this is primarliy due to a faulty way of thinking, these patients are trained to recognise and alter these negative cognitions.

Interpersonal Therapy — This aims at finding out the immediate interpersonal problems which the patient is facing. These are dealt with psychotherapeutically.

Different workers use different psychotherapeutic approaches which are useful if the patient's depression is associated with real life problems, and when it is mild.

PERSISTENT DEPRESSION

Some patients have a prolonged depression lasting 2 years or more; ordinarily, a depressive episode lasts between 6-12 months. The chronic depression can be of the following types :

- Chronic major depression
- Dysthymia
- Cyclothymia

Chronic Major Depression

When a depressive episode fulfilling the criteria of major depression persists for two year or more, without an intervening period of normalcy of a minimum of two months, it is called chronic major depression: It is to be treated as described earlier.

Dysthymia

This is a type of chronic depression which usually starts in late adolescence. Patients are usually only mildly depressed, show lack of interest, have poor appetite, a low energy level, lowered self-esteem, and are indecisive and hopeless. Patient usually has only a few of these symptoms. The patient often appear indifferent to various life situations. For a diagnosis of dysthymia, this state should persist continuously for 2 years or more and the patient should not have had mania or any other psychiatric illness in the past.

This illness is not very uncommon. It is found in nearly 3% of the population, and twice as commonly in women than in men.

Etiology

Some patients show features similar to major depression with a similar etiology, while in others, psychological factors play a major role. Repetitive traumatic or catastrophic experiences can lead to a chronic depressive transformation.

Clinical Features

The characteristic features of this chronic illness are : (ICD-X)

The patient generally feels sad most of the time continuously for 2 years or more (one year in children and adolescents). They complain of lack of interest, may complain against others and blame their luck for their misfortune.

Poor appetite or overeating
Insomnia or hypersomnia
Low energy or fatigue
Low self esteem

Poor concentration or difficulty in making decisions

Feeling of hopelessness.

In addition to the first, two more symptoms from the rest must be present. If a large number of symptoms are present, it may be difficult to differentiate dysthymia from major depression.

These patients should have none of the following :

Any symptom-free period of two months or more

Any evidence of major depression in the first two years of the illness

Any evidence of manic or hypomanic episodes

Any evidence of underlying schizophrenia or an organic disorder.

These patients may turn to drug or alcohol abuse, to help manage their psychological distress.

Dysthymia can be primary (when it develops de novo) or can be secondary to any prexisting non-mood disorder illness.

Course and Prognosis

Most patients develop this disorder before the age of 25 years. The illnes generally runs a chronic course. A few may develop major depression, anxiety disorder or drug abuse.

Management

It is basically psychotherapeutic. The cognitive and interpersonal psychotherapies are useful. In a few, antidepressants are helpful. In secondary dysthymia, treatment of the primary disorder can be of help.

Cyclothymia

Cyclothymia is characterized by swings of mood ranging from elation to sadness alternately. The illness is diagnosed when the duration is of two or more years . The mood swings, however, are not severe enough to qualify for a diagnosis of bipolar disorder. The swings can cause severe interpersonal difficulties specially at home and in job because of the unpredicatable behaviour of the patients. The illness is considered to be a partial expression of bipolar disorder and responds well to lithium.

OTHER TYPES OF BIPOLAR AFFECTIVE DISORDERS

Seasonal Pattern

Some affective disorders have a specific temporal relationship of recurrence with a particular season. It is usually observed as recurrent patterns of depression during winter seasons in countries having shorter daylight hours in winters. It is uncommon in our country, although it is interesting to note that a reverse pattern is usually observed in India. To make a diagnosis of Seasonal Affective Disorder (SAD), one has to establish a regular temporal relationship between the onset of an episode of bipolar disorder (or recurrent major depression) on a particular 60-day period of the year, taking care to rule out any obvious effect of seasonally repeated psychosocial stressors. At least 3 episodes of such mood disturbances in 3 separate years should be observed, at least 2 of the years being consecutive and such seasonal episodes should outnumber any non-seasonal ones by more than a 3:1 ratio.

Such patients often present with atypical depressive features (hypersomnia, hyperphagia and carbohydrate craving), though such symptoms are not exclusive to SAD.

This syndrome requires a different approach of treatment. High intensity light (in the intensity of 2000-2500 lux) over a period of several days in the morning or evening is associated with beneficial effects. This treatment can also be used prophylactically throughout winters in a patient with marked SAD.

Rapid Cycling Disorders

Rapid cyclers are arbitarily defined as those patients of bipolar disorder having four or more episodes per year. Though they show a poor response to lithium, they are clinically indistinguishable from the rest of the bipolar group with respect to age of onset, duration of illness prior to lithium treatment, type of symptoms and family history.

Many factors have been proposed to induce rapid cycling — tricyclic antidepressants therapy, MAO inhibitor therapy and even lithium therapy, L-dopa, cyprohepatadine, propranolol, as also subclinical hypothyroidism, neurological disease or insult specially multiple sclerosis and an intrinsic periodicity of specific circadian pacemakers.

Treatment options include drug discontinuation if any drug is identified as the offending agent, institution of lithium or ECT for manic states and lithium, carbamazepine or ECT for depressive states. The combination of lithium with carbamazepine may be suitable alternative for lithium resistant and possibly carbamazepine resistant rapid cyclers, despite reports of untoward neurotoxic side-effects of this combination. A role for thyroid hormone supplementation in the disorder has been proposed, especially in depressives showing an augmented TSH response to TRH. A family assessment and perhaps continued family counselling, may assist in relieving stressors and conflict and improving medication compliance. The spouse and family may also help in monitoring the course of illness as well as the response to treatment.

NEUROTIC, STRESS RELATED AND SOMATOFORM DISORDERS

This group of disorders include most of those conditions which were earlier called neurosis. The term neurosis implied a causative mechanism, wherein it was presumed that the psychological disturbances are responsible for these disorders. However the modern classifications have abandoned the etiological approach and have mainly takeup descriptive approaches.

The conditions included in this section may not be related to each other.

The following categories are included in this section.

Phobic Anxiety Disorders
Agoraphobia
Without panic disorder
With panic disorder
Social phobias
Specific (isolated) phobias
Other phobic anxiety disorders
Phobic anxiety disorder, unspecified

Other Anxiety Disorders
Panic disorder [episodic paroxysmal anxiety]
Generalised anxiety disorder
Mixed anxiety and depressive disorder
Other mixed anxiety disorders
Other specified anxiety disorders
Anxiety disorder (unspecified)

Obsessive-compulsive Disorder
Predominantly obsessional thoughts and ruminations
Predominantly compulsive acts (obsessional rituals)
Mixed obsessional thoughts and acts
Other obsessive-compulsive disorders
Obsessive-compulsive disorder, unspecified

Reaction to Severe Stress and Adjustment Disorders
Acute stress reaction
Post traumatic stress disorder
Adjustment disorders
Brief depressive reaction
Prolonged depressive reaction
Mixed anxiety and depressive reaction
With predominant disturbances of other emotions
With predominant disturbances of conduct
With mixed disturbances of emotion and conduct
With other specified predominant symptoms
Other reaction to severe stress
Reaction to severe stress unspecified

Dissociative (Conversion) Disorders
Dissociative amnesia
Dissociative fugue
Dissociative stupor
Trance and posession disorders
Dissociative motor disorders
Dissociative convulsions
Dissociative anaesthesia and sensory loss
Mixed dissociative (conversion) disorders
Other dissociative (conversion) disorders
Ganser syndrome
Multiple personality disorder
Transient dissociative (conversion) disorders occurring in childhood and adolescence
Other specified dissociative (conversion) disorders
Dissociative (conversion) disorders, unspecified

Somatoform Disorders
Somatization disorder
Undifferentiated somatoform disorder
Hypochondriacal disorder
Somatoform autonomic dysfunction
Heart and cardiovascular system
Upper gastrointestinal tract
Lower gastrointestinal tract
Respiratory system
Genito-urinary system
Other organ or system
Persistent somatoform pain disorder
Other somatoform pain disorder
Somatoform disorder, unspecified

Other Neurotic Disorders
Neurasthenia
Depersonalization-derealization syndrome
Other specified neurotic disorders
Neurotic disorders, unspecified

PHOBIC ANXIETY DISORDERS

Phobia is defined as an irrational fear towards an object, activity or situation which ordinarily does not evoke fear. These fear producing situations could be; fear of going out, spiders, lizards, going on stage, meeting people, etc. These patients are always preoccupied with avoidance of phobic siutations. The anxiety starts building up whenever they are expected to encounter such a situation which is known as anticipatory anxiety. The anxiety will show both psychological, as well as autonomic symptoms.

Phobias are subclassified as follows :
Agoraphobia
Social phobias
Specified (isolated phobias)

AGORAPHOBIA

Agoraphobics fear going into situations or places from where they cannot escape to a safe place (usually home). It includes the following situations :

a) Fear of leaving home alone. However they may be able to go out if accompanied by an attendant, who may even be a child ;

b) Fear of entering shops, crowds or public places; and

c) Travelling alone in trains or buses.

The symptoms may progress to such an extent that the patient may not venture out of his home.

Epidemiology

The exact nature of epidemiology is not known. It is largely because most agoraphobics do not seek help. Recently, this condition has been redefined although a large scale epidemiological data is still not available. One year prevalence is estimated to be around 3%. The onset of the illness is usually in twenties. The Western researchers indicate that it is more common in women. In clinical practice in India, most patients seen are men.

Etiology

The majority of patients develop agoraphobia in association with panic disorder. Some patients may have agoraphobia without panic disorders. There are many etiological speculations regarding its development but none have been confirmed as yet.

Genetic Factors — The first degree relatives of these patients show a much higher prevalence of agoraphobia (15% to 20%). Monozygotic twins also show a high concordance rate.

Neurophysiological Factors

These patients may have a biological vulnerability for development of this disorder. This biological vulnerability could be a biophysiological instability or defect. Though no such consistent defect has been identified but alteration in the Nor-adrenaline / 5HT / Gaba-ergic systems are postulated.

Psychosocial Factors

The development of the individual may be effected both by the internal cues and the external events. Life experiences may modify the individual's personality due to which his self-esteem may be seriously impaired. He may need external support or approval for proper functioning. Whenever such persons come across a biological or psychological stressor, they may develop a phobic illness. The strength of the stressor required will be inversely proportional to the personality strength.

Psychoanalytic workers assume that such patients have been separated from their parents (one or both) in childhood. This separation anxiety becomes manifest whenever they go out and the fear of being abandoned can produce panic like symptoms.

The behaviourists explain this disorder on the basis of the conditioning paradigm. According to them whenever a patient experiences severe anxiety in a particular situation, that situation may later become a phobic situation. For instance, if a person experienced anxiety while travelling in a train, he may develop phobic avoidance of travelling in a train which may later become generalised to other modes of travel. This hypothesis, however, does not explain why anxiety was initially aroused. Thus conditioning paradigm does explain development of agoraphobic symptoms in panic disorders.

Patients with phobic disorder may generally feel insecure within themselves, though many of them may put forward a brave facade.

Clinical Picture

These patients usually avoid situations which produce phobia. The anxiety starts building whenever they come to know of their impending encounter with phobic situations. For instance, a patient with phobia of travelling in a train will start getting anxious as soon as the travel plans are made to travel and the anxiety will reach at its peak when he has to start for the railway station and may attain highest levels as soon as he enters the train. He may feel anxious, apprehensive and may the even develop various autonomic symptoms of anxiety. Many patients might try to escape this situation by making excuses. These symptoms could be controlled if someone is accompanying the patient.

The disorder may be mild in which the patient can fulfil most of his daily activities without much difficulty but develops anxiety only while going out alone or travelling. Exposure to the phobic situation may produce any of the following symptoms : extreme anxiety, restlessness, a feeling of impending death, and a need to escape. Common autonomic symptoms are palpitation, trembling, dryness of mouth, frequency of micturition and motor restlessness.

Illness can sometime become so disabling that the patient may not venture out of their home for many years. One patient of agoraphobia had not gone out of his house for nearly twenty years. His shop was just two kilometers from his home but he could not even go there, neither could he go out for treatment.

Case example

M is a 26 year old salesman. He has developed a fear of travelling for the past one year. Whenever he went to the railway station, he became so apprehensive that he had to return home. A year back he had quarrelled with his wife in which she threatened to commit suicide. He was quite apprehensive and anxious but because of his duty he went on tour by train. As soon as the train started moving he felt acute anxiety. He could somehow travel that day. Since that day his symptoms continued to get worse and he could not even travel by bus or train. He was treated with Imipramine 75 mg/day and behaviour therapy to which he responded very well.

Diagnosis (I.C.D.-X)

a) The psychological or autonomic symptoms must be primary manifestations of anxiety and not secondary to other symptoms, such as delusions or obsessional thoughts.

b) The anxiety must be restricted to (or occur mainly in) at least two of the following situations: crowds, public places, travelling away from home and travelling alone; and

c) Avoidance of the phobic situation must be, or have been, a prominent feature.

Differential Diagnosis — The diagnosis in a typical case is quite clear. Sometimes the patient may have other symptoms like depression, obsessions, depersonalisation. These do not invalidate the diagnosis provided they are not prominent. Sometimes, a depressive episode may precede agoraphobia, and in such situations depression may be a more appropriate diagnosis.

Agoraphobia should be further classified into :
Without panic disorder
With panic disorder.

Course and Prognosis

When agoraphobia is secondary to panic attacks, it resolves with improvement in panic disorder, but when agoraphobia has developed de novo, then the course can be quite chronic.

Management

Agoraphobia with panic disorder is treated for panic disorder and the agoraphobia automatically disappears (details under panic disorder).

Agoraphobia without panic disorders

The role of pharmacotherapy in this disorder is not firmly established but the following drugs could be tried :

a) Antidepressants — Imipramine in dosage of 75 to 150 mg/day. Drugs should be started gradually from 25 mg per day because these patients often fear the side effects of the drug. Fluoxetine 20 mg/day has also been found effective in some cases.

b) Benzodiazepines have also been used. Alprazolam in dosage of 1 to 4 mg/day could be effective.

Psychological Treatment

This is the main stay of treatment in agoraphobia. Most effective results have been obtained by behaviour therapy and cognitive therapy. The aim of the treatment is as follows :

1. To change the faulty cognitions.
2. To help the patient to stay calm in agoraphobic situations.

The technique used are :
Cognitive restructuring
Relaxation
Desensitisation-in vitro and in vivo

The details of these methods are given in Chapter on psychotherapy.

SOCIAL PHOBIAS

Social phobia is characterized by fear of

encountering other people, usually in small groups or doing certain acts in a public place (like eating, urinating in public toilets, public speaking). These people fear that others may not approve of them or may consider them inferior.

Epidemiology

The prevalence of social phobias is not properly known. Some Western researchers estimate that it may effect 3% to 5% of the population. The problem usually starts in the teens and affects both the sexes equally.

Etiology

The etiology of these disorders is explained on the basis of psychological development. Many of these patients exhibit poor self confidence, show anxiety on trifles and may be very conscious of some physical or psychological defects in themselves. They feel anxious whenever they have to interact with other people, more so, with the opposite sex or superiors. They gradually start avoiding these situations. Later, whenever they are expected to go in these situations, they develop severe anxiety. Psychological formulations are similar to those given under agoraphobia.

Clinical Picture

These patients usually present with irrational fears and avoidance of one of the following situations:

Talking to the opposite sex,

Speaking on stage or to small groups, and/or

Eating in public.

Whenever they are expected to go into the phobic situation, they develop severe anticipatory anxiety. They may utilise various excuses to avoid the phobic situation. This avoidance usually effect their lives quite adversely and they may develop secondary depression.

Case Example

A 25 year old Ph.D. scholar found it difficult to face people for the last few years. He felt that somehow his behaviour gets altered whenever he is talking to other people, specially to members of the opposite sex or while facing interviews. He stated that he tried to face the situation himself but as soon as he encountered these situations he felt dumb. Even when he continued talking, he felt that what he was saying was not proper or correct. He felt that his life has been badly restricted by this problem. He was the first born in a sibship of four. He had a consistently good academic record. He did not play any games and had very few friends.

Course and Prognosis

Majority of social phobias diminish with the advancement of age. Sometimes it can become chronic.

Diagnosis (I.C.D.-X)

a) The psychological, behavioural or autonomic symptoms must be primarily a manifestation of anxiety and not secondary to other symptoms such as delusions or obsessional thoughts,

b) The anxiety must be restricted to or predominate in a particular social situation; and

c) The phobic situation is avoided whenever possible.

Treatment — Similar to other phobias.

SPECIFIC (ISOLATED) PHOBIAS

These include all other phobic situations which are not covered either in agoraphobia or social phobias.

Common phobic situations are :

Fear of particular animals (lizards, worms, etc)

Heights

Lightening and thunder

Darkness

Flying

Closed spaces

The sight of blood or injury

Fear of certain diseases (HIV infection, tetanus, syphilis, etc.)

Epidemiology — Specific phobias are quite common. They seldom come to the notice of the clinicians because the patients usually avoids them.

Etiology — Similar to as described in other phobias.

Clinical Picture

This is characterized by anticipatory anxiety whenever there is a chance of coming in contact with a phobic situation. The situation can induce symptoms of severe anxiety or panic. The patients generally avoid the phobic situations.

Course and Prognosis

The majority of the person can lead a fairly normal life by making various changes in their life style, so that they are able to avoid the phobic situation.

Diagnosis

The diagnostic features are similar to the social phobias.

Management

Same as in other phobias.

OTHER ANXIETY DISORDERS

This group of disorders are predominantly present with anxiety symptoms. Though, they may exhibit symptoms of depression, phobia or obsession, these are not prominent.

Following conditions are included :
Panic disorder
Generalized anxiety disorder
Mixed anxiety and depressive disorders.

PANIC DISORDER

The panic disorder is characterized by episodes of acute and severe anxiety which is not in response to any external or internal stress or due to any other disease. Panic symptoms can commonly occur in phobias or in states of severe terror but they are not part of panic disorders.

Epidemiology

The diagnosis of panic disorder has been separated from anxiety disorders only recently, therefore, the older epidemiological surveys did not mention it separately. Recent surveys from the West indicate a life-time prevalence of about 1-3% The disorder starts in young age and it is said to be more common in the females.

Etiology

Genetic — There is strong evidence of a genetic basis for panic disorders. The first degree relatives of these patients show similar disorder in about 15%. Monozygotic twins show a concordance rate of 80%-90% for panic disorders.

Brain Neurophysiology — It is hypothesised that following regions of the brain may show disturbances of function in this disorder :

a) Locus coeruleus which has strong Noradrenergic connections.

b) Limbic system and prefrontal cortex is involved with cognitive aspects of panic. The cereberal blood flow increase has been observed in nondominant (right) parahippocampal area in the panic disorder patient, who showed panic on lactate infusion.

c) Increased sympathetic tone and slow adaptation to repeated stimuli.

Hyperventilation and CO_2 inhalation — Hyperventilation as well as CO_2 inhalation has been found to induce panic attacks.

Lactate infusion test — It is hypothesised that excess of lactate production may be responsible for development of panic. In some patients, panic may be associated with high lactate production but it is not a general finding in panic disorders. On the other hand, 90% of the panic disorder patients develop panic, when they are infused with sodium lactate while panic will be induced in only in 5% of normal population. This indicates that sodium lactate has a panicogenic property, but how it is associated with panic disorders, is not yet clear.

Mitral Valve Prolapse (M.V.P.) — M.V.P. is seen in nearly 50% of patients of panic disorder, but many persons may have M.V.P. without panic disorder. In some patients M.V.P. also improves with improvement of panic. Some researchers believe that M.V.P. may be a symptom of panic and not its cause. The exact relationship between M.V.P. and panic disorder is as yet not clear.

Psychosocial Factors — Panic episode appears to be primarily of biological origin. The psychosocial factor may play a role in sensitising the patient to develop a panic episode and may also act as precipitating factors.

Psychological theories can explain the development of anxious apprehension and agoraphobia in these patients. The psychological experience during a panic episode is so terrifying that a person develops apprehensions of developing a second attack. Agoraphobia is a direct derivation of this anxious apprehension. The patient fears going out because he is apprehensive of developing a panic attack and fears that he may not be able to get immediate help, if the symptoms develops when he is away from home.

Clinical Picture

The first episode of panic usually starts spontaneously. However, it may be precipitated by a state of emotional arousal (by heated arguments, by chronic mental tension, physical exhaustion or any other physical or psychological stress). Main symptoms of a panic attack are :

a) **Psychological Symptoms**

There is an intense fear and the patients feel that

they are not going to survive. They may feel that they are going to become mad or crazy.

They may fear that they are going to have a heart attack or respiratory failure (inability to breathe/ choking).

There is severe apprehension and anxiety. Few patients may feel as if they are changing (depersonalisation), or the world has changed (derealisation).

b) **Autonomic Symptoms** — These may refer to any system :

Palpitation, choking sensation and chest pain

Dizziness, vertigo or unsteady feelings

Abdominal symptoms — Feeling of sinking in the pit of stomach, diarrhoea

Motor tension, restlessness

Frequency of micturition

Sweating, cold and clammy limbs.

These symptoms develop within minutes and reach their peak between 10-15 minutes and usually subside within an hour.

These attacks may occur repetitively after a few days or weeks. Many patients develop anxious foreboding about the development of these attacks and may remain anxious all the time.

The history will reveal that these patients repeatedly rush to medical emergency, where they are investigated for cardiac problems or other physical diseases.

Case History

A 32 years old police constable sought consultation because he had not been able to do his duty for the past one year. The illness started with a panic episode which occurred one evening after he returned home from his work. He was talking to his wife when he suddenly felt severe chest pain and felt as if he was dying. He was acutely anxious and he rushed to a nearby doctor. The doctor did an E.C.G. and gave a bottle of I.V. glucose. He felt better after few hours. He did not go for his work the next day. Later, he went to the police station but felt apprehensive that he might have another attack and returned home after a few hours. Later, he stopped venturing out due to the fear of getting a panic attack. He had multiple panic attacks during the last one year and each time he was infused with a bottle of glucose. He came for consultation accompanied by six people. They were carrying water and medicines so that these could be given if he gets an attack. The patient was put on imipramine 75 mg/day in divided dosage. Within a month his panic attacks ceased and he was gradually encouraged to go out. Later, his agoraphobia also disappeared. The treatment was continued for one and a half years.

Comments

This young man gave a typical history of panic disorder with agoraphobia. There were no clear cut psychological factors associated with his problem. He was a policeman very much liked both by his superiors and colleagues. Family history also did not reveal any clear cut stress.

Diagnosis

Panic attacks should show the symptoms described earlier. These symptoms should occur : (I.C.D.-X)

a) In circumstances where there is no objective danger ;

b) Without being confined to known or predictable situations ; and

c) With comparative freedom from anxiety symptoms between the attacks (although anticipatory anxiety is common),

At least 4 attacks should occur in a month or anticipatory anxiety should persist even if there are less than four attacks.

Differential Diagnosis

Panic symptoms can be seen in phobias, depression schizophrenia and other organic conditions (dementias, pheochromocytoma). All these conditions will also have symptoms characteristic of these conditions and the panic episode will not fulfil the criteria described earlier.

Course and Prognosis :

The majorty of patients with panic disorders improve on long term follow up. Nearly 20%-30% may run a chronic course. Modern methods of treatment are able to provide help to nearly ninety percent of these patients. Some of these patients may develop depressive illness.

Management

The patients of panic disorders are usually very anxious and are certain that they suffer from a very serious illness. It is essential to take a proper history, undertake a detailed examination and order relevant investigations.

Once the patient has been fully assessed, he must be explained the following :

a) He has been thoroughly examined and investigated and there is no evidence of any physical disease.

b) These symptoms sometime occur in some individuals and the precise reasons for their development are not known. It is presumed that there are certain biochemical changes in the body which may be reponsible for development of these attacks.

c) Psychological and social problems may play some part in their development but they are not essential.

d) The patient need not rush to a doctor, if he gets a subsequent attack because these attacks are never life threatening and will cease within an hour.

e) The disorder can be easily treated by some medicines and psychological help.

f) The treatment is likely to take a year or more.

Pharmacotherapy

Antidepressants — Imipramine has been found to be quite effective in panic disorders. Other antidepressants can also be used. These patients usually fear taking drugs and are very sensitive to the side - effects.

They should be clearly explained the common side effects like dryness of mouth, constipation and dizziness. The drug should be started gradually. Imipramine may be given 25 mg twice a day. The dosage should be increased gradually. They may require full antidepressant dosage of 150 mg to 300 mg/day. Drugs should be continued for six months before tapering is considered.

Fluoxetine — This drug has also been found quite effective in panic disorders. It has fewer side effects and dosage is 20mg/day. It will be more easily accepted by the patients.

Benzodiazepines — Alprazolam is quite effective in these patients and it provides immediate and quick relief. The dosage required are 1-4 mg/day. The drug may produce sedation. The biggest problem with this drug is its dependence producing potential. Whenever this drug is withdrawn there, are chances of relapse and rebound anxiety is common. The drug should be gradually withdrawn.

Some clinicians use a combination of alprazolam and imipramine, take off alprazolam after one month and maintain the patient on imipramine.

Psychological Treatment

Support and encouragement, as described earlier are essential for the treatment. If the patient is very much preoccupied with his symptoms, cognitive behaviour therapy is required.

The majority of patients will improve within a month. The treatment should be continued for six months to one year and then the drugs should be tapered off.

GENERALIZED ANXIETY DISORDER

This condition is characterized by chronic anxiety which is not directly related to any object or situation. These patients are anxious or apprehensive about everything and they will exhibit some of the autonomic symptoms of anxiety. Quite often this condition is confused with anxiety due to situations like marriage, examination, jobs, etc. But whenever anxiety is related to a particular object or situation, then it will require to be classified elsewhere (E.g. phobias, reaction to stress or adjustment disorders).

Epidemiology

Older epidemiological data indicate that this disorder is quite common (prevalence 2%-5%). But most of these studies did not take into account current restricted definition of this disorder. Many workers feel that this disorder is not as common as was earlier thought. It is more common in females (F : M = 2:1). It usually starts in the twenties but can start earlier or later. It is often associated with multiple stresess.

Etiology

Genetic Factor — It is thought that this disorder may have a genetic basis as nearly 15% of the first degree relatives of the patients show this disorder.

Neurophysiological Abnormalities — It is presumed that noradrenergic, gama aminobutyric acid system, and serotonergic systems are involved. The exact nature of disturbance has not been so far demonstrated.

The frontal and limbic lobe are considered to be the areas where various neurophysiological changes may take place.

The EEG shows multiple non specific abnormalities. Sleep EEG shows multiple discontinuity and reduced delta sleep, REM sleep and Stage I sleep.

Psychosocial Factors — Various psychosocial stresses play a predominant role in the development of this disorder. These patients may have a vulnerable personality. They undergo multiple and repetitive stress which makes them chronically anxious. A student who does badly in examinations even after putting in his best effort may become repeatedly anxious about everything. Similarly, house wives who get continuously unpredictable responses from their inlaws and husband may become chronically anxious.

Clinical Picture

The clinical picture is characterized as follows :

The patients are chronically anxious. This may be expressed as nervousness (uljhan).

They are apprehensive that some calamity may befall them. (Whenever anybody goes out they may feel that something unforeseen will happen to them, they may fear that their projects will not succeed etc.)

Sleep is often disturbed. They may find it difficult to fall asleep and there may be repeated awakenings and anxiety provoking dreams. Some can also have increased sleep.

They complain of trembling, shakiness, muscle tension, restlessness and easy fatiguability.

Weight loss may be present.

Autonomic Symptoms

Shortness of breath or smothering sensation

Palpitation

Sweating or cold clammy hands

Dry mouth

Dizziness or light headedness

Nausea, diarrhoea or abdonminal distress

Loss or increase of appetite

Flushes

Frequent urination

Trouble in swallowing (lump in throat)

Vigilance or Scanning— Feeling keyed up or on edge

Exaggerated startle response

Difficulty in concentration due to anxiety, it is often complained as poor memory

Irritability

The patient will experience some of the above symptoms. His working capacity is impaired. His social relationships are also affected.

Case History

A thirty-five year old female was brought for the complaints of poor sleep, anxiety, weight loss and irritability. Her symptoms have gradually developed during the past two years, after she delivered her third female child. She belonged to a middle class joint family where she was living with her mother-in-law, husband, three daughters and a sister-in-law. She was being continuously blamed for producing three daughters, for not doing work properly, for being slow and sloppy. She gradually lost self confidence and began worrying over trifles. She would always be worried whether she had cooked food properly or not or what should she do to make her inlaws happy. Her appetite decreased and she had lost weight. She had some depressive symptoms but they did not fulfil the criteria of the depressive episode.

Comments

This patient developed chronic anxiety in face of multiple and repetitive stresses. Though, one may think that the problem developed after the birth of the third daughter it is associated with a specific situation. But the anxiety was neither due to having three daughters nor she was markedly concerned about it.

Course and Prognosis

Anxiety disorder is a chronic condition. The patient's improvement will depend on changes in life stresses. Some patients may develop panic disorders or depression.

Diagnosis (I.C.D.-X)

The sufferer must have primary symptoms of anxiety most days for at least several weeks at a time and usually for several months. (DSM III R requires a time period of 6 months) These symptoms should usually involve elements of :

a) Apprehension (worries about future misfortunes, feeling on edge, difficulty in concentrating, etc.) ;

b) Motor tension (restlessness, fidgeting, tension, headaches, trembling, inability to relax) ; and

c) Autonomic overactivity (light headedness, sweating, tachycardia or tachypnoea, epigastric discomfort, dizziness, dry mouth, etc.).

In children, the frequent need of reassurance and recurrent somatic complaints may be prominent.

Differential Diagnosis — Anxiety is a very common symptom and can occur in large number of psychiatric and physical disorders.

Almost every psychiatric disorder can have anxiety symptoms. The typical constellation described under the diagnosis will help to rule out all other conditions. In each case of anxiety, the following conditions should be ruled out :

Endocrinal Disorders

Addison's Disease
Cushing's Syndrome
Diabetes
Hyperthyroidism
Hypoglycaemia
Hypoparathyroidism
Menopausal syndrome
Pheochromocytoma
Premenstural tension

Cardiovascular System

Severe anaemia
Angina
Congestive heart failure
Hyperactive beta-adrenergic states
Mitral valve prolapse
Myocardial infarction
Paradoxical arterial tachycardia

Respiratory System

Asthma
Hyperventilation
Pulmonary Embolism

Neurological

Cerebrovascular accident
Dementia
Epilepsy
Infections of CNS
Meniere's Disease
Migraine
Multiple sclerosis
Neoplasms

Drug Intoxication

Amphetamine
Anticholinergics
Hallucinogens
Marijuana
Nicotine

Drug Withdrawal

Alcohol
Antihypertensives
Opiate
Sedative

Other

Anaphylaxis
B_{12} Deficiency
Electrolyte disturbances
Systemic infections
Systemic lupus erythematosis

Psychiatric Disorders

Anxiety could be a manifest symptom in the following :

Phobia
Obsession
Dissociative disorders
Adjustment reaction
Reaction to stress
Depression
Schizophrenia

In each case of anxiety, direct questions should be asked to rule out the symptoms of these disorders.

Management

These patients usually are very anxious and have develop a low self-esteem. The main stay of treatment is psychotherapy.

Psychotherapy

It is aimed at following :

a) Therapeutic relationship

The patient and therapist should develop a relationship of trust and understanding.

Ventilation

The patient should be able to verbalise his problems and anxieties. This by itself, causes tremendous emotional relief.

Support — The patient should be provided psychological support in facing daily life situation.

Environmental Manipulation — If environmental stressor are effecting the patient, then environmental manipulation could be attempted. The family should always be involved in treatment. In our country, the most common family stressors are conflicts with mother-in-law, father-in-law, husband and wife. There could be other stressors like job, education, social position, financial condition, etc.

Cognitive therapy may be indicated in some long standing cases.

Meditation and Yoga Therapy — Meditation and yoga often help to reduce anxiety and may help the patient to reorient his life. This is suitable for those persons who believe in detachment as the ultimate goal in life.

Pharmocotherapy

Anti-anxiety drugs can be used. One has to be cautious in their use, because most of them produce dependence and withdrawal anxiety after long term use.

The following are commonly used minor tranquilizers in this country :

Long Acting Drugs	Dosage (in mg per day)
Diazepam	2 - 30
Chlordiazepoxide	10 - 80

Short Acting Drugs	Dosage (in mg per day)
Oxazapam	30 - 120
Lorazepam	1 - 6
Alprazolam	5 - 4

These drugs should be given in a fixed dosage. The patient should not be given the option of increasing or decreasing the drug because it is likely to cause anxiety, as they will be struggling all the time to reduce the dosage. They must be warned that sudden stoppage may cause reemergence of anxiety. When the drugs are to be withdrawn they should be tapered off in 10-15 days.

These drugs often produce very positive effects in the individual. Their confidence increases and they are able to face situations more boldly.

Buspirone

This is a new anti-anxiety drug. This has very low abuse potential. Its antianxiety effects are apparent only after 1 - 2 weeks. This drug is not effective in panic disorder. The dosage is from 10-60 mg/day. It may be preferable to Benzodiazepines for long term use.

Antidepressants — These drugs are now considered quite effective in treating the psychic component of anxiety. Muscle tension, palpitation, etc. may not be helped. The dosage required is lower than antidepressant dosage.

Propranolol — Beta-adrenergic blocking drugs have been found effective in treating autonomic symptoms of anxiety.

Antihistaminics have also been used in treating anxiety.

MIXED ANXIETY AND DEPRESSIVE DISORDER

This is a new category used in this classificatory system. These patients have symptoms of both anxiety and depression but none is severe enough to merit the diagnosis of either condition. It is said that, this is a common condition in general practice.

It should be treated with psychotherapy and antidepressants or antianxiety drugs.

OBSESSIVE COMPULSIVE DISORDER

This disorder is characterized by repetitive ideas or acts which have the following quality :

The idea, image or act, though recognised as one's own, is considered unwanted and repetitively intrudes into one's conscious.

The patient recognises the absurdity of it (sometimes specially in obsession of cleanliness, the patient may feel that it is not absurd).

There is a strong desire to resist them but any attempt at resistance increases anxiety. (Cleanliness compulsions may not be resisted as they are culturally approved). After some time the resistance to various obsessions and compulsions may decrease.

Epidemiology

Earlier it was thought to be a rare disorder. Recent epidemiological studies in the West estimate its lifetime prevalence between 2% to 3.0%. A large number of these cases do not consult a psychiatrist because most of the obsessives are very secretive and do not reveal their illness. Clinical experience in India also indicates that this disorder is quite common. The disorder starts in adolescence. The male-female ratio is nearly equal.

Etiology

Genetic — O.C.D. is seen in 5% to 7% of first degree relatives which is much higher than its prevalence in general population. But genetic factors alone are not able to explain the etiology.

Neurophysiological Factors — There is evidence to indicate that, there are some abnormalities in the frontal lobe and basal ganglion of these patients. These patients exhibit higher local glucose metabolism in these areas.

Neurochemical Factors — Drugs effecting 5HT system seems to be effective in treating this disorder. Therefore some abnormality of 5HT system is presumed. Other neurotransmitter systems like dopaminergic or cholinergic system may also be implicated.

Personality Factors — This disorder often develops in persons who have preexisting anankastic (obsessional) personality. This personality is characterized by orderliness, punctuality, cleanliness, parsimony (miserliness) and meticulousness. They get anxious or agitated whenever the set routine of their life is disturbed.

This disorder can develop in other personality types also.

Psychosocial Factors — In a large number of patients (50% or more) the disorder usually starts acutely, in a stressful situation. It is hypothesised that emotional arousal gets associated with a particular act or thought. For instance, a young lady observed that brown ants were crawling near her infant. She became very apprehensive and started fearing that brown ants may harm her child. She later became obsessed with the idea that sugar may be lying on the floor and started excessive cleaning.

Similarly, one man was in a state of sexual arousal when his daughter entered the room. He became severly apprehensive that he might have sexual thoughts about his daughter. He started having sexual thoughts whenever he saw his daughter, which made him feel very guilty. After some time, these sexual thoughts were generalised to other close relatives like his mother and sister.

Psychoanalytical writers have emphasised the use of following defense mechanisms in obsession : isolation, undoing and reaction formation. These psychological processes are involved in obsessive symptom formation but the underlying psychoanalytic presumptions have not been proved.

In earlier example one can visualise the usage of these three defense mechanisms. When there is chance association of a thought or impulse in emotionally aroused state, the person tries to isolate the ideas from its affect, e.g. in the example quoted above the person having sexual arousal will try to isolate the affect from the thought to make it innocuous. To make this thought more ineffective, he may start doing certain acts which might undo its effect. He may start repeating God's name or may touch an object and so on (undoing). To completely overcome this sexual thought he may develop antisexual ideas and may become a reformist (reaction formation).

These three defence mechanisms explain development of OCD, without utilising psychoanalytic assumptions.

Clinical Picture

The illness usually starts in adolescence but the patients often seek consultation many years after the development of illness. The presenting symptoms are: somatic aches and pains, depression, and inability to perform social and occupational functions properly. The symptoms of obsession are often revealed on direct enquiry.

The common symptom patterns are :

Obsessions of contamination asociated with compulsive cleaning : These patient feel that they have become dirty and to remove this feeling, they repetitively clean themselves.

A young lady developed doubts of contamination. She required buckets of water to clean herself in the toilet. After washing she would get a doubt that some droplet of dirty water might have spluttered on her. She would also wash her hands repetitively. Bathing also took place for many hours. She did not allow her husband or children to get into the house without cleaning themselves.

Obsessions of doubt with checking is also quite common. A young man had developed a doubt that he might speak or write obscene or wrong words. After talking to anyone, he needed repetitive assurances that he has not said anything wrong. He sent a letter to a university and became anxious that he might have written the address wrong. He even went to the post office to check whether the address was written correctly or not.

Few patients develop aggressive or sexual thoughts. One patient developed the fear that he might stab his friends and relatives. To avoid this thought, he started keeping all sharp objects away from home and kept his hands in the pocket.

Another patient developed the thought that someone might have sexual relations with her. She could not sleep with the windows and doors open. She avoided all kinds of contact with males. Many a times, she did not sleep at all due to the fear that someone may have sexual relations with her.

Some patients may be involved in repetitive ritualistic behaviour, e.g. while walking they must not put their feet on any crack or feel they must touch every electricity pole, etc. Even after following their thoughts properly, they will develop a doubt whether they have done it correctly or not. Such persons may take hours to walk a short distance.

These patients can have many other kinds of doubts ideas or images.

The sleep is usually not disturbed.

They may have associated affect of anxiety or depression. Many such patients may attempt suicide.

Attention, concentration, speech, thinking, intelligence, memory, insight and judgement are intact.

Course and Prognosis

Earlier, it was thought to be a chronic illness which was refractory to treatment. It has now been shown that nearly 25% cases may have complete remission while another 50% improve and nearly 25% may become chronic. Recent advances in treatment have changed the prognosis of this condition.

Diagnosis (I.C.D.-X)

For a definite diagnosis obsessional symptoms or compulsive acts or both must be present on most days for atleast two successive weeks and be a source of distress to the patient and interfere with his activities. The obsessional symptoms should have the following characteristics.

a) They must be recognised as individuals with own thoughts or impulses ;

b) There must be at least one thought or act that is still resisted unsucessfully, even though others may be present which the sufferer no longer resists ;

c) The thought of carrying out the act, must not in itself be pleasurable (simple relief of tension or anxiety is not regarded as pleasure) ; and

d) The thoughts, images or impulses must be unpleasantly repetitive.

Differential Diagnosis — It has to be differentiated from depression. If obsessive symptoms came first or are present when there are no depressive symptoms, then O.C.D. should be diagnosed. If obsessive symptoms occur only in presence of depression, then depression should be diagnosed.

Management

The O.C.D. patient is usually severely disturbed by his problems and it is essential to explain to him the nature of illness and to infuse in him the hope that the treatment is likely to improve his condition.

The treatment requires pharmacotherapy and psychotherapy.

Pharmacotherapy

Most of the drugs which increased 5 H.T. transmission have been found effective in this disorder.

Clomipramine — This is effective in the dosage of 150-300 mg/days. The symptom relief may occur after a month or two. It has been seen that improvement continues to occur even after one year or more. It is not certain as to how long the drug should be continued. However, the dosage can be safely reduced to 40% after symptom relief has occurred.

Fluoxetine — This is also effective in dosage of 20-60 mg/day. It has less side-effects and it is more easily tolerated.

Patients who do not respond to the above drugs may need augmentation by the following :

Buspirone — This is a 5 HT agonist. It may be added along with the previous drugs in dosage of 10-30 mg/day.

Pimozide — It has also been found effective as an augmenting agent. Dosage is 4-8 mg/day.

If anxiety is severe, other Benzodiazepines can be added.

Psychosurgery

Earlier psychosurgery was considered as an effective treatment of O.C.D., but now this treatment has been nearly abandoned.

Psychotherapy

Cognitive behaviour therapy has been found effective in the treatment of O.C.D.. The main techniques used are :

a) Cognitive restructuring

b) Exposure

c) Response prevention

d) Flooding

The results are usually very satisfactory (details in chapter on psycotherapy).

REACTION TO SEVERE STRESS AND ADJUSTMENT DISORDERS

This group of disorders are temporally related to stress, e.g. an exceptionally serious stress or significant change in life situations may lead to symptom formation. The symtomatology can be of any type. These disorders could develop at any age. The role of stress is paramount in these disorders.

It should not mean that stress is not associated with

other psychiatric disorders, but in most of these conditions, the presence of stress is neither essential nor significant enough.

Acute Stress Reaction

This is a transient disorder which develops in an individual, without any psychiatric disorder, in response to a severe stress.

The stress should be overwhelming, e.g. the death of a loved one, natural catastrophe, accident, battle, criminal assault, rape, sudden change in social status, being involved in charges of moral turpitude, etc.

Disorder is more likely to develop in people who are physically exhausted, are at the extreme ages (childhood and old age), in people who have poor coping skills, and is found more commonly in females. These patients may have a history of mental disorder.

Clinical Picture

The disorder usually starts with a condition of daze during which the patient develops some constriction of the field of consciousness, narrowness of attention, inability to comprehend stimuli and disorientation. This state may lead to stupor, agitation or overactivity. Signs of acute anxiety with autonomic symptoms like palpitation, dryness of mouth, diarrhoea, sweating and trembling may be present.

Symptoms usually start within a few moments of the event and may last from a few hours to a few days.

Diagnosis (I.C.D.-X)

There should be a clear temporal correlation between exceptional stress and onset of symptoms. In addition, the symptoms :

a) Show a mixed and usually changing picture ; in addition to the initial state of daze, depression, anxiety, anger, despair overactivity and withdrawal may all be seen, but no one type of symptom predominates for long ;

b) Resolve rapidly (within a few hours at the most) in those cases where removal from stressful environment is possible, in cases when the stress continues or by its nature cannot be reversed, the symptoms usually begin to diminish after 24-48 hours and are usually minimal after about 3 days.

This diagnosis does not include exacerbation of preexisting psychiatric disorder except personality disorder. They may however have a history of previous psychiatric disorder.

Management

As the illness is transitory, the management aims at helping the patient to pass through the crisis. Removal from stressful situation, if possible, is helpful. If the patient is hyperactive, benzodiazepines can be used. These drugs can also be given by intramuscular injection if patient is very agitated.

POST TRAUMATIC STRESS DISORDER

This disorder develops as a consequence of a severe and unusual stress which is likely to cause pervasive stress in almost anyone. The symptoms may develop immediately after the stress or may be delayed up to six months or more. The symptoms of this syndrome are specific.

Epidemiology

The symptoms may occur in nearly 60-70% of people who have survived a major disaster. In general population, the lifetime prevalence is between 1.3% to 2.6% in Western countries. There are no studies available in India. The Bhopal gas leak disaster was a major tragedy which affected a large population. Unfortunately PTSD was not a prevalent diagnosis at that time but a large number of victims suffered from neurotic disorders.

Etiology

This disorder is more likely to be associated with the following :

People in childhood and old age

More common in females

People who had already suffered from a mental illness or had behavioural problems in childhood

People who have poor coping skills

Severity of the disaster and intensity of experience

Lack of timely support

Poor social support system

The following factors tend to reduce the risk of this disorder :

Male sex

Previous experience with similar situations

Good psychosocial adjustment

Low anxiety

Disaster training

Major situations which have resulted in PTSD are :

Combat experience

Concentration camps of Nazis

Volcano eruptions

Train disasters

Earthquakes

Typhoons, etc.

In recent times, we have witnessed many major disasters, e.g. The Bhopal Gas Tragedy, Uttarkashi Earthquake, Bihar Coal Mine Collapse, etc.

Clinical Picture

The disorder arises after an unusual and pervasive stress.

The onset of symptoms could be soon after the event or may be delayed upto six months or more.

The typical symptoms are :

Recurrent or intrusive reexperiencing of the traumatic event either in memory flash-backs or dreams. There could be hallucinatory experiences of the event.

Intense distress at exposure to events that resemble the original events. After Bhopal gas tragedy, threat of repeated gas leakage were often rumoured and the people responded with panic.

Effort are made to avoid thoughts and feelings associated with the trauma.

Partial or complete amnesia for the event.

Feeling of numbness and detachment from other people and unresponsiveness to other people.

Anhedonia — Inability to feel pleasure.

Increased arousal, there is usually hypervigilance, and enhanced startle reaction.

There may be depression, anxiety or persistent panic with autonomic symptoms.

There may be insomnia.

Case Report

A 40 - year old bank manager witnessed a bank raid by armed terrorists, during which two persons were killed. He did not show any symptoms soon after the attack. Few days later, he was called to the police station to identify the terrorists and as soon as he returned from there, he became markedly apprehensive. He left his home and wandered around for two weeks. He used to get repetitive flash backs of the shoot out and raid. He was markedly anxious and hypervigilant. He would scan the environment for any Sikh and would go into panic on seeing them. He had grown a beard and hair to look like one. The condition lasted for nearly six months after which he was transferred from the area and he could resume to his duties.

Comments

This patient underwent an unusual and traumatic experience. Symptoms emerged when he was called to identify the persons, which aroused in him the feeling that they may also kill him. After this event, he went into a state of daze and wandered off without informing anyone. He showed typical relieving of the experience with hypervigilance.

Course and Prognosis

The majority of the patients of P.T.S.D. show complete recovery. Few may become chronic and their recovery may continue for many years, as seen in the Vietnam war soldiers. Some may show complete personality change. The change seen in King Ashoka after the Kalinga war were indicative of the personality change after the devastating experience of war.

Diagnosis (I.C.D.-X)

This is based on the following :

1. Devastating and unusual traumatic event.

2. Development of symptoms within 6 months of the event.

3. The typical symptoms are :

Reliving of the experience either in flash-back or dreams ;

Feelings of numbness, poor relatedness, anhedonia

Increased vigilance and scanning ;

Other symptoms of anxiety, depression or panic may be present.

Differential Diagnosis — This should not be a worsening of pre-existing psychiatric illness.

Many studies have shown that almost all the patients of P.T.S.D. can be given a comorbid diagnosis of alcohol dependence, atypical depression and pathological grief, anxiety disorder, somatization disorder, dysthymia, panic disorder, etc. Due to this reason many investigators doubt the independent existence of P.T.S.D..

Management

The experience of various disasters have helped to develop some guidelines for the management of this problem.

Predisaster Management — In situations where the likelihood of disaster are high, predisaster training and planning is very helpful. (Factories, coal mines, railways, earthquake prone areas, army, airways, etc.) There should be specific planning as to who does what in these situations. The role of each should be specified and the second order of people should also be identified as to who takes over if the key person has been hurt or is not available.

Disaster drills are very helpful.

Postdisaster Management — Speed of help is of utmost importance. The help should reach soon after the event. The availability of social, financial and medical support will allay anxiety. The person should feel reasonably secure that he will not be abandoned and reasonable help will be available.

Psychotherapy

The mainstay of treatment is psychotherapy. It could be individual or group. The aims of the psychotherapy are :

Ventilation of anger, guilt, frustration. This will help the individual to view the situation more realistically. Irrational thoughts, fears and guilt are to be removed.

Realistic evaluation of damage to self, family members, group and property. One should try to compensate and minimize these losses.

Individuals may have many personal fears and anxieties which need to be dealt with in psychotherapy.

Often, group treatment with survivors of other disasters or the same disaster as group leader may be very effective.

One of the major cause of continued disability often is the difference between the help promised and the help received. In Bhopal as well as in Uttarkashi, the majority of the victims are grossly dissatisfied with the help offered and the way it was disbursed. The charges of corruption are often made against the help giving individuals which further heightens the anxiety and disillusionment of the victim. It is essential that in such situations the maximum possible honesty is practiced.

Pharmacotherapy

Those patients who show depressive or anxiety symptoms respond well to antidepressants. Antianxiety drugs are best avoided because they may lead to dependence as the symptoms are likely to be present for sometime.

ADJUSTMENT DISORDERS

This group is characterized by disturbing psychological symptoms which effect the personal, social or occupational life of the individual and are directly related to a significant life change. Epidemiology of these conditions have not been systematically studied but they are quite frequent.

Etiology

The problems usually occur in persons who are predisposed to a psychological break down. These people may show different personality disorders or difficulty in coping with stresses. The stresses usually are :

Serious physical illness

Separation from spouse or family

Death of near and dear ones

Refugee status

Migration to a new area or a new country.

Clinical Picture

The patient may show a variety of symptoms and the condition is further subdivided according to predominant symptoms.

Brief Depressive Reaction

This is characterized by a transient mild depressive state of duration not exceeding one month.

Prolonged depressive reaction :

A mild depressive state occurring in response to a prolonged exposure to a stressful situation but of duration not exceeding two years.

Mixed anxiety and depressive reaction :

Both anxiety and depressive symptoms are prominent but at levels no greater than mixed anxiety and depressive disorders.

With predominant disturbances of other emotions :

The symptoms usually involve several types of emotions such as anxiety, depression, worry, tension and anger. This category is also used for children who show regressive behaviour such as bed wetting and thumb sucking after exposure to stress.

With predominant disturbances of conduct :

These patients exhibit conduct disorders in the form of aggression or dissocial behaviour like stealing, lying, etc.

With mixed disturbances of emotions and conduct :

Both emotional disturbances and disturbances of

conduct are prominent.

With other specified prominent symptoms :

When symptoms other than those mentioned above are present, this category could be used.

For diagnosis of this group the following conditions should be fulfilled : (I.C.D.-X)

1. Form, content and severity of symptoms should be as described earlier ;

2. The previous history and personality may show vulnerability ;

3. Stressful event should be clear and temporally related to symptoms.

Management

The mainstay of management is psychotherapy. The aim is to realistically evaluate the situation and help the patient to cope with the situation effectively. Imaginary fears, false assumptions have to be clarified

Pharmacotherapy

For short lasting problems benzodiazepines (diazepam, lorazepam, alprazolam) can be given for short periods. Patients showing depressive symptoms should be treated with antidepressants. The dosage required are low (Imipramine 25-75mg/day).

DISSOCIATIVE (CONVERSION) DISORDERS

This disorder was previously called Hysteria. This term is now no longer used as it was often used, in multiple ways and often has prejorative connotation. Later, this disorder was called conversion hysteria or conversion disorder which indicated that psychic energy has been transformed into bodily symptoms, but this is not scientifically acceptable. This latter term has also been given up.

It is now conceived that this disorder is characterized by a partial or complete loss of normal integration between memories of the past, awareness of identity, immediate sensations and control of bodily movements, hence the term dissociation is used. The symptoms of this disorder are characterized by amnesias, fugue, trance, disorder of movements and sensations, and convulsions. All of these could be produced by poor integration of various aspects of psychological functioning.

There has been a continuing debate whether this loss of control is conscious or unconscious. The symptoms in this disorder may vary from hour to hour or may differ by change in situation which may make one feel that this is a conscious phenomenon. On the contrary, the symptoms quite often may persist inspite of severe discomfort and disability to the patient. This controversy is still unsettled and it can be safely said that these symptoms are more subtle than those seen in malingering and appear to be a result of severe psychological stress, which affects the normal integrative mechanism. These symptoms are at least partly not under voluntary control. These patients may also have a biological vulnerability for dissociation.

Epidemiology

Detailed epidemiological studies are not available. It is said to be more common in underdeveloped and developing countries. It is also more common at a the uneducated and the lower socioeconomic groups. It is much more common in females. It is more common in younger age and in early youth (15-35 years). The disorder is quite common in clinical practice in India, specially in general practice.

Etiology

The illness is more common in individuals with hysterical personality, but it can develop in any other personality.

The characteristics of hysterical personality are :

Attention seeking — They like to be the centre of attraction. If they do not get attention they feel insecure. They will dress flashily or act in a manner which will attract others.

Emotionally immature — They often appear highly emotional. They laugh, cry or get angry easily due to which such persons can become good actors. Their relationships are characterized by superficiality. One dissociative disorder patient who was being treated for dissociative disorder due to failure in a love relationship developed strong infatuation with her treating doctor. This indicates that their emotional relationship can change easily.

Impulsive — They are often impulsive and wish to gratify their needs immediately. Due to this trait they may get into many psychological and social difficulties. If they like someone they may become too friendly only to regret their decision later.

Sexuality — They are overtly seductive and appear to be sexually inclined. Quite often they may not be able to enjoy sex or may suffer from various sexual problems.

The disorder is usually precipitated by life stresses which the patient is unable to solve or face and feels that he or she may have a loss of face if the situation is not solved. Common situations seen in the clinical practice are :

Anxiety about examination or studies

Marriage being arranged with person not liked by the patient

Familiar disputes and disturbances ;

Threat of loss of face or honour ;

Sexual problems ;

Others ;

This list is not complete but it provides an idea about the nature of situations. The common characteristics of these difficulties are :

a) The patient cannot control or alter the situation;

b) The situation if allowed to continue is likely to cause immense psychological pain ;

c) The failure to solve the situation may lead to loss of face or prestige.

Patients faced with problems of this nature tend to get a temporary respite by developing these symptoms. It is expected that in due course of time this situation will change. This is called primary gain.

These patients are given many advantages by their family members because of their illness, e.g. (not asked to work, fulfiles, their demands or wishes, everybody is more attentive, etc.) These benefits help to maintain the illness and are called secondary gains.

Recently attempts are being made to identify biological factors associated with this illness. No factor has been identified so far.

Clinical Picture

Patients of dissociative disorders can develop multiple symptoms. The following are common features seen in most of the patients :

The onset of symptoms is acute and dramatic,

The patient usually is not very concerned about his symptoms (la belle indifference). However few patients may exhibit anxiety or depression,

The symptoms usually belong to those areas which are under voluntary control,

The symptoms can show variability,

The symptoms usually do not occur during sleep,

The symptoms usually refer to loss of a function, e.g. paralysis of a limb, loss of complete memory, etc. This loss will not be related to anatomical and physiological functions, e.g. a patient may not be able to walk but may have full movement while lying down,

The symptoms are associated with a stress, though it may not be apparent in initial interviews,

The patients generally deny any psychological causation.

Some specific symptoms are described below :

DISSOCIATIVE AMNESIA

These patients forget a part of their lives. This forgetting is not similar to day-to-day forgetting. The amnesia is usually for a traumatic event or situation. The patients are seldom disturbed by this memory loss. This is often seen in young boys and girls. Other psychological functions are unimpaired.

This must be differentiated from organic amnesia. Organic amnesia are usually characterized by recent memory loss or inability to remember recent happenings. This will include all recent events. Some remote memory is intact. They are usually distressed by their memory loss.

Dissociative amnesia is usually sharply localised. All other memories are retained.

Case History

A young married woman suddenly stopped recognizing her husband, father-in-law and parents. She could recall all the events that happened in the past. She said that her husband and father in law ill-treated her and did not allow her to meet her father. But, while referring to her husband she would call him that young man, and her father in law as a dirty old man. She could recall how she has come to the clinic and remembered all other events, but refused to identify all close relatives.

Comments

This patient demonstrated the development of partial amnesia for husband, father-in-law and father. She could recall all the other events. The illness was clearly precipitated by severe marital difficulties.

DISSOCIATIVE FUGUE

These patients show all the signs of dissociative amnesia and in addition they undertake a purposeful journey away from home or place of work. During this journey their behaviour is normal, they take care of themselves, will buy tickets and follow rules. No evidence of mental confusion is seen. A few patients may assume a new identity.

This condition is quite rare.

It has to be differentiated from organic fugue specially post-ictal fugue state. These patients will show a confusional state, their behaviour is more fragmented and they may exhibit in inappropriate behaviour.

DISSOCIATIVE STUPOR

The patient becomes immobile, does not respond to external stimuli such as light touch. Speech and spontaneous purposeful movements are almost lost. However, breathing, muscle tone, eye movements are such that, it is clear that the patient is neither unconscious nor asleep.

This condition usually arises suddenly following an emotional upheavel. It may last for some time and may recur with another emotional disturbance.

Differential Diagnosis — The stupor should be differentiated from catatonic schizophrenia, depressive stupor, manic stupor and organic stupor. History of previous schizophrenic, manic or depressive symptoms can differentiate them from dissociative stupor. Organic stupor will show disturbances of consciousness, neurological findings and history of some neurological disorder.

TRANCE AND POSSESSION DISORDERS

In this disorder, there is a temporary loss of both the sense of personal identity and full awareness of the surroundings. In some instances individual acts as if he has been taken over by another personality, spirit, deity or force. Attention and awareness may be limited to or concentrated upon one or two aspects of the immediate environment and the person may repeat a few acts or words or maintain special postures.

Case Example

A 24 year old lady started behaving oddly one afternoon. She started saying that she is goddess Durga. She often raised one hand, as if blessing others. She told her mother-in-law that you have not fulfilled the promise made to her (the goddess). She also told her husband that you should work harder and look after your children well. Many people gathered around her and she blessed them and answered their questions. This state lasted for one hour. She got repeated attack every second or third day. History revealed that her husband was an alcoholic who did not work properly. Her mother-in-law used to blame her for not working and for her son's alcoholism.

Comments

The case clearly demonstrates a posession state by goddess Durga which developed in a state of psychological tension. This was a culturally approved way of communicating her distress.

Trance and posession states are very common in India. Few people induce a trance deliberately during a religious ceremony or for therapeutic purposes. Self induced trance states are not included here. People assemble and in some religious places may pass into group trance states. They may exhibit shaking head and swaying their body or making noises according to the custom. These are also not included indissociative stupor.

Sometime posession state may occur as part of schizophrenia or other illness. These should be differentiated by eliciting specific symptoms of that disorder.

DISSOCIATIVE MOTOR DISORDERS

The patient develops complete or partial weakness of any or all the limbs. The weakness may be complete or some movements may be possible. They can also develop involuntary movements of any limb. They may show difficulty in walking or standing. The illness may mimic ataxia, apraxia, akinesia, aphasia, dysarthria, dyskinesia or paralysis.

This has to be differentiated from organic diseases. The differences are :

Dissociative Motor Disorder	Organic Disease
1) Loss of a function, e.g. paralysis of lower limb will extend only upto thighs.	Loss follow distribution according to spinal segments or nerve distribution.
2) Some movement may be possible in some situations	Weakness is same in all situations.

3) The neurological examination will be normal.	Neurological examination will show altered reflexes or other positive findings.
4) Disease is acute in onset and may show a fluctuating course.	Disease can be acute or insidious. The course is usually either steady worsening or steady improvement. Moment to moment variations will not be present.
5) General characteristics of dissociative disorders described earlier will be present	Absent.

DISSOCIATIVE CONVULSIONS

This is a very common presentation in our country. The clinical features are : sudden loss of consciousness which is seldom complete. The patient can often hear what is being talked about. They may show bizarre movements of body, limbs and head. They may also speak few words or sentences during the fit. The fit usually starts suddenly and may continue for hours. Later the patient will become normal. The fit can occur many times a day. The patient is usually fully normal between the attacks. Attacks are often preceded by emotional disturbances.

These fits are to be differentiated from epileptic seizures.

Dissociative convulsions	Epileptic convulsions
Consciousness is partly impaired	Complete loss of consciousness.
Partial or full recall of fit is possible.	Complete amnesia for the fit.
Body and limb movements are bizarre and may change from one fit to another.	Sequence of events follow a stereotype pattern. Aura, cry, tonic state and clonic movements
Duration of fit may range from minutes to hours.	Fits usually last for 3-5 min.
Fits do not occur at night or when alone.	Can occur at anytime.
Serious injury or tongue bite does not occur.	Tongue bite or serious injury can occur.
Incontinence of urine and faeces do not occur	Can occur.

Sometimes, epileptic patients can also develop dissociative convulsions due to stress. It may be very difficult to differentiate the two. If the pattern of seizure has changed or is inconsistent, then dissociative seizures should be suspected.

Case History

A 16-year old girl was having repeated fits from past seven days. The fits started one morning while she was going to school. As soon as she got ready to go to school, she fell down on the ground. She started shaking her limbs and was uttering 'Ashok is very bad'. She continued in this state for nearly 20 minutes. After which she became normal. She started having similar fits twice or thrice a day. There was no history of tongue bite or bladder or bowel incontinence.

History revealed that she was having a friendship with a boy named Ashok who has lately become friendly with another girl.

Comment

This patient started having dissociative fits in a state of emotional turmoil. Her utterances during the fit provided some idea of conflict.

DISSOCIATIVE ANAESTHESIA AND SENSORY LOSS

Some patients may develop sensory loss of some

part of the body. They usually complain of loss of sensation in one half of the body. This sensory loss can also be associated with paraesthesias.

Some patients may complain of loss of vision. This loss of vision is seldom complete. The patients are usually able to walk about unaided and they seldom hurt themselves. Dissociative loss of hearing and smell is very uncommon.

These conditions have to be differentiated from organic sensory loss. Organic sensory loss follows a dermatome distribution while functional sensory loss is confined to layman's concept e.g. functional sensory loss of half of body will be in a straight line dividing the body while the organic sensory loss cannot be mid-line because the dermatome overlap at the midline.

OTHER DISSOCIATIVE (CONVERSION) DISORDERS

GANSER SYNDROME

This syndrome is characterized by approximate answers. If the patient is asked the sum of 2+2, his answer would be 3 or 5, indicating that he knows the answer but is giving an approximate reply. They may exhibit other dissociative symptoms. This condition is seen in situation of acute stress (Prisoners awaiting trial or sentencing). It is very rare.

MULTIPLE PERSONALITY DISORDERS

In this condition the patients assumes one more additional personality. Both the personalities are unaware of each other. The functioning of each personality is normal. It is also a very rare condition. Some investigators in Canada claim that it is common there.

Course and Prognosis

Nearly 90% of the patients may get spontaneous relief from their symptoms, or improve with treatment. But the symptoms have tendency to recur. Thus the disorder can produce perpetual tensions in home life. Some patients can also become chronic. It is said, that if the symptoms persist for two years or more then the chances of improvement are much less.

Management

The dissociative disorders are characterized by the following

a) Personality of the patient is such that he needs constant emotional support and reacts with dissociation, whenever this support is not available.

b) The disorder is precipitated by certain adverse life circumstances which the patient is not willing to admit.

c) The family exhibits extreme concern which is providing secondary gain to the patient and thus helps in maintaining the illness.

The management has to be psychological. The role of pharmacotherapy at its best is suggestive.

A detailed history should be obtained. One should always try to look for any immediate stressors which may be responsible for the condition. The stressors are often denied or concealed by the patient. A detailed physical examination should always be done. Once the examiner is sure of the diagnosis, the following steps should be undertaken :

1. Assure the family members that there is no evidence of a physical disease in this patient, which could be life threatning. This illness is psychogenic in origin, which does not mean that the patient is feigning or malingering. Psychological problems can produce disabling symptoms. This could be further illustrated by examples, e.g. showing, relationship of anxiety to loss in appetite, frequency of micturition or trembling, etc. The family has to be explained that they should neither show excessive concern for the patient's illness nor fulfil his unwanted demands. This will help to remove the secondary gain.

The patient has to be similarly reassured that these problems have developed mainly because of his inability to cope with their situations. There exact nature could only be revealed by him. He should also be communicated that, quite often this relationship between situation and symptoms is not in the conscious awareness of the patient. If the patient is able to acccept the relationship between situations and symptoms then the symptom relief may occur.

Sodium pentothal narcosis — Some patients who are unable to reveal their problem in a fully conscious state can do so under Sodium pentathol narcosis. .25 gram of pentathol is dissolved in 10 cc of distilled water. This solution is injected very slowly, so that the patient develops slurring of speech but does not go to sleep. In this state the normal conscious inhibitions are lost and the patient may be able to reveal the conflict. This state can also be used for giving suggestions for the removal of symptoms. If the symptom is removed, then it is always better to invite the relatives in the consultation chamber and demonstrate to them the improvement.

Once the symptom is removed, then the effort is made to resolve the conflicting situation. Sometimes it may not be possible (E.g. failure in exam or love). In such situations the patient is helped to cope with them. The majority of the patients will respond to this treatment programme.

Pharmacotherapy — Benzodiazepines are often prescribed to reduce the anxiety. They also act as face saving devices and provide an excuse for the patient to give up their symptoms. They should be used for short periods only.

SOMATOFORM DISORDERS

These disorders are characterized by the following :

a) Repeated presentation with somatic symptoms which do not have any physical basis. Even if some organic disorder is present, it does not explain all the somatic symptoms ;

b) A persistent request for medical investigations and treatment inspite of repeated assurances by the doctors that there is no physical basis for these complaints.

These patients may have associatied anxiety or depression but the patient will usually state that these symptoms are a consequence of physical problems and not their cause. Psychogenic etiology is often denied by the patient.

Epidemiology

These symptoms occur quite frequently in primary care. In the American Hospital Association survey of nearly 2,60,000 patients, 5.2% were kept in ill-defined condition category. Indian workers have primarily studied somatic complaints in psychiatric outpatient setting and the rate of somatization varied from 29% to 80%.

However, the differentiation of somatoform disorder from other psychiatric diagnosis is of recent origin and not many studies have been done after this conceptual change.

Etiology

Many hypothetical models have been proposed for explaining somatization.

Psychological state by itself may induce certain somatic symptoms like fatigue or loss of appetite. Psychological states may also produce bodily symptoms by different patterns of arousal, it may also affect the monitoring of bodily sensations. Somatization may also be a way to draw attention, or may be a pattern of communication of distress. Somatization may be a result of the demands of health care system, where only persons with bodily symptoms are allowed care.

Many neurophysiological aspects of somatization are being studied. These patients may have abnormal perception of pain and discomfort. Their arousal system may also be faulty.

In general, it can be said that this group of disorders have not been properly understood so far and need much more research.

SOMATIZATION DISORDER

This syndrome is characterized by multiple, frequently changing physical symptoms of long duration. These patients have had repeated contacts with physicians with no relief.

Epidemiology

This condition is more common in females. Lifetime prevalence is not known. These patients are commonly seen in general practice.

Etiology

The illness is seen much more frequently in the first degree relatives of somatization disorder patients. A hereditory basis is proposed. The illness usually starts before 20 years of age. Neurophysiological instability is presumed but the exact nature is not known.

Psychosocial Factors — Most of these patients will exhibit life long patterns of maladjustment, repetitive stresses and difficult life circumstances. But the patients steadfastly deny any relationship between psychosocial factors and their symptoms.

Clinical Picture

The patients usually reach the psychiatrist after many years of consultations with different specialists. The symptoms are usually changing. Symptoms like headache, weakness, sexual symptoms, pain in other body parts, etc. are seen.

The patients usually seek help from various doctors and specialists and carry their prescriptions and investigations as prized possessions.

Many patients might have undergone multiple operations without any relief. The course of the disorder is chronic and it usually affects the social and personal life of the patient.

Diagnosis (I.C.D.-X)

A definite diagnosis requires the presence of all of the following :

a) At least 2 years of multiple and variable physical symptoms for which no obvious physical explanation has been found ;

b) Persistent refusal to accept the advice or reassurance of several doctors that there is no physical explanation of the symptoms ;

c) Some degree of impairment of social and family functioning attributable to the nature of the symptoms and resulting behaviour.

Hypochondriacal Disorders

The differences from are as under :

Somatization Disorders	Hypochondriacal Disorders
The emphasis is on individual symptoms	The emphasis is on underlying disease and its deleterious consequences
Symptoms are changing	Usually restricted to one or two systems
Patient demands treatment and removal of symptoms	Wants investigations to settle diagnosis
Excessive drug use with noncompliance	Fear drugs and their side effects

Delusional Disorders

Sometimes patients with somatic delusions can be confused with somatization disorder. They can be differentiated by their fixed and bizarre nature. Somatic delusions are usually few in number.

Management

A large number of these patients may have a hysterical personality and they react to day-to-day stresses adversely. The therapist should develop a stable relationship and should be able to help the patient to deal with the day-to-day problems. Relaxation therapy with graded physical exercises is usually helpful.

Patients who have comorbid depression should be treated with antidepressants. Antianxiety drugs should be avoided as the patients are likely to become dependant.

Differential Diagnosis

Physical Disorders

These disorders should be carefully differentiated from other physical disorders. However, multiplicity of symptoms, chronic course and lack of any evidence in favour of physical disease are quiet diagnostic.

Almost all patients of somatization disorders quite often fulfil the criteria for depressive or anxiety disorders. Generally these symptoms emerge after the onset of somatization and fluctuate with the severity of somatization. A comorbid diagnosis of these disorders can be made. However, if symptoms of somatization develop for the first time after 40 years of age, then a possibility of depressive disorders should be strongly suspected.

UNDIFFERENTIATED SOMATOFORM DISORDER

When patients have multiple somatic symptoms without any physical cause but do not fulfil the criteria of duration of illness or forceful and dramatic presentation, or social and work impairment, then this category is used. These patients may be less chronic and may be more amenable to treatment.

HYPOCHONDRIACAL DISORDER

This disorder is characterized by :

Persistent preoccupation with the existence of one or two progressive physical disorders, even though investigations and doctors have repeatedly advised the patient that there is no such possiblity.

The patients go from doctor to doctor seeking fresh investigations to identify and confirm the diagnosis. The symptoms are not variable.

The patient usually have marked depression or anxiety.

Epidemiology

Though its prevalence in general population is not known, it is estimated that around 5 to 10 percent population in primary health care suffers from it. The male female ratio is similar. It is more common in the, 50's and 60's.

Etiology

Etiology of this disorder is not well understood. Heredity may play some part. These patient seem to misinterprete normal physiological signals as pain and discomfort.

Psychosocial factors seem to play an important role. This illness may often start after acute stress like fatal sickness in close relatives. The patient may also take cues from social situations and may copy a sick role.

Diagnosis (I.C.D.-X)

The following are required :

a) A persistent belief in the presence of at least one serious physical illness underlying the presenting symptoms, even though repeated investigations and examinations have identified no adequate physical explanation, or a persistent preoccupation with a) presumed deformity or disfigurement.

b) A persistent refusal to accept the advice and reassurance of several different doctors that there is no physical illness or abnormality underlying the symptoms.

Differential Diagnosis

These patients have to be differentiated from somatization disorders and physical disorders. Many of these patients may have comorbid depressive or anxiety disorders. If the symptoms of depression antedates the symptoms of hypochondriasis, then the diagnosis of depression should be made.

Course and Prognosis

The majority of patients run a chronic course. However, hypochondriacal children tend to remit with increasing age. Proper treatment often produces change.

Treatment

The mainstay of treatment is psychotherapy. But psychotherapy should not focus on psychological factors initially. The doctor should develop a stable relationship with patient where his somatic symptoms should be checked from time to time so that he is reassured that the illness is not progressing further. The patient should be provided regular programme of exercise and relaxation.

If the patient has depression or anxiety then appropriate pharmacotherapy should be done.

The majority of patients may be helped to cope with the illness by psychosocial support.

SOMATOFORM AUTONOMIC DYSFUNCTION

The symptoms in this category refer to organ systems, directly under autonomic control, e.g. cardiovascular, respiratory , gastrointestinal and genitourinary systems. Symptoms usually refer to one organ system and they may have the characteristic autonomic symptoms of that organ system or vague symptoms referring to that organic system.

C.V.S. :

Palpitation

Heavyness in praecordium

Weakness

G.I.T. :

a) Upper :

Psychogenic aerophagy, hiccups dyspepsia, pylorospasm,

b) Lower :

psychogenic flatulence, irritable bowel syndrome and diarrhoea gas syndrome.

Respiratory System

Psychogenic cough and hyperventilation.

Genitourinary System

Psychogenic increase of frequency of micturition and dysuria.

Other organ system can also be involved.

Epidemiology is not well known. The symptoms are quite common. They are often transient.

Etiology

It may differ from patient to patient. In few instances, psychogenicity may be apparent and in others it may be strongly denied.

Instability of autonomic nervous system may be a factor. This disorder is more akin to a syndrome and various etiological factors have to be identified.

Diagnosis (I.C.D.-X)

Definite diagnosis requires all of the following :

a) Symptoms of autonomic arousal such as palpitation, sweating, tremors and flushing which are persistent and troublesome ;

b) Additional subjective symptoms referred to a specific organ or system ;

c) Preoccupation with and distress about the possibility of a serious (but often unspecified) disorder of the stated organ or system, which does not respond to repeated explanations and reassurances by doctors.

d) No evidence of a significant disturbance of structure or function of the stated organ.

Differential Diagnosis — The disorder has to be differentiated from anxiety disorder. In the latter, apprehension and baseless fear of future predominate the picture, the autonomic symptoms are not the focus of attention. In S.A.D. the autonomic disturbances predominates and anxiety is secondary.

Somatization disorders can also have autonomic symptoms but they are not prominent.

Management

Management should mainly rely on psychotherapy. This will have to vary according to the personality of the patient and etiological factors.

Benzodiazepines, beta-blockers (propranolal) and antidepressants have been used with some success.

PERSISTENT SOMATOFORM PAIN DISORDER

This disorders is characterized by severe, persistent and distressing pain which cannot be fully explained by a physiological process or a physical disorder.

The pain is usually associated with a conflict or psychosocial problem which is severe enough and can explain the pain.

This condition has not been sufficiently studied.

Diagnosis (I.C.D.-X)

The pain should be dominant, persisting and disabling.

It should not be explained on the basis of physical disorder.

Clear psychogenic factors should be present.

Management

The management is basically psychotherapeutic. The immediate conflict and psychosocial stresses should be analysed. The patients generally respond well to psychological help.

Analgesic should be generally avoided. They may lead to dependence. Antidepressants are sometimes helpful.

SOMATOFORM DISORDERS, UNSPECIFIED

This is a category which includes miscellaneous conditions which present with somatic symptoms of psychogenic etiologies but do not fulfil the requirement of categories specified above. This includes following :

a) Globus hystericus (or feeling of lump in the throat causing dysphagia and other forms of dysphagias).

b) Psychogenic torticollis and other disorders of spasmodic movements excluding Tourette's syndrome.

c) Psychogenic pruritis (excluding specific skin lesion such as alopecia, dermatitis, eczema or urticaria of psychogenic origin.)

d) Psychogenic dysmenorrhea (but excluding dyspareunia and frigidity)

e) Teeth grinding.

Management and course will differ from condition to condition. The general principles of this treatment are the same as for other somatoform disorders.

OTHER NEUROTIC DISORDERS

This is characterized by the following : (I.C.D.-X)

a) Either persistent and distressing complaints of increased fatigue after mental effort or persistent or distressing complaints of bodily weakness and exhaustion after minimal effort.

b) At least two of the following :

Feeling of muscular aches and pains

Dizziness

Tension headaches

Sleep disturbances

Inability to relax

Irritability

Dyspepsia

c) Any autonomic or depressive symptoms present

are not sufficiently persistent and severe to fulfil the criteria for any of the more specific disorders in this classification.

The independence of this entity is doubtful. Many of these cases can fall into other categories.

DEPERSONALISATION — DEREALISATION SYNDROME

This syndrome is characterized by feelings of unreality or changes in the self or outside world. All these changes are qualified with the word 'as if'. It indicates that the patient retains insight into this phenomenon. He will complain as if his thoughts and emotions are not his own or as if his body parts have changed. He may also complain that the people outside or the world in general also appears changed. At the same time, he will state though there is no real change, everything appears to be changed to him.

Epidemiology

Complete depersonalisation syndrome is rare but transitory feelings of depersonalization and derealization are quite common.

Etiology

The etiology of complete syndrome is not known. These symptoms can be seen in any of the following situations :

During a state of acute anxiety
After a devastating experience
In depression
Schizophrenia
Post traumatic stress disorders
Dissociative disorders
Drug intoxication
  Marijuana
  Alcohol
  Amphetamine
  Cocaine
  L.S.D.
  Opium
  Others
Neurological conditions
Epilepsy
Any condition involving the frontal lobes

Toxic and metabolic disorders :
Hypoglycaemia
Hypoparathyroidism
Hypothyroidism
Carbon monoxide poisoning
Hyperventilation

All these conditions can give rise to depersonalization, derealization experience but not to the full syndrome.

Diagnosis (I.C.D.-X)

The diagnosis of this syndrome requires either or both of a and b, plus c and d.

a) Depersonalization symptoms i.e. the individual feels that his or her own feelings and/or experiences are detached, distant, not his or her own, lost, etc. ;

b) Derealisation symptoms, i.e. object, people and/or surroundings seem unreal, distant, artificial, colourless, lifeless, etc. ;

c) An acceptance that this is a subjective and spontaneous change, not imposed by outside force or other people, (i.e. insight) ;

d) A clear sensorium and absence of toxic confusional states or epilepsy.

The syndrome has to be differentiated from depersonalisation phenomenon and delusions of depersonalisation and derealisation encountered in conditions enumerated under etiology.

Management

No specific management plan has been documented. The treatment should be of associated symptoms like depression and anxiety. Psychotherapy could be useful.

OTHER SPECIFIED NEUROTIC DISORDERS

This group include various conditions seen in different cultures. Three conditions which are seen in India are described :

Dhat syndrome,
Koro,

DHAT SYNDROME

This syndrome is characterized by preoccupation and excessive anxiety about true or presumed loss of semen. The patients complain of various psychological and somatic symptoms.

Epidemiology

Exact prevalence is not known. But it is quite common in young adolescent males. Occasional female patients are also seen.

Etiology

The condition is presumed to be due to culturally

approved beliefs regarding the energy aspect of semen. It is widely believed that a drop of semen is produced from hundred drops of bone narrow and one drop of marrow is made from hundred drops of blood. Thus in each emission precious energy is lost. Similarly, it is also believed that sexual energy is fixed in quantity and one who has wasted his manhood by repetitive ejaculations is likely to become impotent, and physically weak. These beliefs are reinforced by the literature on sex as well as by religious texts.

The young boys who are more impressionable or who may have inborn tendency to be more suggestible, become acutely anxious about true or presumed semen loss and develop various symptoms. Education, religious beliefs, peer reinforcement and inherent vulnerability plays a role in the development of this syndrome.

Clinical Picture

Young adolescent boys usually consult the primary care doctors or quite often, self advertised specialists who treat problems of semen loss. Their fears are often exaggarated by these self-styled specialists and non-allopathic physicians (Hakims and Ayurvedic doctors).

Common complaints are :

Excessive masturbation

Repetitive nocturnal emissions

Discharge of whitish dhat or jelly-like substance with urine or at the time of defaecation.

They feel that it has caused them irrepairable harm and following group of symptoms emerge :

a) Psychological Symptoms

Anxiety

Depression with or without guilt feelings

Suicidal thoughts

Memory loss and inability to concentrate.

b) Somatic Symptoms

Sleep difficulties

Weight loss

Erectile difficulties or early ejaculation

Aches and pains in various parts of the body

Diagnosis

The diagnosis is based on the following :

a) Preoccupation with real or imaginary semen loss (masturbation, nocturnal ejaculation or with urine) ;

b) Conviction (usually not of delusional intensity) that this has caused irrepairable harm ;

c) Presence of various psychological or somatic symptoms affecting the social or occupational life of the patient.

Management

The management is primarily psychotherapeutic. The patient has to be explained that masturbation, nocturnal emission are almost universal in adolescents and youth. If semen loss causes weakness, it should occur in all young people, as also in married persons who may have frequent sexual intercourse. They should also be explained that the jelly-like substance with urine or whitish residue with urine is not semen but secretion of various glands opening in urethra and the whitish substance is generally a precipitate of phosphates.

The religious emphasis on not wasting semen was based more on control of one's desire. It was presumed that people who can control their bodily desires can concentrate more on their studies or work and will turn out to be more mature individuals. Thus, the emphasis in our scriptures was on control of desires which has now been literally translated into loss of semen. Semen ejaculation, per se, will not cause any weakness but the anxiety generated by it, produces various symptoms which they are now experiencing.

They should also be educated about normal physiology of semen formation, erection and ejaculation.

The majority of patients can get over their symptoms by this counselling. Few may be resistant and may become chronic.

KORO

This condition is characterized by a sudden fear that the penis is shrinking into the abdomen and the patient develops symptoms of panic. Some patients may even try to tie a rope around their penis to stop it from shrinking into the abdomen. Few instances of Koro have been detected in the North-eastern part of our country. Sporadic cases have been seen elsewhere also.

Treatment lies in psychological help and management of panic with antianxiety drugs. The majority of patients respond to treatment.

CHAPTER 10

BEHAVIOURAL SYNDROMES ASSOCIATED WITH PHYSIOLOGICAL DISTURBANCES AND PHYSICAL FACTORS

This group of disorders is characterized by disturbances in physiological functions, which are attributable to psychological factors. Some of them may not have direct psychological causation but the behavioural symptoms are associated with physical disorders.

Following is the detailed classification :

Eating Disorders

Anorexia Nervosa

Atypical Anorexia Nervosa

Bulimia Nervosa

Atypical Bulimia Nervosa

Overeating associated with other psychological disturbances

Vomiting associated with other psychological disturbances

Other eating disorders

Eating disorders unspecified

Non-Organic Sleep Disorders

Non-organic insomnia

Non hypersomnia

Non disorders of the sleep-wake schedule

Sleep walking (Somnabulism)

Sleep terror (Night terrors)

Nightmares

Other non-organic sleep disorders

Non-organic sleep disorders unspecified

Sexual Dysfunctions, Not Caused By Organic Disorders Or Disease

Lack or loss of sexual desire

Sexual aversion and lack of sexual enjoyment

Sexual aversion

Lack of sexual enjoyment

Failure of genital response

Orgasmic dysfunction

Premature ejaculation

Non-organic vaginismus

Non-organic dyspareunia

Excessive sexual drive

Other sexual dysfunctioning not caused by organic disorder or disease

Unspecified sexual dysfunction, not caused by organic disorder or disease

Mental And Behavioural Disorders Associated With Puerperium, Not Elsewhere Classified

Mild mental and behavioural disorders associated with puerperium, not elsewhere classified

Severe mental and behavioural disorders associated with puerperium, not elsewhere classified

Other mental and behavioural disorders associated with puerperium, not elsewhere classified

Puerperal mental disorders unspecified

Psychological Or Behavioural Factors Associated With Disorders Or Diseases Classified Elsewhere

Abuse Of Non-Dependence-Producing Substances

Antidepressants

Laxatives

Analgesics

Antacids

Vitamins

Steroid Hormones

Special herbal or folk remedies

Other substances that do not produce dependence

Unspecified

Unspecified Behavioural Syndromes Associated With Physiological Disturbances And Physical Factors

EATING DISORDERS

These include all those conditions where eating is influenced by psychological factors. Psychogenic vomiting is also included here.

ANOREXIA NERVOSA

This disorder is characterized by deliberate attempt at weight loss either by restricting food intake or by increasing exercise or by use of purgatives. The appetite is generally not reduced but the patient deliberately reduces food intake. Thus the use of term anorexia for the disorder is inappropriate as the appetite is not lost.

Epidemiology

Anorexia Nervosa is more common in developed countries where the prevalence is around 0.5% to 1% in adolescent girls. It is not as common in our country but the prevalence is likely to increase with improvement in economic conditions. It is much more common in females and rare in men. Disorder usually starts in ea y teens, quite often by 10 to 11 years of age and may persist throughout life. It is more prevalent in upwardly mobile section of population where thinness has greater premium.

Etiology

Genetic factors may play some part. Biochemically, it has been demonstrated that some of the anorexic patients show reduced 3 Methoxy-4 hydroxy phenyl glycol (MHPG) in urine and CSF indicating that norepinephrine turnover is low. There is also some evidence indicating that endogenous opioid may also be responsible for denial of hunger. Opiod antagonists tend to induce weight gain in these patients.

Starvation produces many changes in Hypothalamic-thyroid-pituitary-gonadal axis. Most of these patients develop amenorrhea. If the illness starts before secondary sex characters develop, then the secondary sex characters may also not develop fully.

These patients usually belong to higher socioeconomic strata with both parents working. These patients are usually preoccupied with their gender identity. They avoid looking like mature females. They may often gaze at the mirror to repeatedly confirm non development of breasts. Any signs of plumpishness in the body makes them more averse to food intake.

Clinical Picture

The disease usually starts around 13-14 years of age. These patients avoid eating high calorie foods. They may not take sugar, chapati, fatty foods, etc. They may hide or throw the food given to them. Physically they are very active and inspite of their low weight they may continue all their normal activities. Their weight is usually 15% or more lower than the normal weight for their age and sex.

These patients usually develop amenorrhea. Breast may stop developing. There body looks thin and emaciated. When weight loss is too much, the patients develop giddiness and weakness.

Some patients show complete lack of interest in sexuality while others may retain this interest and can be sexually provocative.

Symptoms of depression and anxiety may develop in some patients. Sleep may be disturbed if the patient is anxious.

These patients can develop various complications due to severe weight loss, vomiting or diarrhoea, like confusion, tetany, cramps. They may develop dehydration, severe electrolyte imbalance. They should be carefully monitored whenever there is severe cachexia.

Course and Prognosis

The course is variable. Some patients may show spontaneous recovery and majority show a chronic course. Mortality is quite high ; 5%-18% patient may die on long term follow-up.

Case example

An 18-year old girl was brought for consultation for weight loss and increased irritability. History revealed that she had been avoiding fattening food from the age of 11 years and she has lost weight. Her present weight was 32kg. She had been a good student and she had consistently performed very well in studies. She had poor social relationships and could not get along with others. Both her parents were working and belonged to upper middle class. This patient had been in treatment for more than a year. Her weight has stabilised around 37kg. She is having mensturation. She has now started showing sexually precocious behaviour and wants to marry soon.

Comments

This patient is a typical patient of anorexia nervosa. She has not responded much to treatment. Her relationship with the therapist is stable which has helped her to some extent. Her preoccupation with food has not changed.

Diagnosis (I.C.D.X)

For a definite diagnosis all the following are required :

a) Body weight is maintained at least 15% below that expected (either lost or never achieved) or Quetlets body mass index is 17.5 or less. Prepubertal patients may show failure to make the expected weight gain during the period of growth.

$$\text{Quetletes body mass index} = \frac{\text{weight in (kg)}}{\text{height in (M)}^2} \quad \text{(to be used for age 16 or more)}$$

b) The weight loss is self-induced by avoidance of "fattening foods". One or more of the following may also be present : self-induced vomiting, self-induced purging, excessive exercise, use of appetite suppresants and/or diuretics.

c) There is body image distortion in the form of a specific psychopathology, whereby a dread of fatness persists as an intrusive, over valued idea and the patient imposes a low weight threshold on himself or herself.

d) A widespread endocrine disorders involving the hypothalamic - pituitary - gonadal axis is manifest in women as amenorrhoea and in men as loss of sexual interest and potency. (An apparent exception is the persistence of vaginal bleeding in anorexic women who are receiving replacement hormonal therapy, most commonly taken as contraceptive pill). There may also be an elevated level of growth hormone, raised level of cortisol, changes in the peripheral metabolism of the thyroid hormone, and abnormalities of insulin secretion.

e) If onset is prepubertal, the sequence of pubertal events is delayed or even arrested (growth ceases; in girls the breasts do not develop and there is primary amenorrhoea; in boys genitals remain juvenile). With recovery, puberty is often completed normally but the menarche is late.

Differential Diagnosis

The clinical picture of the disease is quite typical but it should be differentiated from other chronic debilitating diseases.

Management

The majority of these patients resist treatment. They neither want to consult a doctor nor are ready to be admitted in a hospital. The treatment revolves around the following :

a) Psychotherapy

b) Pharmacotherapy.

a) **Psychotherapy**

The doctor should make sustained efforts to develop a trusting relationship with the patient. These patients often feel lonely and neglected by their families because nobody is able to appreciate their inner compulsions of avoiding food. This situation can be therapeutically utilised by communicating to the patient, that the therapist understands her inner compulsions. She may further be encouraged to express her anxieties regarding her body, sexuality, mensturation and other daily psychological problems. The patient may then start trusting the therapist.

Management of weight loss — The patient will require supervised feeding at frequent interval. The therapist and the patient may decide on target weight. Their anxieties regarding weight gain should be discussed.

b) **Pharmacotherapy**

Cyproheptadine has been found useful in inducing weight gain. Experimentally the following drugs could be tried :

Fluoxetine/Clomipramine may effect the obsessive need to avoid food intake.

Opiod antagonist like Trexon can be tried.

ATYPICAL ANOREXIA NERVOSA

This category is used when the clinical picture is of anorexia nervosa but one or two key elements are missing (Amenorrhoea, weight loss, etc.)

BULIMIA NERVOSA

This disorder is characterized by episodic excessive eating which is followed by excessive guilt and anxiety over food intake and the patient may induce vomiting and diarrhoea to control weight. Their preoccupation with eating and weight loss is similar to anorexic patients.

Epidemiology

This is said to be more prevalent than anorexia nervosa in the West. Obesity in the family members or the patients could be a precipitating factor. The disorder usually starts in the late teens or during early adulthood. It could also be a consequence of anorexia nervosa. It is quite rare in this country so far.

Etiology

These patients tend to respond to antidepressants so the possibility of disturbances in norepinepherine and serotonin metabolism are presumed. Endogenous opioids may also play some role.

Psychologically these patients are high achievers and ambitious. They are more an extrovert than an anorexics.

Clinical Picture

The syndrome is characterized by repeated bouts of binge eating in which disproportionate amount of fattening foods are ingested. The bout is usually terminated by feeling of bloating or nausea due to excess food intake. These patients later induce vomiting or use purgatives to nullify the effects of excessive eating. Every binge also induces feeling of guilt and depression. The patients of bulimia are excessively concerned about their body and are often worried as to how they may appear to others.

They may have heterosexual interest and they may be sexually active.

Their weight could be normal, lower or excessive.

Course and Prognosis

The course is often fluctuating but this disorder does not restrict the patient's life very much.

Diagnosis (I.C.D.-X)

For a definite diagnosis the following are required :

a) There is persistant preoccupation with eating, and an irresistable craving for eating, in which large amounts of food are consumed in short periods of time.

b) The patient attempts to counteract the "fattening" effects of food by one or more of the following : self induced vomiting ; purgative abuse, alternative periods of starvation, use of drugs such as appetite suppressants, thyroid preparations or diuretics. When bulimia occurs in diabetic patients they may choose to neglect their insulin treatment.

e) The psychopathology consists of morbid dread of fatness and the patient sets herself or himself a sharply defined weight threshold, well below the premorbid weight that constitutes optimum in the opinion of the physician. There is often , but not always, history of earlier episode of anorexia nervosa, the interval between the two disorders ranging from a few months to several years. This earlier episode may have been fully expressed or may have assumed a minor cryptic form with a moderate loss of weight and/or transient phase of amenorrhoea.

Differential Diagnosis

These patients are to be differentiated from upper G.I. tract disorders which can present with vomiting and weight loss. The psychological constellation is quite specific in bulimia and should not be difficult to diagnose.

This should also be differentiated from atypical depression with excessive eating by eliciting compulsive nature of eating in bulimia and preoccupation with body image.

Management

These patients are managed with psychotherapy and antidepressant drugs. Psychotherapy has to be aimed at their preoccupation with body image and binge eating. Behaviour therapy can be useful in some cases.

Pharmacotherapy

Antidepressant drugs like imipramine are useful. Fluoxetine may be more effective, as it causes loss of appetite along with an antidepressant action.

ATYPICAL BULIMIA NERVOSA

When the clinical picture though typical for bulimia does not have one or two key elements like weight loss, then this category is used.

OVEREATING ASSOCIATED WITH OTHER PSYCHOLOGICAL DISTURBANCES

When obesity is a reaction to psychological events like bereavement, accidents and emotionally distressing events, then it has to be coded here. Obesity induced by drugs or endocrinal factors or due to constitution, is not included here.

The management will be mainly on psychological lines. If associated depression is present than antidepressants can be used.

VOMITING ASSOCIATED WITH OTHER PSYCHOLOGICAL DISTURBANCES

This condition includes vomiting induced by psychological causes. This is a common condition. The patients can have associated dissociative disorder or other eating disorder.

The management is based on etiology. When no etiological factor can be found, behaviour therapy can be useful. Amytriptiline in low dosage is often effective.

SLEEP AND NON-ORGANIC SLEEP DISORDERS

Sleep is the normal requirement of a healthy individual. It is regular, recurrent and easily reversible state a, which is characterized by a state in which the organism does not respond to external stimuli as easily as in waking state. All human beings do not require same amount of sleep. Some could be called short sleepers who require around six hours of sleep per day, others are called long sleepers who require around 9 hours or more of sleep per day. Short sleepers are usually more efficient, forward looking and self-contented individuals while long sleepers are more anxious, lack ambitions and are socially withdrawn.

The sleep in the whole night is not of similar nature. It can be broadly divided into the following types :

1) Non rapid eye movement sleep
2) Rapid eye movement sleep.

Non Rapid Eye Movement Sleep (NREM Sleep) - This sleep is characterized by restfulness, low B.P. slow and reduced rate of breathing and episodic body movements. There are no rapid eye movements. On electro encephalogram, the NREM sleep can be divided into the following stages.

Stage I — It is characterized by theta waves of 3-7 cycles per second.

Stage II — After few minutes of Stage I, the individual passes into the second stage characterized by spindle shaped waves of 12 to 14 cycles per second which are called sleep spindle and slow triphase waves which are called K complexes.

Stage III — The record now shows high voltage delta wave (.5 to 2.5 c/s) which occupy less than 50% of record.

Stage IV — The delta waves occupy more than 50% of the record.

If a person is awakened during Stage III or IV of sleep he may show disorientation and confusion for some time. Sleep disorders like somnambulism, night terrors occur in Stage III or IV of NREM sleep.

Rapid Eye Movement Sleep (REM, Paradoxical sleep) — This stage is quite similar to waking state and that is why it is also called paradoxical sleep. REM sleep is characterized by the following :

Rapid eye movements — Eyes show scanning movements.

Physiological functions like heart rate, blood pressure and respiration rate are similar to waking state and may be slightly increased.

Muscular activity is reduced and a person may find it difficult to move his body. Many a time when a person is dreaming he may want to get up or move during the dream but he often finds the movement impossible. This is due to motor paralysis during this stage. This paralysis helps to maintain sleep during dream. Sometimes if a person wakes up during this period he may experience momentary paralysis.

Penile Erection — Penis is usually fully or partially erect during this phase. This observation is utilised to differentiate organic from functional impotence.

Dreams — Most persons dream during this period.

Temperature Control — Normal temperature control which occurs during the waking stage and NREM sleep, is lost during this phase. The individual cannot maintain temperature during this phase.

Sleep Architecture — Normally sleep starts with NREM phase and first REM phase occurs after 90 minutes of sleep onset. The first REM phase lasts for 10 minutes. Later, every 90 to 100 minutes, one REM phase lasting for 15-40 minutes occurs.

Children have more REM sleep and as they mature to adults the REM sleep is reduced and replaced by adult pattern.

Control of Sleep — Sleep is controlled by many areas in the brain stem. Dorsal Raphae nucleus which contain the cell bodies of almost all serotonergic cells appears to be involved. Any reduction of serotonin effects sleep. Other neurotransmitters like norepinepherine and acetyl-choline are also involved in sleep regulation.

Functions of Sleep — Sleep is not only a restful period for the body but it also has restorative functions. Many hormones are secreted during sleep. Sleep deprivation can lead to debilitation, increase irritability and at times to psychosis.

Sleep-Wake Rhythm — Normally sleep-wakefulness follows a cycle. People sleep during fixed hours at night and may take a nap in the day. The sleep rhythm develops only after 2 years of age. The sleep-wakefulness cycle is disturbed by jet travel from east to west or by any other disruption of sleep-wake cycle, e.g. in shift workers, psychosis, etc.

When this cycle is advanced, people sleep later than their normal sleeping time and may wake up much later. This may sometimes happen in students who study till late in night for long periods. Their sleep rhythm is advanced and they may not be able to sleep till early morning.

This rhythm may sometime be retarded. In such

situations person gets sleep much earlier than the usual sleeping time and may also wake up earlier than usual.

NON-ORGANIC SLEEP DISORDERS

This group includes disorders of sleep which are primarily of emotional origin. However, some of the disorders included may have a major role of non-psychogenic factors. This section excludes syndromes which are primarily of organic origin like Kleine Levin syndrome, narcolepsy, disorders of sleep- wake schedule, sleep apnoea and episodic movement disorders of sleep including nocturnal myoclonus. As these are important disorders for differential diagnosis they will be discussed at the end of this section.

NON-ORGANIC INSOMNIA

Insomnia is characterized either by inability to get sleep or to maintain sleep for average duration. Most of the sufferers remain preoccupied with sleep difficulties. Insomnia generally effects their daily life adversely.

Epidemiology

Insomnia is a very common disorder. Nearly 20% of the population suffers from insomnia in a year. However, most of the insomnias are transient and may not need medical attention. Insomnia is very common in females and the elderly people.

Etiology

The majority of insomnias occur due to medical or psychiatric conditions. The common conditions are :

Symptom Organic Psychitric Conditions

Symptom	Organic	Psychitric Conditions
Difficulty in falling asleep	Any painful condition Hyperpyrexia CNS lesions Intake of stimulants (Tea, coffee, amphetamines)	Anxiety disorder Depression Schizophrenia Mania Tensions of daily living
Difficulty in remaining asleep	Sleep apnoea Nocturnal myoclonus Drug withdrawal Painful conditions Brain stem or hypothalamic lesions	Environmental change Dreams Conditions mentioned above

Most of the conditions named above are usually not coded as sleep disorders, unless the sleep disorder is prominent and is a presenting symptom. But there is a large group of patients who complain of insomnia but may have none of the abovementioned factors. These patients do not complain of anxieties, fear or any other symptoms but complain only of insomnia and all other problems appear secondary to insomnia. The etiology of this condition is not clearly known. But following factors may be contributory :

Tension about somatic aches and pain
Chronic anxiety or tension
Severe loss
Change in life pattern
Chronic dissatisfaction

Often the patients deny all the above reasons.

Clinical Picture

These patients present with difficulty in falling asleep or of only a few hours of sleep or of unrefreshing sleep interrupted with dreams and/or repeated awakening. One should not measure these symptoms in terms of hours of sleep because different persons have different requirements of sleep. Short sleepers may require only six hours of sleep, while long sleepers may feel uncomfortable even with nine hours of sleep. The complaint of insomnia should be asessed on the basis of personal discomfort caused by this problem.

These patients may also complain of poor concentration, tiredness, lack of interest, sadness and anxiety. It may also be associated with anorexia. They are usually preoccupied with the thought "How can I get sleep, will I be able to sleep tonight". This preoccupation peaks at bed time and further reduces their sleep.

Diagnosis (I.C.D.-X)

The following are essential clinical features for a

definite diagnosis :

a) The complaint is either of difficulty in falling asleep or maintaining sleep or of poor quality of sleep;

b) The sleep disturbance has occurred at least three times per week for at least one month ;

c) There is preoccupation with sleeplessness and excessive concern over its consequences at night and during the day ;

d) The unsatisfactory quality and/or quantity of sleep either causes marked distress or interferes with ordinary activities in daily living.

Whenever insomnia is the primary complaint, it should be coded here. The presence of symptoms of anxiety and or depression does not invalidate the diagnosis. If the symptoms of depression, anxiety or any other condition fulfil the diagnostic criteria of that condition additional diagnosis can be given.

Differential Diagnosis

Conditions referred to under etiology should be cautiously differentiated. If the symptoms of these conditions predominate then they should be diagnosed.

Management

Insomnia is a chronic condition and should be treated preferably by non-pharmacological measures as these patients are likely to become drug dependant and may require more and more drugs to maintain sleep.

The following non-pharmacological measures may help :

a) Sleeping at fixed time. In case sleep does not come, do not force yourself to sleep but start doing something monotonous like repeating the name of a god or counting mangoes on a mango tree, etc.

b) Wake-up at fixed time even if sleep has been short and unsatisfactory.

c) Do all the activities like eating, working, etc. at fixed times.

d) Avoid emotionally arousing situations specially in evenings and at night.

e) Avoid stimulants like tea, coffee, smoking, alcohol or other drugs.

f) Do not take naps in the day.

g) Evening should be spent in a non-stimulating way.

h) Evening walk may be useful.

i) Take light evening meal.

j) Listen to instrumental music at bed time.

k) Sleep at the same place every night.

l) Relaxation exercises may be done at night.

These steps may help majority of the patients. One has to the look for specific psychological factors affecting the individuals and these should be dealt with psychotherapeutically.

NON-ORGANIC HYPERSOMNIA

This is characterized by excessive sleep in the day time which cannot be accounted for by lack of sleep at night. This may also present as prolongation of waking up time from sleep. These patients may need long time to become fully alert on waking up.

Epidemiology

It is quite a rare disorder.

Etiology

Hypersomnia is usually associated with the following :

a) Depression

b) Narcolepsy

c) Encephalitis and other brain disorders.

Hypersomnia associated with the above conditions is not included here. Here, we include only those hypersomnias where no definite organic or psychiatric condition can explain this phenomenon. It is often associated with difficult life circumstances.

Clinical Picture

This is characterized by excessive day time sleep or difficulty in waking up. These patients will often complain of excessive sleep. It will effect their normal day to day activities. It can be associated with lethargy, depression and anxiety.

Diagnosis (I.C.D.-X)

The following clinical features are essential for a definite diagnosis :

a) Excessive day time sleepiness or sleep attacks not accounted for by an inadequate amount of sleep and/or prolonged transition to the fully aroused state upon awakening (sleep drunkenness) ;

b) Sleep disturbances occurring daily for more than one month or for recurrent periods of shorter duration causing either marked distress or interference with ordinary activities of daily living ;

c) Absence of auxillary symptoms of narcolepsy

(cataplexy, sleep paralysis, hypnogogic hallucinations) or of clinical evidence for sleep apnoea (nocturnal breath holding attacks, typical intermittent snoring sounds, etc) ;

d) Absence of any neurological or medical condition, of which day time somnolescence may be symptomatic.

Differential Diagnosis

Non-organic hypersomnia should be differentiated from the following :

a) **Narcolepsy** — It is characterized by the following :

Irresistible desire to sleep — The patient can fall asleep anywhere and at anytime. These sleep attack may last for few minutes or longer. These sleep attacks are usually refreshing.

Cataplexy — They develop a sudden loss of muscle tension, which may manifest as jaw drop, head drop or patient may slump on the ground. The patient is usually awake at such times.

Hypnogogic hallucinations — These patients can develop vivid auditory or visual hallucinations which occur either at the time of going to sleep or while awakening from sleep. They can last for one to two minutes.

Sleep paralysis — It usually occurs on waking up from sleep. The patient is awake but cannot move his body. This state may last for many seconds.

Epidemiology

This is seen in around 3-4 per 1,000 population. It can occur at any age but usually starts in adolescence.

Etiology

This is characterized by the disturbances in the control of REM sleep. There is REM phase at the time of sleep onset. Day time sleep episodes also generally show REM sleep.

Management

Forced nap at specific times may help to resolve the condition. Methylphenidate is the drug of choice. It can be given in the morning and at noon.

Antidepressants are also sometimes useful.

SLEEP APNOEA

This is characterized by cessation of air flow at mouth or nostrils. If cessation of respiration lasts for 10 seconds or more, it is called sleep apnoea. These patients may have hundreds of apnoeic episodes per night.

This is a dangerous condition and can even lead to death if apnoea is prolonged. These patients wake up repetitively due to these attacks and this results in hypersomnia in the day. The patient himself may not complain of any sleep abnormality but the spouse will complain of loud intermittent snoring which may be associated with gasping for breath.

This is a common clinical condition. It is usually seen in the obese and the elderly.

Management

No drugs are effective. Sedatives and alcohol should be avoided.

KLEINE LEVINE SYNDROME

This is a rare syndrome which is characterized by hypersomnia and hyperphagia. These patients get bouts of sleep which may last for days. During this period they may be wakened up but like to return to bed immediately. They may also have excessive appetite. They often show psychotic features like hallucinations, delusions and thought disturbances.

The legendary 'Kumbhkarna' of Ramayan may be a prototype of this illness.

Organic illness associated with hypersomnia are :

a) Withdrawal of stimulant drugs may result in hypersomnia

b) Some types of encephalitis may be associated with hypersomnia

c) Other neurological conditions which involve the area around third ventricle can also lead to hypersomnia.

All these conditions can be differentiated by history and clinical examination.

Management

Primary or idiopathic hypersomnia is a rare condition. No definite treatment has been specified. Antidepressants and methylphenidate can be tried.

NON-ORGANIC DISORDER OF THE SLEEP-WAKE SCHEDULE

This is characterized either by advancing or delaying of the sleep wake schedule. This could occur either due to intrinsic malfunction of the circadian oscillator or due to abnormal processing of the time cues that drive the biological clock. The latter problem could be due to emotional and/or cognitive disturbances.

The condition is often seen in people who undertake frequent jet travel, or in people doing shift duties or sometimes in people who have severe emotional problem due to which they do not attend to time cues. It is often seen in schizophrenia and depression/ mania.

Diagnosis (I.C.D.-X)

The following clinical features are essential for a definite diagnosis :

a) The individual's sleep-wake pattern is out of synchrony with the sleep wake schedule that is normal for a particular society and shared by most people in the same cultural environment.

b) Insomnia during the major sleep period and hypersomnia during the waking period are experienced nearly every day for at least one month or recurrently for shorter periods of time ;

c) The unsatisfactory quantity, quality and timing of sleep, cause marked distress or interferes with the ordinary activities in daily living.

The presence of other psychiatric symptoms does not invalidate the diagnosis, provided these symptoms are not prominent. The additional diagnosis of other conditions can also be made.

Management

If the sleep-wake pattern shift has occurred due to an emotional problem, then the treatment should aim at that problem and it will help in normalising the sleep wake pattern.

In situations where no emotional factor is evident the following steps may be useful.

a) Unorganised sleep schedule should be avoided. Frequent changes of sleep pattern due to shift duty and long working hours (more than 24 hours) should be avoided. Frequnt jet travel should be avoided.

Patient should wake up at normal waking time.

Naps in the day should be avoided.

Patient should sleep at normal sleeping hours even if he does not get sleep.

Relaxing exercise may be tried.

Sedative drugs should be avoided.

SLEEP WALKING (SOMNAMBULISM)

This disorder is characterized by : a) Walking during sleep, b) The patient is neither fully awake nor asleep, c) The patient becomes normal after he awakens from sleep d) He has no memory of the sleep walking episode.

This disorder is commonly seen in young children and adolescents. It may sometime occur in adults also. It is considered to be a maturational disorder. Sleep waking generally occurs in Stage III or IV (NREM) sleep. Some minor neurological abnormality may be associated with it. It may become more frequent during the periods of emotional crisis.

Clinical Picture

The person gets up from sleep, appears dazed, does not respond to stimuli, may perform complex acts like opening a door and walking out. Usually, they return to their bed unaided and go to sleep again. Sometimes, they may go to some other persons bed and sleep. Occasionally, these patients may get involved in an accident. A 22 year old boy did frequent sleep walking. One night, he got up from bed while he was sleeping on the terrace and fell down from the terrace during sleep walking.

Diagnosis (I.C.D.-X)

The following clinical features are essential for a definite diagnosis :

a) The predominant symptom is, one or more episodes of rising from bed usually during the first third of nocturnal sleep and walking about ;

b) During an episode, the individual has a blank staring face, is relatively unresponsive to the efforts of the others to influence the event or to communicate with him or her and can be awakened with great difficulty ;

c) Upon awakening from the episode, the individual has no recollection of the episode ;

d) Within several minutes of awakening from the episode, there is no impairment of mental activity or behaviour, although there may initially be a short period of some confusion and disorientation ;

e) There is no evidence of an organic mental disorder such as dementia or a physical disorder such as epilepsy.

Differential Diagnosis

Temporal lobe epilepsy — These patients may show similar symptoms but their activities are more fragmented and they may exhibit other symptoms like chewing movements, swallowing and rubbing of hands. Dissociative disorders may also show such symptoms. Dissociative patients will behave like normal person and will respond to others. They may not remember their earlier identity.

Management

The problem usually disappears with advancing age. Precaution should be taken to avoid injury. Such patients should not be allowed to sleep on the terrace. Their rooms should be locked and sharp objects should be removed. Diazepam at night generally relieves this problem.

SLEEP TERRORS (NIGHT TERROR)

These are very closely related to sleep walking and both may occur in the same patient. They are characterized by a sudden scream. The patient wakes up in intense fear, he does not respond to external stimuli and usually goes back to sleep after a few minutes. This is also a disorder of Stage III and IV of (NREM) sleep.

Diagnosis (I.C.D.-X)

The following clinical features are essential for a definite diagnosis :

a) The predominant symptom is that one or more episodes of awakening from sleep begin with a panicky scream and are characterized by intense anxiety, body mobility, and autonomic hyperactivity, such as tachycardia, rapid breathing, dilated pupils and sweating;

b) The repeated episode usually last one to 10 minutes and occur in the first third of nocturnal sleep ;

c) There is relative unresponsiveness efforts of others to influence the sleep terror event and such efforts are almost invariable, followed by at least several minutes or disorientation and perseverative movements ;

d) Recall the event, if any, is minimal (usually limited to one or two fragmentary mental images) ;

e) There is no evidence of a physical disorder, such as brain tumour or epilepsy.

Differential Diagnosis

They must be differentiated from nightmares. The patients having nightmares can be easily awakened and they can vividly recall the dream content.

Management

Usually the night terror remits with advancing age. Therefore, no treatment is required. If they are too troublesome then diazepam 5 mg may be given at bedtime for short periods.

NIGHTMARES

Some individuals get frightening dreams which may lead to awakening. During the dream there is little or no vocalisation or body movements. However, the person may exhibit signs of autonomic arousal like sweating, dilated pupils, increased heart rate, etc. The person can vividly recall these dreams. A few patients may have the nightmares of same theme repetitively.

Nightmares are often associated with emotional difficulties, specially in adults. Children's nightmares may be related to difficulties in their maturational process.

Nightmares can also occur due to use of certain psychotropic drugs such as chlorpromazine, thioridazine, imipramine and other antidepressants and benzodiazepines. Sometimes withdrawal of drugs which cause REM suppression may lead to rebound increase of REM sleep and development of nightmares.

Diagnosis (I.C.D.-X)

The following clinical features are essential for a definite diagnosis :

a) Awakening from nocturnal sleep or naps with detailed and vivid recall of intensely frightening dream usually involving threats to survival, security or self esteem. The awakening may occur at anytime during the sleep period, but typically during the second half ;

b) Upon awakening from the frightening dream, the individual rapidly becomes oriented and alert ;

c) The dream experience itself and the resulting disturbances of sleep causes marked distress to the individual.

Differential Diagnosis

It has to be differentiated from the nightmare which has been detailed earlier.

Management

Usually the patient needs to be assured that no permanent harm will occur and the person can tolerate them. If there is an associated emotional problem, that should be treated psychotherapeutically. Few persons continue having nightmares chronically, specially after severe traumatic experiences like accidents, dacoity and involvement in life threatening situation.

Sexual Dysfunction Not Caused by Organic Disorder or Disease

These group of disorders are described together

with other sexual problems in the chapter on Human sexuality, so that the reader may be able to get a comprehensive idea of this problem.

Mental and Behavioural Disorders Associated with Puerperium, Not Classified Elsewhere

Puerperium (child birth) is associated with a number of psychiatric and neurological disorders. The reasons for the development of these problems include :

Changes in hormonal profile after child birth ;

Stress of child birth (pain and physical exhaustion) ;

Increased responsibility of motherhood ;

Pre-existing personality difficulty ;

Pre-existing marital difficulties ;

Neurological problems can arise due to embolic phenomenon.

Puerperium includes a 6 weeks period after child birth. The following psychiatric problems can be observed during this period.

Organic delirium
Schizophrenia
Mania
Depression

Whenever the symptoms fulfil the diagnostic criteria for a specific category that disorder should be diagnosed. Quite often the mental symptoms arising after puerperium may not fulfil the diagnostic requirements of above mentioned disorders than one of the categories listed below could be diagnosed.

MILD MENTAL AND BEHAVIOURAL DISORDER ASSOCIATED WITH THE PUERPERIUM NOT ELSEWHERE CLASSIFIED

This condition generally presents as mild depression. The patient shows lack of interest in the child as well as herself. This may also be associated with the feelings of apprehensiveness. This is usually a transitory condition and passes of after a few weeks.

SEVERE MENTAL AND BEHAVIOURAL DISORDERS ASSOCIATED WITH PUERPERIUM NOT ELSEWHERE CLASSIFIED

When the patient shows psychotic behaviour which cannot be classified in any other category, then this category is used.

Management

These disorders have to be managed with psychological support to the mother. Her fears and apprehensions are allayed. If there are marital or family difficulties, they should also be attended to.

Pharmacotherapy

If symptoms are of anxiety then antianxiety drugs can be used. If depression or psychotic symptoms predominate then appropriate antidepressants or antipsychotics can be used for short time.

Breast feeding should be encouraged and the mother should be helped to look after the child.

PSYCHOLOGICAL AND BEHAVIOURAL FACTORS ASSOCIATED WITH DISORDERS OR DISEASES CLASSIFIED ELSEWHERE

This category is used when psychological factors seem to play an important part in the genesis of a physical disorder. e.g. asthma, gastric ulcer, eczema, etc. These disorders exhibit physiological change in the effected organ or system. Disorders where there is no physiological change such as somatoform disorders are not included in this group.

These disorders were earlier called psychosomatic or psychophysiological disorders. These terms indicated a more direct relationship between psychological factors and physical disorders. The present nomenclature indicates the association and direct etiological relationship is not emphasised.

Etiology

These disorders were earlier presumed to be either occurring in a specific personality type or due to a specific unconscious conflict. However, repeated investigations could not establish either of these hypotheses. The following factors seem to play an important role.

Organ Vulnerability

Some of these disorders show genetic predisposition. It is presumed these genetic factors may alter the autonomic or endocrinal response in such a way that any stress or conflict may affect that particular organ or system.

Organ vulnerability may also be induced by repeated trauma or disturbances of that organ due to the external or internal factors. This may make that organic system vulnerable.

Personality

Personality develops by interaction between innate qualities and the environment. The personality to a large extent determines how a person will cope with stress. Some of these disorders tend to develop in personalities which are characterized by type A personality. Such persons are always on a go, they are intensively competitive, they are always in a hurry to keep time schedules and they often show competitive hostility. They have ever changing set of goals. Such persons are more prone to develop coronary artery disease. Current researchers are trying to establish links between various personality traits and biological parameters. Current researches are also trying to identify specific traits, which may be associated with a particular disease.

Stress

A stress is defined as a situation which puts extra pressure on the system. In the human context, stress refers to various traumatic events, to which the individual cannot adequately respond. These are also called life events, e.g. death of near one, failures in exam, child birth, promotion, disease, etc. It has been shown by many researchers that these disorders show multiple stresses prior to their onset.

Conflict

Conflicts are characterized by two or more options which forces one to make a choice. Conflict between deciding to marry a girl A or B or to decide between higher education or job, etc. These conflicts can produce arousal in autonomic nervous system and hypothalmic endocrine axis and may result in these disorders.

Common disorders having psychological or behavioural disturbances ; associated with them are following.

CARDIOVASCULAR SYSTEM

Coronary Artery Diseases (C.A.D.)

This has been a comprehensively studied disorder both from behavioural and biological viewpoint. These patients exhibit type A personality with increased amounts of low density lipo-proteins triglycerides and raised serum cholestrol. They may also have associated risk factors like smoking which is also dependant on personality.

Along with the pharmacological management most of these patients are also managed psychologically by their physicians. Usual advices are :

Go slow
Stop smoking
Stop worrying
And take diazepam

However, such advices are either not followed by the patient or themselves become a source of conflict for the patient.

Instead, it is essential that each patient should be evaluated individually regarding the following :

a) His aims and goals in life
b) Types of stressesor or conflicts he is undergoing
c) How he has been coping with stresses so far.

He has to be helped to identify realistic goals. He should be encouraged to identify alternative strategies to cope with stresses or conflicts, e.g. if there is a pressure to finish a particular task at 9 AM tomorrow which he finds it difficult or impossible to do, he may be advised to split the task into two or three and finish the part which is possible to be done today. When he is angry or frustrated he may be advised to go for a brisk walk, etc. These strategies will have to be individualised so that they are acceptable to the individual. Relaxation excercises and meditation may be helpful for some.

Hypertension

This is a common disorder. Though genetics seems to play a major part, psychological factors may also be contributory. The patients will have to be convinced for the need of taking drugs regularly. Relaxation excercises and biofeed back have been found useful. Psychotherapy as described under C.A.D. may also be helpful.

RESPIRATORY SYSTEM

Bronchial Asthma

This disorder is characterized by chronic recurrent obstruction of the respiratory pathways. The disease occurs due to interaction of genetic factors, allergic factors, infections and stress.

Exact psychological factors are not known. However, some patients show a dependant personality and react to stresses with helplessness. Psychological support during crisis may be helpful.

GASTROINTESTINAL SYSTEM

Peptic Ulcer — These patients may have gastric or duodenal ulcers. These ulcers have also been produced by non specific stress (for example in burns). Psychological factors may play am important role in some patients. Psychological factors should be identified and dealt with as indicated under CAD.

Ulcerative Colitis

This is a chronic ulcerative disease of colon. It is characterized by bloody stools. Etiologically genetic factors play an important role. Psychological factors are also thought to be contributory. The personality is generally of obsessive type (excessive punctuality, cleanliness, orderliness and excessive control of emotions).

Along with the medical treatment, appropriate psychological help may produce better improvement.

Obesity

This is characterized by excessive accumulation of fat and body weight that exceeds 20% of the standard weight.

Obesity could be genetic or due to environmental factors. Usually, both play a part. Adult obesity is caused due to increase in size of fatty cells while adolescents obesity is due to multiplication of fat cells. Psychological factor play an important role specially when obesity is associated with excessive eating.

Excessive eating could be a consequence of rejection by others, anxiety, depression or some other factors. These will have to be dealt with while treating obesity. Some patients may also have disturbances of body image.

MUSCULO SKELETAL SYSTEM

Rheumatoid Arthritis

These patients develop chronic progressive inflammation of the joints which leads to deformities. This disorder has a hereditary disposition. Immunological factors and psychological factors play an important role.

Psychological problems should be looked along with medical treatment to provide maximum relief.

Headache

This is a common symptom. It is estimated that nearly 80% of the people have at least one headache in a year. Millions of rupees worth headache pills are sold over the counter. The majority of headaches are transitory yet a substantial population suffers from persistent headaches.

Headaches could occur in any of the following conditions.

Intracranial pathology (raised intracranial tension) common causes are Trauma, Tumor, Meningeal infections

Systemic diseases

High pyrexia

Electrolyte imbalance

Endocrinal disorders

Pituitary adenoma

Hypoglycaemia

Thyrotoxicosis

Myxoedema

Opthalmic-squint, high refractory error

Vascular headaches

Migraine

Tension headache

Excessive heat

Worries

Tiredness

Sleeplessness

Psychiatric Causes

Anxiety

Depression

Schizophrenia

Somatoform disorder

Differentiating features of neurological headache :

It gets worse on coughing or straining for defaecation.

The patient may wake up in the middle of the night with headache.

It is associated with vomiting.

It may be associated with other neurological findings including papillaedema.

Headache associated with other systemic diseases :

It will show other symptoms of that disease.

The headache will increase or decrease with changes in primary illness.

Headaches due to tiredness, worry and sleeplessness will be transitory and a clear association can be established.

Headaches due to psychiatric disorders will show symptoms of basic disease, often the headache may be expressed as burning, light headedness, emptiness of head, in these disorders. Sometimes the patient may have delusions of headache.

MIGRAINE

This disorder occurs in bouts and it is characterized by unilateral bursting headache. It is often associated with nausea, vomiting and eye symptoms like darkness in front of eyes, star dancing or at times blindness. The illness is usually caused by disturbances in cranial circulation. This disorder has a tendency to run in the family. Psychological factors often play an important role. These patients often have obsessoid, perfectionistic personality and they react to various stresses with suppression of anger. Any stress may precipitate an attack.

Course and Prognosis

Often the illness runs an episodic course. Each episode lasting from few hours to few days. The illness runs a chronic course but as age advances many patients lose these attacks.

Management

These attacks can be aborted if ergotamine tartarate is given at the time of the onset. If one tablet is not enough to abort the attack, a second tablet may be given after 30minutes. Once full blown headache has developed, then ergotamine does not help but other analgesics can provide symptom relief.

If the attacks are recurrent then Propranalol 80-120 mg per day can be given. Other patients may respond to Phenytoin sodium 100 mg twice a day

The patient needs to change his reaction to daily stresses and problems. This can be achieved by cognitive behaviour therapy.

TENSION (MUSCLE CONTRACTION) HEADACHES

This is the commonest type of headache. It is caused by worry and tensions. These worries make the muscle of head and neck to contract which may cause secondary ischaemia and headache.

Clinical Picture

The headache usually starts as a dull ache in the suboccipital region and later spreads entire the throughout head. The headache is experienced as a tight band around the head. The headache usually starts towards evening after one has undergone the days tension. In females, the headache may start anytime but is usually associated with work or family stresses. The headache may subside with sleep. These patients often exhibit signs of depression or anxiety.

Management

These patients often respond to Amitriyptiline in dosage of 25-50 g/day. In addition, the life problem will have to be tackled. Often, the patients deny any life difficulties. In such cases, details of daily life should be obtained and a better day management plan might be helpful. Relaxation excercises, and meditation have been found useful.

ENDOCRINE SYSTEM

Hyperthyroidism

There is some evidences that the psychological factors may be involved in the precipitation of this problem.

Diabetes Mellitus

These patients may develop secondary psychological problems due to the illness which may require psychological help.

Female Endocrinal Disorders

Premensturał syndrome—This is characterized by feelings of anxiety, sadness, lassitude, emotional lability and lack of interest in work. The patient may also get a feeling of heaviness of body due to water and salt retention. The symptoms may gradually develop after ovulation (14th day) and the peak in the last week prior to mensturation. The symptoms settle down soon after the onset of mensturation.

This syndrome is considered to be due to the changes in oestrogen, progestrone, androgen and prolactin levels. Prostaglandins secreted by uterus may be the cause of pain. Psychological factors like, denial of feminity, fear of pain and anxiety may also play a role.

Management

These patients can be given diuretics to reduce salt and water retention. Analgesics may reduce pain. (Aspirin should be avoided as it may cause excessive bleeding). Psychotherapy may help the patient to tolerate the distress, Antidepressants and minor tranquilisers can be used.

Post-menopausal syndrome

The majority of women attain menopause between 45-50 years. Usually it passes off without any symptoms. A few persons may develop both psychological and physiological symptoms. Psychological symptoms include irritability, anxiety, depression, lassitude and insomnia. Physical symptoms include hot flushes, night sweats and night-flushes.

The physical symptoms are presumed to be due to decreasing levels of oestrogens, progestrone, L.H. and F.S.H. Androgens may also be implicated.

The psychological symptoms are dependant on the personality of patient and her life situations. These patients may exhibit life-long patterns of insecurity and difficulty in coping with stresses which gets accentuated after menopause.

Management

Physical symptoms could be controlled by a combination of oestrogen and progestrone. If the symptoms are not too distressing, these drugs should be avoided as they may produce side-effects. Psychological symptoms should be treated with psychotherapy, which should focus on immediate life problems.

Idiopathic Amenorrhea

Sometimes a women may develop amenorrhea when there are no explainable physiological factors. Often mental stress or worries can cause amenorrhea which may induce marked anxiety in the patient and the family. If she is unmarried this anxiety may further supress mensturation.

Sometimes phenothiazines can also induce amenorrhea which is primarily due to the increase of prolactin and is associated with milk discharge from the breast.

Psychogenic amenorrhea often improves by itself and no treatment is required. Other causes of amenorrhea should be excluded.

IMMUNE DISORDERS

It has now been quite clearly shown that psychological state effects immune responses. Negative emotions and worries effect the immune response negatively while positive emotions lead to positive immune responses. The patients who experience positive emotions like happiness, love and being wanted, show early and prompt recovery while patients who hope, and negative thinking may respond poorly.

These factors can be utilised in the management of the patient with infections and immune disorders.

Chronic Pain

Chronic pain can be either due to psychological problems or due to organic diseases like cancer, arthritis, trigeminal neuralgia and herpes zoster, etc.

It is advisable to differentiate between psychogenic pain disorders and organic pain disorders. The psychogenic pain responds to antidepressants alone and their combination with phenothiazines is often helpful.

The organic pain requires analgesics including opioid analgesics.

The management of organic pain has now become a specialised area where a team of experts from different specialities treat it. The following principles have to be borne in mind.

The patient should be explained clearly that the pain is a part and parcel of his illness but he will get sufficient drugs so that he does not feel uncomfortable. He should not worry about the problems of dependence or side effects because this is the physician's responsibility. The patient should be given adequate dosage of analgesics at a fixed time, so that he is not unnecessarily apprehensive about pain.

Analgesics should be given in sufficient quantity. There is no need to restrict their use because every fresh experience of pain will increase anxiety.

In terminal cases, one should not worry about dependence.

The patient should be seen at fixed times whether he has pain or not. It will increase his confidence.

Thus, he need not have pain to communicate his distress.

CANCER

Cancer is often a dreaded diagnosis and many patients percieve it as a death sentence. Many types of cancer are treatable and in many others, the life can be prolonged reasonably. Every cancer patient should undergo a psychiatric work up for the following :

The patient's personality / coping skills

Previous psychiatric illness if any

Family support system

Financial status

Problems which the patient is currently facing

Problems which the patients are likely to face due to the disease

Availability of proper medical care.

After evaluating all the above, the patient should be apprised of the realistic situation. His worries and anxieties should be discussed. He should be given sufficient time on weekly or fortnightly basis to unburden his anxieties and fears. In India, it is also important to discuss the cost of the treatment vis a vis less efficient treatment or no treatment. Quite often the treatment undertaken may produce very little benefit vis a vis financial and family disruption costs. It is imperative that the treatment, its side effects and its impact on prognosis be clearly discussed.

SKIN DISORDERS

Many of the skin disorders may have an associated psychological disturbance. Many kinds of pruritis, eczema and other skin disorders are associated with psychological problems. It is important to differentiate between psychological problems that were associated with the onset of the disease and that problems that have developed secondary to the disease.

These problems should be managed psychotherapeutically along with specific drug management.

ABUSE OF NONDEPENDENCE PRODUCING SUBSTANCES

Some people develop unnecessary and repetitive use of substances like analgesics, laxatives and antidepressants, etc. These drugs may have initially been prescribed but later the patient continues using them without any need. Many patients may not be able to stop them inspite of the fact that they have produced serious harm like renal dysfunction or electrolyte disturbances. These substances do not induce dependence. There are no withdrawal symptoms on the withdrawal of these substances. The following subtypes of abuses are observed :

Antidepressants
Laxatives
Analgesics (Aspirin, paracetamol, phenacetine)
Antacids
Vitamins
Steroids
Specified herbal and folk remedies
Other substances that do not produce dependence (Such as diuretics)
Unspecified

These substances can be stopped suddenly or gradually, according to the psychological state of the individual. The physician should be able to provide psychological support.

CHAPTER 11

DISORDERS OF ADULT PERSONALITY AND BEHAVIOUR

Personality is defined as an unique organisation of behavioural traits. A behavioural trait includes a group of behaviour, e.g. shyness sociability, hard workingability, etc. The personality is stable and does not ordinarily change in adult life, except after severe traumatic events or after psychiatric or neurological disorders. One can reasonably predict the behaviour of a person in any given situation, if the personality is known.

All individuals have different personalities. Most of the problems described in this chapter may appear in minor form in normal personality. They are called personality disorders, only when they repetitively disrupt or effect the personal life of the individual or show deleterious effects on the society or the family.

Personality disorders are usually identified only after 16-18 years. Earlier, the same behaviour described as temperament.

Diagnosis (I.C.D.-X)

Conditions not directly attributable to gross brain damage or disease or to another psychiatric disorder meeting the following criteria :

a) Markedly dysharmonious attitudes and behaviour involving usually several areas of functioning, e.g. affectivity, arousal, impulse control, ways of percieving and thinking and style of relating to others.

b) The abnormal behaviour pattern is enduring, of long standing and not limited to episodes of mental illness.

c) The abnormal behaviour pattern is pervasive and clearly maladaptive to a broad range of personal and social situations.

d) The above manifestations always appear during childhood, adolescence and continue into adulthood.

e) The disorders leads to a considerable personal distress but this may only become apparent late in its course.

f) The disorder is usually but not invariably associated with significant problems in occupational and social performance.

Personality disorders are often experienced as egosyntonic by the patient and thus they seldom complain about them. It is usually the relatives or society which will bring the patient to clinical attention. Patient with personality problems are capable to modify their behaviour according to situation for short periods of time due to which the examiner may find them normal on clinical interview.

PARANOID PERSONALITY DISORDER

These patients show excessive suspiciousness (not amounting to delusions) in almost all situations and to all persons. They feel that they are being mistreated and are often hostile and angry. They get involved in repetitive litigations and are percieved as complainers.

Epidemiology

The exact prevalence is not known. But the disorder appears to be quiet common. Almost every office will have one or two persons with paranoid personality. It is more common in men. It is frequently seen in the minority groups and immigrants.

Etiology

The disorder does not show familial preponderance. The relationship with schizophrenia is doubtful. People and families which are singled out or have a minority status may feel that they are being discriminated against and may develop paranoid personality because of their need for excessive vigilance.

Clinical Picture

These patients show suspicious behaviour from adolescence. During school, they may blame their teachers for deliberately giving them poor marks. They may feel that they are being neglected by their peers. As they grow up, they become extravigilant. Every scrap of paper is saved. They will suspect their spouse of infidelity, may complain against their chief for dishonesty and partiality. They are very secretive.

Course and Prognosis

The disorder often runs a chronic course. Some people may take up a religious or social cause and may get fully involved in it. They usually have life long interpersonal difficulties.

Diagnosis (I.C.D.-X)

Personality disorder is characterized by :

a) Excessive sensitiveness to setbacks and rebuffs;

b) Tendency to bear grudges persistently, i.e. refusal to forgive insults and injury or slights ;

c) Suspiciousness and a pervasive tendency to distort experience by misconstruing the neutral and friendly acts of others as hostile or contemptuous ;

d) A comparative and tenacious sense of personal rights out of keeping with actual situation ;

e) Recurrent suspicions, without justification regarding sexual fidelity of spouse or sexual partner;

f) Excessive tendency to experience self-importance manifest in a persistent self-referntial attitude;

g) Preoccupation with unsubstantiated "conspirational" explanations of events both immediate to the patient and in the world at large.

At least three of the above should be present for a firm diagnoses.

Management

These patients will not voluntarily seek treatment and often resent treatment. Pimozide in low dosage has been found useful in some people.

Psychotherapy is the treatment of choice. But the therapeutic relationship is stormy as the therapist may also be viewed with suspicion. However, an unemotional approach by the therapist could help to build a relationship. The therapy aims at changing or modifying suspicious constructs.

SCHIZOID PERSONALITY DISORDERS

Schizoid individuals exhibit social withdrawal, poor emotional warmth and avoidance of human contact. These persons are often considerd queer by others.

Epidemiology

The exact prevalence is not known but it is considered to be quite common. More common in men than women.

Etiology

Genetic factors may play some part. The exact relationship with schizophrenia is not clear. Few patients with schizoid personality disorder may develop schizophrenia.

Clinical Features

These patients usually stay aloof and have very few (one or two) friends. They usually shun the company of the opposite sex. They may get married according to the customs but do not show any interest in sex or their partners. They may continue to work but do not show any interest in improving the work or initiating new work. Sleep and appetite is usually not disturbed.

Course and Prognosis

The disorder runs a chronic course. Some persons may show better sociability with advancing age.

Diagnosis (I.C.D.-X)

The patient should fulfil at least three of the following :

a) Few, if any, activities provide pleasure ;

b) Emotional coldness, detachment or flattened affectivity ;

c) Limited capacity to express either warmth, tender feelings or anger towards others ;

d) Apparent indifference to either praise or criticism ;

e) Little interest in having sexual experiences with another person (taking into account age) ;

f) Almost invariable preference for solitary activities ;

g) Excessive preoccupation with fantasy and introspection ;

h) Lack of close friends or confiding relationship (or having only one) and of desire for such relationships;

i) Marked insensitivity to prevailing social norms and conventions.

Management

These patients often do not agree for treatment and establishing a therapeutic relationship is quite difficult. However, if they develop a relationship with the therapist then they can be helped to improve their activities to some extent.

Drugs have not been found useful. Depending on the symptoms, antidepressants or antipsychotics can be used.

DISSOCIAL PERSONALITY DISORDERS

These persons get repeatedly involved in antisocial activites or criminal acts. They are unable to conform to the social norms of the society. These patients should be differentiated from the criminals. The criminal has a motive, plans his act, and avoid detection while the patient of dissocial personality are often impulsive in their behaviour. Their attempts to hide their act appears ridiculous and they do not seem to learn from experience.

Epidemiology

This disorder has been seen in around 1-2% of the population in the west. Males have this problem much more frequently than women. The disorder usually starts in preadolescence.

Etiology

It is not very well understood. The first degree relatives of male patients show a much higher prevalence of this disorder. Many psychological theories were propounded. It was thought to occur more commonly in households where social controls are lax and dissocial behaviour is either accepted uncritically or applauded. Many patients who develop this problem, do not come from such environments or families. It is speculated that these patient somehow do not develop proper moral sense (superego). The majority of these patients show maturational difficulties. Enuresis is quite common during childhood. Lying, stealing and illicit use of drugs starts in childhood.

Clinical Features

These patients are usually brought by their families who have become fed up with the patient's behaviour. They will steal money, or sell household articles. They will take loans from all friends or relatives by telling them convincing stories. One patient's father told the doctor that it is quite likely that he may come to the doctor after a few days with such a convincing story that even he will give him a loan.

They develop multiple sexual relationship. They are quite charming to the opposite sex and they may have multiple affairs simultaneously. They may commit petty crimes like shop lifting. They are habitual liars and they can speak two contradictory lies at the same time. These patients do not experience anxiety, remorse or guilt for their misdeeds. However, when caught they may show repentence, sadness and even suicidal thoughts, but these are momentary and disappear as soon as they overcome the situation. On examination they will appear normal and will not exhibit any positive findings.

Case Example

A nineteen year old boy was brought for consultation for repetitive lying, stealing and promiscuous sexual behaviour. He was the eldest son of a sibship of four. His father was a middle class businessman. He started lying when he was 8 or 9 years of age. He would not go to school and play marbles on the street. Gradually, he started smoking ganja. He was caught copying in high school examination and was debarred. He did not go to school again. He was found to have multiple sexual relations with girls in, neighbourhood. He was caught by some people and was beaten mercilessly. This did not produce any change in him. He used to steal money from home. Once he tried to sell his mother's necklace to the local goldsmith who recognised him and took him to his parents. After this episode he was brought for treatment. He showed marked guilt and anxiety for his acts when confronted, but this lasted only for a short time.

Comments

This patient shows dissocial personality disorder in a a well adjusted household. His behaviour exhibited repeated lying, promiscuity, drug abuse and copying in the examination which is a cognizable offence in Uttar Pradesh.

Course and Prognosis

Dissocial personality disorder runs a chronic course. These symptoms are maximum in late adolescence and early adult life. Later they tend to diminish. Some dissocial acts persist throughout the life.

Diagnosis (I.C.D-X)

Personality disorder usually comes to attention because of a gross disparity betwen behaviour and the prevailing social norms and is characterized by :

a) Callous unconcern for the feeling of others ;

b) Gross and persistent attitude of irresponsibility and disregard for social norms, rules and obligations;

c) Incapability to maintain enduring relationship, though having no difficulty in establishing them ;

d) Very low tolerance to frustration and low threshold for discharge of agression, including violence ;

e) Incapacity to experience guilt or to profit from experience, particularly punishment ;

f) Marked proneness to blame others or to offer plausible rationalizations for the behaviour that has brought the patient into conflict with the society.

These patients may often show conduct disorder in childhood.

Differential Diagnosis — The clinical picture is quite typical and ordinarily there is no difficulty in diagnosis. Some times, antisocial behaviour may arise as a consequence of drug abuse, in such a case drug abuse should be the primary diagnosis. Some times, both drug abuse and dissocial personality disorder can coexist. One should carefully exclude any neurological disorder, which might manifest such symptoms. Occasionally, maturational defects and

E.E.G. abnormalities may be noticed.

Management

Drugs have a very limited role. If there are EEG abnormalities antiepileptics can be tried.

Psychological management is also very difficult, as the patients are unable to form therapeutic relationships. The following guidelines may be used :

The majority of parents and spouses try to hide and minimise the antisocial acts of the patient due to which the patient gets encouragement and he may even blackmail the parents to fulfil his desires ;

The patient should not be bailed out from jail or from difficult situations. He should undergo punishment for his misdeeds.

There should be, limit setting to his behaviour and everytime he transgresses the limit, his privileges should be withdrawn ;

In some cases hospitalization in a special hospital for long term may be the only solution.

EMOTIONALLY UNSTABLE PERSONALITY DISORDER

This disorder is characterized by impulsivity lack of self control and emotional instability. These patients may get into outbursts of violence on little provocation. This personality is further subdivided into :

IMPULSIVE TYPE

These patients are characterized by emotional instability and repetitive outbursts of anger or violence on little provocation.

BORDERLINE TYPE

Borderline personality disorder as a concept had a chequered history. At one time, it was thought to be on the borderline of neurosis and psychosis, later as a type of schizophrenia and now, it is considered nearer to depression. It is characterized by emotional instability, impulsivity, poor self image and unclear goals.

Epidemiology

This disorders is quiet common. Its estimated prevalence is around 1-2%. It is more common in women.

Etiology

The first degree relatives of these patients show a higher prevalence of depression and drug abuse.

Clinical Picture

These patients show instability of mood, which may change from moment to moment. Their interpersonal relationships are stormy. They feel dependant and at the same time angry on the people that are close to them. They seek company and often get into many unfortunate relationships. They may have promiscuous sexual behaviour. These patients may often experience micropsychotic episodes (very short periods of hallucinations, delusions and disordered thinking). These episodes are neither common nor prolonged.

They may often show exhibitionistic suicidal behaviour like wrist slashing, drinking phenyl or taking few tablets of diazepam.

Course and Prognosis

This disorder runs an unchanging course. Thers is some evidence that some of these patients may develop depressive episodes.

Diagnosis (ICD-X)

a) The patient shows marked emotional instability, mood may range from depression, intense irritability to outburts of anger ;

b) There may be chronic feeling of emptiness ;

c) Multiple intense but conflicting relationships which may range from complete idealization to devaluation of the other person ;

d) Sexual promiscuity ;

e) Micro psychotic episodes may be present ;

f) Series of suicidal threats or acts of self-harm.

The status of this pesonality disorder is still uncertain. Few feel that this is a stable syndrome while others deny its existence.

Management

Psychotherapy is the recommended method of treament. The psychotherapeutic relationship is often stormy. The patient is helped to identify the contradictory needs of having a relationship and alongwith, the need to control the relationship by emotional means. Behaviour therapy is also used.

Pharmacotherapy — Antipsychotics are used to control impulsivity and psychotic episodes. Antidepressants may help to control the depressive feelings. Fluoxetine has been found effective by some clinicians.

Histrionic Personality Disorder

These patients are usually extroverts, seeks many and new relationships, but are incapable of maintaining sustained relationships. They often wear flashy dresses and exhibit dramatic behaviour.

Epidemiology

Exact prevalence is not known. It is more common in the females.

Etiology

It is associated with dissociative disorders and somatoform disorders. Heredity may play a role.

Clinical Picture

These patients often take excessive pains to improve their appearance and dress. They will wear fashionable dresses according to their circumstances. A hysterical girl from a village may chew betel leaves, use Kumkum and may comb her hairs well, while a highly placed person may use the latest cosmetics and dresses to produce the same effect. Their behaviour is often theatrical. They will overemphasize simple things and may exhibit excessive display of emotions. If the other person with whom they are talking is in difficulty they may try to impress him. They are unable to form deep emotional relationships. They always want to be the centre of the attraction and if they can not draw attention of others they feel uncomfortable and unhappy.

They often show seductive behaviour but may not be able to respond adequately in sexual relationships. They usually exhibit strong dependency needs. They are often self centered and feel happy if praised.

Course and Prognosis

Histrionic behaviour is at its peak during youth and early adult life. As the person matures, hysterical behaviour diminishes yet, the core of hysterical personality may persist life long.

Management

These patients are best treated with psychotherapy. The aim is to make them aware of their dependency needs and poor emotional relationships.

Drugs should not be used, as such persons are likely to become dependant.

ANANKASTIC PERSONALITY DISORDER (OBSSESSIVE COMPULSIVE)

This disorder is characterized by perfectionism and inflexibility of behaviour. These patients are orderly and punctual. They feel irritable even if others do not follow their wishes.

Epidemiology

Though its exact prevalence is not known, it appears to be quite common. People with obsessive personality are usually quite successful scientists and executives.

Etiology

The first degree relatives of the probands of obsessive compulsive personality show much higher prevalence of similar personality. This personality is associated with obsessive compulsive disorders and a large number of physical disorders, where psychological factors are associated to, e.g. coronary artery diseases, ulcerative colitis, hypertension, etc.

Clinical Picture

These patients are punctual, orderly and perfectionists. They resent any interference in their routine and become irritable or anxious on any disruption. They like to follow rules upto every comma and fullstop. An nankastic bank clerk has kept each cash memo of purchase because it might be required in his income tax return. Their social relationships are poor. They lack humour and cannot tolerate others who are sloppy or unsystematic. They may exhibit excessive doubts in every activity.

Course and Prognosis

A large number of patients may lead productive life with poor social relationships, others may overcome this emotional constriction and may become better socialised as the age advances. Many may develop depression, psychosomatic disorders and a few may develop schizophrenia.

Diagnosis (I.C.D.-X)

This personality disorder is characterized by :

a) Feeling of excessive doubts and caution ;

b) Preoccupation with details, rules, order, organisation or schedule ;

c) Perfectionism that interferes with task completion ;

d) Excessive conscentiousness, scrupulousness and undue preoccupation with productivity to the exclusion of pleasure and interpersonal relationship;

e) Excessive pedantry and adherence to social conventions ;

f) Rigidity and stubborness ;

g) Unreasonable insistence by the patient that others should submit to exactly his or her way of doing things, or unreasonable reluctance to allow others to do things ;

i) Intrusion of insistent though or impulses.

Any three of the above are required for a definite diagnosis. Obsessive compulsive disorder should be excluded by absence of obsessive thoughts or compulsive acts.

Management

The treatment is done by psychotherapy. Cognitive behaviour therapy is useful. It aims at correcting faulty congnitions.

Drugs like Clomipramine or Fluoxetine can be used in severe cases.

ANXIOUS (AVOIDANT PERSONALITY DISORDER)

This disorder is characterized by pervasive fear of rejection by others and these persons are always apprehensive and anxious about being ridiculed by others. In lay language, they are often called as persons suffering from an inferiority complex.

Epidemiology

It is not exactly known but the condition appears to be quite common.

Etiology

These patients may have had a difficult upbringing. They might have undergone rejection or unwarranted comparison by their parents or relatives. One lady was very frequently called as an ugly duckling as she was not as good looking as her sisters. She had been repeatedly rejected by her mother. She developed a severe personality disorder of anxious personality type.

Clinical Picture

These patients avoid making new relationships due to the fear of rejection. They like having many good relationships but this fear makes them shy or timid. They cannot ask for favours because of the fear of denial. They often fear taking challenging assignment due to fear of failure and ridicule by others. They pass their lives in a secluded corner to avoid hurt of rejection.

Course and Prognosis

This is usually a chronic condition. Most such patients marry and hold jobs but their social interaction is limited to their families or close colleagues. They may develop social phobias and depression.

Diagnosis (I.C.D.-X)

Personality disorder is characterized by :

a) Persistant and pervasive feeling of apprehension ;

b) Belief that one is socially inept, personally unappealing or inferior to others ;

c) Excessive preoccupation with being criticised or rejected in social situations ;

d) Unwillingness to become involved with people unless certain of being liked ;

e) Restriction in life style because of need to have physical security ;

f) Avoidance of social or occupational activities that involve significant interpersonal contact becuase of fear of criticism, disapproval or rejection.

Any three of the above are required for diagnosis.

Management

These patients generally do well with cognitive behaviour therapy. They also develop more self confidence with each success.

If associated symptoms of phobia or depression are present, then Clomipramine or Fluoxetine can be given.

DEPENDANT PERSONALITY DISORDER

This disorder is characterized by the need of the individual to depend on others. They are not able to function alone, they cannot take any decision without being guided by others. This dependency need is so compelling that they may tolerate abuse by the person on whom they depend.

Epidemiology

This is a frequently occurring disorder. The exact prevalence is not known.

Etiology

These patients may show a familial pattern. Environmental factor seem to play an important part. Many of the families encourage strict discipline and independent judgements are frowned upon. Dependency relationship are often encouraged in our country and many adults even by the age of forty may find it difficult to take independent decisions. This type of family constellation may be conducive to the development of such a personality.

Clinical Picture

The patient usually develops a dependant relationship on one or two persons. All his/her decision are taken by them. He may undergo many hardships to please these persons. In case they abandon him, he feels very anxious and depressed. These persons avoid positions of responsibility.

Diagnosis (I.C.D.-X)

This disorder is characterized by :

a) Encouraging or allowing others to make the most of one's important life decision ;

b) Subordination of one's own needs to those of others on whom one is dependant and undue compliance with thier wishes ;

c) Unwillingness to make even reasonable demands on the people one depends on ;

d) Feeling uncomfortable or helpless when alone, because of exaggerated fears of inability to care for oneself ;

e) Preoccupation with fears of being abandoned by a person with whom one has a close relationship and of being left to care for oneself ;

f) The limited capacity to make everyday decisions without an excessive amount of advice and reassurance from others.

Any three of the above are required for the diagnosis.

Dependency can be a feature of hysteric, avoidant and borderline personality disorders. But the other features of these disorders will help in differentiating them from dependant personality disorders.

Manangement

These patients can easily form relationship with the therapist. They have to be helped to come out of the self defeating dependency relationship. Behaviour therapy has been found effective.

Drug can be used for symptomatic relief if depression or anxiety are present.

OTHER SPECIFIC PERSONALITY DISORDERS

PERSONALITY DISORDER UNSPECIFIED

MIXED AND OTHER PERSONALITY DISORDER

This group includes those conditions which show a mixed picture and cannot be put in any category of.

MIXED PERSONALITY DISORDER

These patients show a combination of traits of various personality disorders.

TROUBLESOME PERSONALITY CHANGE

Some patients develop a change in personality in association with depressive or anxiety disorders.

These personality change are often persistant and may cause serious difficulties of adjustment.

ENDURING PERSONALITY CHANGES NOT ATTRIBUTABLE TO BRAIN DAMAGE AND DISEASE

These group of disorders are characterized by a profound and persistant change in behaviour and thinking, following a catastrophic stress or multiple repetitive stresses or following a severe or recurrent disorder. This should not be an unmasking of previous personality disorder by repetitive stresses. The personality change should effect normal day to day functioning and should not be a part of chronic mental illness like schizophrenia or chronic depression. Personality changes occurring after brain injury are included in Organic main disorder.

A common example in history is the personality change of king Ashoka after the Kalinga War, when he gave up all worldly interests and became a follower of Buddhism and abjured all kinds of violence.

ENDURING PERSONALITY CHANGE AFTER CATASTROPHIC EXPERIENCE

Some persons may develop severe personality changes after undergoing a catastrophic experience, e.g. disaster, being tortured, kept hostage by terrorist or dacoits, experiences in concentration camps, etc. These patients may show symptoms of post-traumatic stress disorder for a short period and later show enduring personality change. Personality changes occurring after a short term exposure to stress are not included here because they may simply be caused by unmasking of previous personality.

Epidemiology

It is not clearly known.

Etiology

Exposure to severe catastrophic stress which has profound impact on the individual induces this disorder.

Clinical Picture

A large number of people who undergo this type of stress become 'Sadhus' (Saints or monks). They give up normal worldly connections and decide to spend the rest of their lives in prayers and in service to God and mankind. This may not be called a disorder as this state is egosyntonic and does not produce difficulties for themselves but it definitely effects others.

Case Example

A highly educated senior executive aged around 60 years, developed a kidney problem and the nephrologist advised him that except renal transplant there is no other option left for him. He decided that he will not undergo this operation and spend the rest of his life in prayers and service to god. He went to Rishikesh and joined an Ashram. Unexplicably, his kidney functioning improved. Since that day, he had a profound personality change and he is spending his life in the service of others and God.

On the other hand, these experiences may produce a negative change in the individual and they may become hostile and mistrustful of others. They become hypercritical and find fault with everything. They may withdraw socially and may feel hopeless and demoralized. Such people become a constant source of irritation to themselves and to others.

Diagnosis (I.C.D.-X)

The personality change should be maladaptive leading to impairment in personal and social functionig. This personality change should be confirmed by a key informant. The following are the common features :

This personality change should have persisted for at least 2 years and should not be attributable to any other mental disorders except post traumatic stress disorders:

a) Hostile or mistrustful attitude toward the world

b) Social withdrawal

c) Feelings of emptiness or hopelessness

d) A chronic feeling of being on edge as if constantly threatened

e) Estrangement.

This disorder should only be diagnosed, if the personality change is enduring, maladaptive and is not due to other psychiatric or neurological disorders.

Management

The basic approach to treatment is psychotherapy. These patients have to be helped to develop a trust in the world and not to overemphasize on the uncertainities of life. If severly depressed or anxious, then appropriate medications can be used.

ENDURING PERSONALITY CHANGE AFTER PSYCHIATRIC ILLNESS

A few people may experience a personality change after recovering from a psychiatric illness. This change should not be explained by the previous personality nor should it be explained by residual symptoms of the preexisting mental disorder.

This kind of personality change can occur after repetitive bouts of depression or sometimes after acute psychosis. The patients may develop a negative attitude towards self and may start feeling that life is not what it should be after the experience of mental illness. They may feel that others do not approve of them and may ridicule them because of their mental illness.

Diagnosis (I.C.D.-X)

a) Excessive dependence on and a demanding attitude towards others ;

b) Conviction of being changed or stigmatized by the preceeding illness, leading to an inability to form and maintain close and confiding personal relationship and to social isolation ;

c) Passivity, reduced interest and diminished involvement in leisure activites;

d) Persistant complaints of being ill which may be associated with hypochondriacal claims and illness behaviour ;

e) Dysphoric or labile mood, not due to the presence of a current mental disorder with residual affective symptoms ;

f) Significant impairment in social and occupational functioning compared with premorbid situation.

The above manifestation should have lasted for at least 2 years. They should not be due to brain disease or disorder.

This disorder has to be differentiated from dysthymia or post-psychotic depression.

Management

Psychsotherapy is the treatment of choice. The guidelines are same as disented earlier. In this disorder, the effect of earlier psychiatric disorder has also to be kept in mind.

Drugs may be used for symptomatic relief.

OTHER ENDURING PERSONALITY CHANGES

This include enduring personality change after

bereavement or after chronic pain. Other specific situation which have led to enduring personality changes are also included here.

HABIT AND IMPULSE DISORDERS

This category contains heterogenous group of disorders which may have no relationship with each other. Most of these patients exhibit impulsive behaviour which the patient cannot resist. There may also be a feeling of tension release or enjoyment by doing the act. There may be a feeling of remorse soon after the act.

Pathological Gambling

These patients indulge in repetitive gambling which affects their social, personal and occupational life. The urge to gamble is often irresistible and they may be preoccupied with the ideas and images of gambling situations.

They may sometimes steal money, tell lies or do other criminal acts to fulfil their desire for gambling. This condition should only be diagnosed, when gambling is undertaken for its own sake and not to earn money.

Etiology and Epidemiology

It is not well known. We are witnessing a new phenomena of large number of people buying lottery tickets daily and which is affecting their personal and social life. This may be included in pathological gambling, if it fulfills other criteria.

Diagnostic Features

The essential features of this disorder is persistently repeated gambling which continues and often increases despite adverse social consequences, such as impoverishement, impaired family relationships and disruption of personal life.

Differential Diagnosis — This should be differentiated from :

a) Gambling for excitement and earning money. Such persons give up gambling when confronted with heavy losses.

b) Gambling by manic patient. This is episodic.

c) Gambling by person of dissocial personality, where it is a part of wider sociopathic disturbances.

Management

Psychotherapy is the treatment of choice. One has to delineate the factors responsible for this disorder and alternative sources of pleasure have to be developed. Behaviour therapy have been found useful in some cases.

PATHOLOGICAL FIRE SETTING (PYROMANIA)

This disorder is characterized by repetitive acts of fire setting without any apparent motive. These patients may show excessive interest in looking at fire or fire fighting equipment. Its prevalence and etiology are not clearly known.

Diagnosis (I.C.D.-X)

a) Repeated fire setting without any obvious motive such as monetary gain or political extremism ;

b) An intense interest in watching fire burn ; and

c) Reported feelings of increased tension before the act and intense excitement immediately, after it has been carried out.

Differential Diagnosis — Fire setting can be some times due to political or monetory motives. It can also be seen in patients with conduct disorders, schizophrenia and sometimes in organic brain disorders.

Management

These patients may need institutionalisation or continous watch to avoid repetition of behaviour. Psychotherapy is the treatment of choice.

PATHOLOGICAL STEALING (KLEPTOMANIA)

This disorder is characterized by repetitive episodes of stealing articles which are not of much use to the person. These articles may be given away or hoarded. Many persons may steal objects which may have emotional significance. One patient used to steal knives and forks from every hotel where he has stayed or dined. This kind of stealing behaviour is more often reported in the Western countries, where goods are displayed in the departmental stores and the person has more chances of stealing unnoticed.

Diagnosis (I.C.D.-X)

There is an increasing sense of tension before and a sense of gratification during and immediately after the act. There is some effort at concealment but all the precautions are not observed. The theft is always a solitary act and not carried out with the help of accomplice. The individual may express guilt and regret after an episode but repeats the act again.

Differential Diagnosis — This must be differentiated from shop lifting for monetory gains. These are well planned acts and costly item are stolen and accomplice is usually involved.

Sometimes the patients with organic mental disorders may not pay for their purchase because of poor memory which may be mistaken for shop lifting. Some depressive patients may show repetitive stealing only during the episode of depression.

Management

These patients have to be prevented from repeating such acts by advising them to have someone with them. Psychotherapy may be useful.

TRICHOTILLOMANIA

These patients exhibit patches of baldness on their heads and at times on eyebrows and other parts of the body, which are a result of hair pulling by themselves. These patients usually complain of tension before hair pulling and a sense of relief after the act. Many of these patients show lack of concern about hair loss and show no signs of anxiety or depression about their appearance.

Trichotillomania is quiet a common disorder. Sometime, it can be a symptom of schizophrenia. It is more often seen in girls.

Psychotherapy is often helpful. A few cases respond to pharmacotherapy when schizophrenia or depression are associated.

OTHER HABITS AND IMPULSE DISORDERS

This category is used to identify those condition which fulfil the criteria of impulse disorders and are not classifiable elsewhere.

HABIT AND IMPULSE DISORDER UNSPECIFIED

OTHER DISORDERS OF ADULT PERSONALITY AND BEHAVIOUR

ELABORATION OF PHYSICAL SYMPTOMS FOR PSYCHOLOGICAL REASONS (COMPENSATION NEUROSIS)

This group of disorders is characterized by gross exaggeration of physical symptoms and a complaining attitude towards doctors, nurses or other care givers. The physical symptom which might be due to a physical disorder continue to persist, even after the original disorders has been treated. These patients can develop an attention seeking behaviour and sometimes depression. They usually complain that they are not getting better and may even threaten litigation.

Sometimes, there may be a compensation motive when the disease developed due to accident at work place but often the symptom persists even after litigation has been settled. This disorder, is often seen in histrionic persons but other personalities may be involved. It is not as uncommon as was once thought. It is also important to keep this condition in mind, when a patient is not recovering inspite of appropriate treatment. Such patients are likely to drag the doctors to the courts.

INTENTIONAL PRODUCTION OR FEIGNING OF SYMPTOMS OR DISABILITIES EITHER PHYSICAL OR PSYCHOLOGICAL (FACTITIOUS DISORDER) (MUNCHAUSENS SYNDROME)

These individuals feign physical and psychological symptoms and their basic motive seems to get hospitalised. They may even inflict injury to themselves or may take drugs which can produce symptoms. They usually do not have any external motive which differentiate them from malingerers.

Epidemiology

The exact prevalence of this disorder is not known. In some western hospitals quite a few such cases get admitted. It is just possible that hospital admission in India may not be a desirable motive because most of the hospitals are not that comfortable, where one would like to get admitted. Yet, such patients are quite consistently seen in India also.

Etiology

It is not clearly understood. These patients seem to have wish to assume a sick role and be cared by others. There are usually no external incentives. It is postulated that some of these patients may have had very satisfying experience with doctors while they were children and they long to get a similar care. The family atmosphere is often of emotional neglect.

Clinical Features

These patients may present either with physical symptoms or with psychological symptoms and sometimes with both.

They usually develop a good knowledge of hospitals, medicines and diseases. They may present with symptoms of any physical disease. Their history will be quiet convincing and this can decieve even expert clinicians in admitting them into a hospital. They may even get operated repeatedly because of which their abdomen may look like grid iron due to multiple scars. When a doctor or hospital refuses them for treatment, they will go to another doctor and get admitted. They often feign acute illnesses which helps them to get admitted quickly.

Psychological illness can also be feigned. These patients may present with psychotic symptoms, depressive symptoms or suicidal attempts. They often give a very convincing history and may gain admission.

Case Example

An 18 year old girl was referred from a T.B. hospital for psychiatric opinion. She was admitted there with a history of hemoptysis. She had been earlier treated for Tuberculosis. The investigations did not reveal any positive findings and the hemoptysis was caused by a deliberate injury in the throat.

This young girl had been sick off and on from the last six years. She belonged to a middle class family. She had 3 male sibs. The family had got so fed up with her that they did not care much for her and seldom visited her in the hospital. She was treated with psychotherapy. She got herself discharged after a week. She never came for a follow-up thereafter.

Comments

This patient was producing deliberate hemoptysis so that she may be considered sick. She was taking all the antitubercular medications which would only harm her. There was no external motivations. Her family situation was quiet rejecting.

Course and Prognosis

The prognosis of this condition is not well known. The disorder appears to be chronic and it is possible that repeated medications and surgical procedure will shorten their life and some may die due to repetitive medication.

Diagnosis (I.C.D.-X)

The following are required for a firm diagnosis :

a) The individual feigns physical and/or psychological symptoms consistently. There is no evidence of any physical or psychological diseases ;

b) The patient will give a history of repeated consultation and/or hospitalization ;

c) They should have undergone many investigations and treatment ;

d) There is no evidence of any physical or psychological illness ;

e) There are no external motivating factors.

This disorder should be differentiated from :

a) Malingering — Malingering is always resorted to; to avoid certain situation or to obtain some advantages. People may malinger to avoid court appearances or to avoid punishment. Some may feign memory loss to avoid being punished. Patients with factitious disorders do not have any such difficulty.

Somatoform Disorders — These disorders do not exhibit deliberate production of symptoms as seen in factitious disorders. They will not deliberately injure themselves or take drugs to produce symptoms.

Management

No definite guidelines are available. These patients should not be rejected or thrown out of the hospital but they may be encouraged to keep in contact with the hospital and helped to adapt to external world. Their need for psychological support may be fulfilled.

CHAPTER 12
HUMAN SEXUALITY

Sexuality is essential for reproduction and preservation of species. All primates are blessed with innate sexual response so that they can produce offsprings. The sexual behaviour is species is specific and follows a biologically determined developmental sequence. Sexual behaviour in human beings has been influenced by culture and civilisation. Each culture has developed specific 'do's and don'ts' about sex, as to when, with whom, in what situation and with what frequency one can have sex. Most of these 'do's and don'ts' have become parts of moral codes and have also been given legal support. These social restraints have affected human sexuality to a large extent.

Biological, psychological and social factors are closely interwoven in sexual behaviour. Any alteration in either of the three can produce sexual disturbances.

RELIGION AND SEX

Almost all religions of the world condemn excessive sexual indulgence and prescribe sexual codes which have usually become part of an individual's psyche and act as internal censors. Hinduism exhibits a highly ambivalent attitude towards sex. Sex is permitted only during grihasth stage (householder) that is between 25-50 years. The main aim of sex is procreation. The pleasure aspect of sex is underplayed. On the other hand, temple sculptures of Khajuraho and Konark exhibit all varieties of sexual activities on the walls of the temples. Some of these temples even today are important places of pilgrimage for the Hindus. It appears that sex during the period when these temples were built, was neither considered sinful nor dirty but was considered an important and beautiful part of human existence. One of the oldest treaties on sex is Vatsayan's Kama Sutra which very clearly describes all kinds of sexual activities, sexual problems and their cures. Thus sex, amongst the Hindus, had been considered as a desired activity which could be perfected to a fine art. However, this concept of sexuality somehow has now become riddled with dogmas and superstitions and sex has became a desirable but dangerous activity.

Christianity, on the other hand, had much more condemning attitude towards sex. All sexual indulgences were considered sinful and it was thought that if one cannot control sexual desires then it was better to marry than to burn in sin. However, recently the church is also showing a significant change in its attitude towards sex.

PSYCHOSEXUAL DEVELOPMENT

Foetal Life

Every foetus is basically female and its growth as a male is dependant on the availability of foetal androgen from 6 to 12 weeks of intra uterine life. Androgen administration to a mother can effect the development of a female child and such a child may develop male external genitalia with ovaries.

Infancy and Childhood — Early sexual exploration of the body starts during infancy. The child accidentaly touches genitals and once this touch gives him pleasure, he tends to repeat the act. This infantile genital exploration is a normal step in psychosexual growth. If children do not get any other stimulation or pleasure they may derive pleasure only by self stimulation. Such stimulation may lead to abnormal development.

Gender Identity

Genitalia, internal sex organs and hormonal profile are the basis of sexual identity. Usually, most children accept their sexual identity and accept their maleness and femaleness. In some cases, the child may not be partially or fully able to accept their sexual identity. In extreme forms it may result into Transsexualism. These persons feel that they have been born with the wrong sex and they consult doctors for sex change operations.

Gender Role

Each culture prescribes male and female roles. Part of the male and female behaviour is innately determined and the rest is culturally conditioned. Males are supposed to be muscular, aggressive, take part in masculine games and dress in a particular manner. Similarly, females are expected to be more passive, to have interest in female games and dress in appropriate clothes. Most people have congruous sexual identity, gender identity and gender role, but a few may not. A female child, may consider herself female but may take on male gender role, while other females may have male gender identity but may follow a female gender role.

In most of the individuals, the infantile sexual

touching gives way to preadolescent sexual behaviour which may include genital caressing. Preadolescent sexual play may include masturbation without sexual fantasy.

Masturbation

This is a predominant sexual activity in boys during adolescence. Masturbation in this age is associated with heterosexual fantasy. This is an acceptable libidinous discharge mechanism. The adolescent is fully developed for heterosexual coitus but most societies do not permit sex at this age; so masturbation is often practised. The individual can explore his sexuality without any fear during masturbation. In most societies, masturbation is considered sinful and harmful and is also considered to be the harbinger for many future maladies like physical weakness, impotence and madness. This view is not at all based on scientific facts. However, when masturbation becomes the sole source of sexual gratification and leads to avoidance of heterosexual desire or contact, then it has to be considered abnormal. Masturbation usually persists throughout life and people often masturbate whenever a sexual partner is not available or when heterosexual relationships are not satisfying.

Homosexual Relationship

Quite a few adolescent boys do develop transitory homosexual relationships. Masturbation may be taught by one boy to another and may lead to mutual masturbation. There may also be homosexual sex contact in normal boys which may last for a short time. This is not abnormal and is part of normal sexual development.

Sexual developments in girls takes a slightly different course. Genital touching may be completely given up by five to six years of age. Later, they may have few or no sexual thoughts or activities till pubertal years. During the pre-pubertal years more emphasis is placed on the development of the body, breasts and physical appearance. Female masturbation is not as common as male masturbation. Kinsey reported that about 3/4th of all women masturbated. In a few studies done in India, the rate of female masturbation was hardly 10% - 15%. This could be a manifestation of cultural differences. In the western culture, sexual behaviour is encouraged in adolescence. Most people go out on dates which arouses the females and may lead to masturbation. The general atmosphere in schools in the West is also more sexually permissive while in India the females are specially taught to avoid all sexual talks or contacts. Virginity is highly prized and the girls are taught that this is the best gift they can offer to their husbands. All these attitudes suppress masturbatory behaviour in females. It also appears plausible that the female sexuality is different from male sexuality. Male sexual desire seems to force him to obtain an outlet. The females sexuality needs fulfillment only when aroused either by external or internal cues. Female sexuality does not by itself force the individual to seek a sexual discharge.

Sexual Behaviour in Marriage

Sexual needs of the couple widely differ. There can be few who require many sexual outlets per day while others may require sex only once a week or even less.

Female sexual requirement have not been well studied. There are no doubt different grades of sexual requirements in females. Females in their youth can enjoy a large number of sex acts/day. The sexual demands decrease substantially with age and many females complain of excessive sexual needs of their husbands. They could however enjoy sex tremendously when they were relaxed and in a happy mood. This also tends to confirm our earlier hypothesis that female sexuality is different from male sexuality and they are capable of enjoying sex to any extent provided. They are physically and mentally satisfied and find the partner desirable.

HUMAN SEXUAL RESPONSE CYCLE

It is only in the last three decades that the human sexual response has been adequately studied. Masters and Johnson studied the physiology of human sexual response. Psychiatrists divide the human response cycle into the following :

Phase 1 Appetitive
Phase 2 Excitement
Phase 3 Orgasm
Phase 4 Resolution

Phase 1 : Appetitive

This phase sets the sexual cycle in motion. In this phase the person develops a desire for sex and may have sexual fantasies.

Phase 2 : Excitement

This phase is brought about by fantasization or by actual contact with desired object by kissing, touching and stroking. It continues into coitus or masturbatory behaviour. The physiological changes that occur in this phase are as follows :

In Males — It leads to penile erection, testes increase in size and are lifted up, 2 to 3 drops of mucoid fluid is secreted from cowper's glands which contains viable sperms, (this may lead to pregnancy even without ejaculation) skin may show maculopapular rash on chest or neck. There could also be mytonia of facial and abdominal muscles. The heart rate may go upto 160/minute, blood pressure increases by 20-40 mm of Hg. The respiratory rate increases. The phase usually lasts for 30 secs. to 3 minutes.

Orgasmic Phase — It is characterized by seminal ejaculation in 3 to 5 spurts at an interval of.8 sec. In this phase the heart rate and blood pressure are further increased. Rectal sphincter also shows rhythmic contractions. There is also an intense feeling of enjoyment.

Resolution Phase — During this phase the body reverts back to the resting phase. The resolution may be completed in 10 - 15 minutes if orgasm has taken place but may take many hours if orgasm was not achieved. Erection is maintained for some time even after ejaculation during the younger age but may be lost quickly as age advances. All other bodily changes gradually subside. All men show a refractory phase after ejaculation during which a second excitement cannot occur. This refractory phase may last for minutes in the young but increases in duration with advancing age. People at the age of seventy may not have a second erection for one week or more.

FEMALE SEXUAL RESPONSE CYCLE

Excitement Phase — It may last from several minutes to several hours but heightened excitement prior to orgasm may last from 30 secs. to 3 minutes. The major physiological changes are :

Labia major becomes elevated and flattened in nullipara and becomes congested and edematus in multipara. Labia minora increases in size and the colour may change to deep red. Clitoris gets swollen and just before orgasm shaft retracts into prepuce. Vagina becomes swollen and elongated. A transudate appears within 10 to 30 secs. of arousal. Lower third of vagina develops orgasmic platform and contracts just before orgasm. Uterus lifts into false pelvis and uterine contractions start occurring before orgasm.

Breast enlarges in size, nipples become erect. Skin may show maculopapular rash on abdomen and breast. Blood pressure and heart rate increases.

Orgasm

During orgasm lower third of vagina develops 3 - 5 contraction at an interval of 8 secs. The contraction of external sphincter also occurs. The uterus shows labour like contractions.

There will usually be hyperventilation and further rise in heart rate and blood pressure. There is an intense feeling of pleasure.

Resolution

All bodily organs return to resting stage in 10 - 15 minutes if orgasm has taken place other wise it may take much longer. Females do not show refractory phase and can have multiple orgasms.

Frequency of Coitus

In average marriages, the frequency of coitus may range from 1-2 coitus per day during the first few months of marriage and later settles down to one coitus/day. After a few years of marriage it may be reduced to alternate days to twice a week which may continue till around 45 years when the frequency further decreases.

COMMON SEXUAL ANXIETIES

Males

Size and shape of penis : A large number of adolescents are worried about the size and shape of their penis. The average length of the penis ranges from 8-12 cms. A few people may have a very small penis in flaccid state while others may have a much bigger flaccid penis. Smaller flaccid penis enlarges much more on erection and after erection most penis will be in the normal range.

An erect penis in young male makes a 45 degree angle with stomach but with advancing age this angle may increase. Slight curve of penis to either side is immaterial.

Thickness of Semen

Many persons worry that their semen has become thin due to excessive ejaculations. The consistency of semen does not affect sexuality or the procreation ability.

Duration of Intercourse

Many people worry about for early ejaculation. While it is a problem in a few, the majority of times this anxiety is based on false expectations, that the sexual act should last for hours. Average duration ranges from 30 secs. to 3 minutes.

Female Sexual Anxieties

They are worried about physical appearance,
Shape of their breasts,
Their ability to respond sexually to their partner,
Their ability to have orgasm,
Their ability to conceive,
Fear of pain during intercourse, and
Fear of pain of childbirth.

SEXUAL DISTURBANCES

These have been included in the following sections of I.C.D.-X classification :

a) Sexual dysfunction, not caused by organic disorder,

b) Gender identity disorder,

c) Disorders of sexual preference,

d) Psychological and behavioural disorders associated with sexual development and orientation.

These disorders will be described in their developmental sequence.

PSYCHOLOGICAL AND BEHAVIOURAL DISORDERS ASSOCIATED WITH SEXUAL DEVELOPMENT AND ORIENTATION

This group includes those disorders where sexual orientation which can be either heterosexual, homosexual or bisexual leads to disturbances either for the individual or in the relationship. Any type of orientation by itself, whether it is homosexual or bisexual, if it does not produce intra or interpersonal problems, is not considered a disorder.

SEXUAL MATURATION DISORDER

These individuals are not certain whether they are homosexuals, hetrosexuals or bisexuals. This uncertainity can cause severe anxiety. It can also be sometime seen in individuals who after a prolonged relationship feel that their sexual preference is changing.

Quite often, this situation arises out of ignorance when a casual homosexual relationship may be considered to be the result of homosexual orientation. Sometimes an unsatisfactory relationship may be misinterpreted as being caused by a wrong orientation.

Management

The patient is helped to identify his natural orientation and his anxiety is thus reduced.

EGODYSTONIC SEXUAL ORIENTATION

In this situation, the patient does not accept his sexual orientation and may wish to be different. This is commonly seen in homosexuality.

Homosexuality connates sexual attraction for the same sex partner. (male to male, female to female). Female homosexuality is also called lesbianism.

The American Psychiatric Association has excluded homosexuality from the list of sexual disorders because it was thought that a small group of people develop different sexual orientation and it is in no way abnormal and a majority of them do not seek treatment.

Homosexuals who seek treatment are also called egodystonic homosexuals. They are not able to accept their homosexuality. Usually most of this discomfort disappears with time.

Epidemiology

Homosexuality is seen in around 4% of men and 2% of women. Another five to ten percent may show bisexual orientation.

Etiology

Homosexuality may have a genetic basis. Monozygotic twins show a high concordance rate. Sexual preference is dependant on foetal hormones and it is presumed that some disturbances occur at that time to produce homosexual behaviour. Homosexuals have not shown any consistent pattern of hormonal disturbances so far. A few studies have shown that they have lower testoserone levels than heterosexuals.

Many psychological theories were earlier postulated but none could be generally validated. Environmental factors may play some part. Non-availability of heterosexual partners, critical and censoring attitude of the females may to some extent be responsible for its development. But all these speculations have not been proved.

Clinical Picture

Homosexual behaviour starts appearing in early adolescence. These boys and girls like the company of the same sex. Their masturbatory fantasies and dreams will also show homosexual contents.

Homosexuality is socially unacceptable in India and most homosexuals have to develop celandestine relationships due to which their life becomes very restricted. They like to choose work where members of the same sex will be available (like school teachers). They also avoid positions of responsibility where the behaviour may be closely scrutinised.

Some homosexuals are forcibly married by their parents and this leads to relationship difficulties.

Manangement

Some homosexuals request treatment because they feel that this orientation is a hurdle in their advancement. One young intern approached for treatment of homosexuality because he felt uncomfortable treating or examining young boys. He was treated with aversion therapy. He showed good response. Many times wives bring their husbands for treatment of homosexuality which seldom suceeds. The patient's motivation is the prime factor in the therapy.

SEXUAL RELATIONSHIP DISORDER

This includes those situations when sexual preference is responsible for difficulties in maintaining a relationship with a partner.

This situation often arises when a homosexual is forced to marry a member of the opposite sex.

A 32-year old lady was brought for marital problems because she did not permit her husband to have sex because of her homosexual orientation. She submitted for sex in the initial one year of marriage and also gave birth to a child. She complained that each sex act was emotionally painfully and equalled them to rape. She later developed a homosexual relationship. The couple could not be helped as the wife did not agree for treatment for her homosexual tendencies.

GENDER IDENTITY DISORDER

These persons do not except their gender identity and wish to be different. Common disorder in this group is Transvestism.

TRANSVESTISM

These persons do not accept their autonomical sex and desire sex change operation to the opposite sex. They usually wear the clothes of the opposite sex and also use the same gender in their talks. This desire becomes manifest in early adolescence.

Many of these patients undego operative treatment for getting their sex changed but the results are equivocal.

DISORDERS OF SEXUAL PREFERENCE (PARAPHILIAS)

This group of disorders are characterized by some repetitive acts or fantasies which become more important for the person than the sexual act itself. These wishes are repetitive in nature and may often bring the person in conflict with law or society.

Epidemiology

These are rare disorders. But the individual repeats these acts so often that the incidents become numerous and that is why they attract public attention.

Etiology

Such individuals might have been sexually assaulted as a child which may have lead to an alteration in sexual preference. Sometimes earlier sexual acts or fantasies of particular object or action may have been experienced as pleasurable which later becomes essential for sexual arousal. Pornographic literature also seems to reinforce such behaviour and may also provide experimental models. Masochism and sadism are seldom seen in India and Indian poronographic literature also does not describe them. Organic factors have been studied but nothing has been clearly identified. Major areas of study are hormonal profiles, minor neurological abnormalities, E.E.G. defects, etc.

FETISHISM

Fetishes are inanimate objects which are essential for sexual arousal and gratification. Fetish objects are usually women's clothing (underwears, bras and shoes). Other articles like a rubber clothing, etc. may also be preferred.

Fetishism is only diagnosed if object of fetish is essential and of paramount importance for sexual gratification. Use of certain objects to enhance sexual pleasure will not be diagnosed as fetishism.

FETISHISTIC TRANSVESTISM

These persons attain sexual arousal by dressing in the clothes of opposite sex. They should be differentiated from transvestism where an individual feels that he has the wrong sex and they dress in clothes of the opposite sexes. This cross dressing is to fulfil their desire to belong to that sex. This cross dressing is not sexually arousing. Fetishistic transvestism may not create any problem if the spouse can acccept it.

EXHIBITIONISM

These patients have a persitent tendency to exhibit there genitalias to member of opposite sex or in public places. There is usually but not invariably a sexual excitement at the time of committing the act which is followed by masturbation.

Exhibitionism is only seen in males. They are generally hetero-sexual. It is often seen in elderly males who do not have regular sex partners. A few exhibitionists may feel distressed by their exhibitonistic behaviour.

VOYEURISM

This is characterized by a repetitive tendency, to peep at people engaged in sex act or naked females. This act is done in secrecy and the persons looked at are not aware of it. It is usually followed by masturbation.

PAEDOPHILIA

This is characterized by sexual preferences for pre-adolescent girls or boys. This disorder is also generally seen in man. Adolescent boys having sexual relations with preadolescent aged boys or girls are not included. Paedophilics often indulge in oral sex or caressing.

This is a common disorder and it is estimated that 10 - 20% young girls are sexually molested by paedophilic men. It is common in our country also, where domestic servants, drivers, rickshaw pullers and elderly males in the house may be involved in such a behaviour. Often such cases are not brought to the notice of the police because the families wish to avoid disgrace. Incest, though not included under pedophilia, is closely related to it.

SADOMASOCHISM

These persons get sexual arousal either by inflicting pain, torture or humilation on the partner or by getting these inflicted on them. Mild pain produced by teeth bites or pinching is normally used to heighten arousal and should not be considered abnormal.

The pain and torture is usually excessive, e.g. beating by hunters, piercing parts of the body, etc. This may even sometimes lead to death. Such cases have not been reported in India.

MULTIPLE DISORDERS OF SEXUAL PREFERENCE

Quiet a few paraphilics may have multiple paraphilias. They are to be classified here. The most common combination is fetishism and sadomasochism.

OTHER DISORDERS OF SEXUAL PREFERENCE

There are a large number of disorders of sexual preference which are quiet uncommon. They can be coded here : Frotteurism is charaterized by rubbing ones genitalia against the back of other persons in crowded places. Simlarly, there could be many other specific paraphilias.

Management

Most of these patients have to be treated when they come in conflict with the law. They are usually not cooperative. The cooperative patients can be treated with behavioural therapy. Psychotherapy is the treatment of choice.

SEXUAL DYSFUNCTION NOT CAUSED BY ORGANIC DISORDER OR DISEASE

This group of disorder covers all those difficulties which an individual may face while participating in a sexual relationship. The disorders in this category are classified according to the sexual response cycle. E.g. lack of desire, failure of excitement phase or failure of orgasmic phase.

Though this group is called non-organic but because the sexual response is psychophysiological in nature, it may often be difficult to precisely identify whether the problem is primarily psychological or biological.

Though these disorders have been sub-categorised according to disturbances in sexual response cycle many patients may exhibit more than one disturbance. Men with premature ejaculation often develop erectile impotence. Women with orgasmic difficulty may find all aspects of love making distasteful.

LACK OR LOSS OF SEXUAL DESIRE (FRIGIDITY-HYPOACTIVE SEXUAL DESIRE)

This is characterized by deficiency or lack of sexual desire or activity. These persons lack desire but may be able to enjoy sex when it happens.

Epidemiology — No reliable estimates are available. It is said to be present in about 10% of the population. It is many times more common in females then males. It's prevalence increases with age.

Etiology — The problem could be caused by biological or psychological factors :

Biological :

Hypogonadism.

Hyper prolactinaemia.

Chronic debilitating diseases.

Antihypertensive drugs.

Psychological :

Psychological factors play an important role in causing of hypoactive sex desire.

Marital disharmony.
Fear of pregnancy.
Undesirable partner.
Tiredness and exhaustion.
Unsatisfactory sexual experiences
(Premature ejaculation in males).

Clinical Picture

Few men complain of hypoactive sexual desire. This could be either seen in primary/secondary hypogonadism or in old age. Men continue to have sexual desires inspite of various sexual or interpersonal difficulties. Females on the other hand commonly present with hypoactive sexual desires.

Diagnosis

This condition should be diagnosed keeping in mind the normal range of sexual desires. Few people may need very infrequent sex. It is essential to demonstrate that sexual desire has decreased from the baseline.

Females in Indian are encouraged to supress their sexuality. Therefore, many women may not complain of personal distress but the distress will be felt by the husband.

Course and Prognosis

Most of the psychologically produced symptoms of lack of sexual desire fluctuates with psychological situation and they may improve when psychological distress is less.

SEXUAL AVERSION AND LACK OF SEXUAL ENJOYMENT

SEXUAL AVERSION

The prospect of sexual interaction is associated with strong negative feelings and produces sufficient fear or anxiety and sexual activity is avoided.

This situation is usually a resultant of either primary fear of sexuality which could have arisen after hearing negative experiences of others or by sexual molestation in childhood or due to culturally induced negative attitudes about sexuality.

It can also arise because of earlier painful or unsatisfactory sexual experiences.

LACK OF SEXUAL ENJOYMENT

The sexual response occurs normally including orgasm but they do not experience psychological pleasure.

This condition arises primarily due to psychological inhibition when inspite of normal physiological functioning the psychic component is suppressed. It is seen more often in females but can occur in males also.

A twenty eight year old man consulted for inability to enjoy sex. The couple were married two years ago. A year ago he came to know that his wife had a premarital relationship with someone. The wife also accepted the relationship. Later the husband started suspecting that the relationship might still continue. At this point he lost pleasure in sex. He had normal erection and ejaculation but did not feel any pleasure which was experienced as painful by him.

FAILURE OF GENITAL RESPONSE

This condition is characterised by failure of erection in men and absence of lubrication response in women. Very few women complain of dryness of vagina except in post-menopausal phase.

Epidemiology

Male erectile dysfunction (impotence) is a common disorder. Primary impotence (never able to obtain erection sufficient for penetration of vagina or completion of sex act) is quiet rare and seen in less than 1% of the population. Secondary impotence is quiet common and its prevalence is around 10%.

Incidence of impotence increases with age and at about 70 - 80 years nearly 75% persons are impotent. However, those man who have regular sex may not loose their potency for a very long time.

Etiology

This disorder can be caused by organic or psychological factors and usually by a combination of both.

The following diseases can cause erectile dysfunction :

Infections
Filariasis
Mumps
Cardiovascular diseases
Atherosclerosis
Cardiac failure
Renal and urological diseases
Peyronie's disease
Chronic renal failure
Cirrhosis of liver
Kline-Felter's Syndrome
Diabetes Mellitus

Other endocrinal disorders effecting Pituitary-thyroid-adrenal- gonad axis

Any disease affecting the spinal cord and nerves supplying the penis.

Drugs :

Alcohol, opioids

Psychotropic drugs

Anti depressants

Antihypertensives

Estrogens

Anti-androgens

Surgical Procedcure, e.g. prostatectomy

Radical surgery in pelvic area

Traumatic Pelvic fracture

Psychiatric disorders :

Depression

Schizophrenia

Anxiety

Psychological factors :

Following are some of the major psychological factors which may affect erectile functions :

Fear of sexual inadequacy

Ignorance about sex and its physiology

Anxieties about size and shape of penis

Guilt about masturbation or nocturnal ejaculation or adolescent sexual practices

Marital disharmony

Anxiety about performance

Failure in the sexual act either due to anxiety or fear

Anxiety generated by premature ejaculation

Marked anxiety due to any cause

Hostility towards spouse.

Clinical Picture

These patients present with a difficulty to obtain erection during heterosexual coitus or inability to maintain erection till satisfactory completion of coitus. These patients are usually very anxious and depressed. They often express suicidal intents and may even attempt suicide.

Diagnostic Features

Repeated and peristent difficulty in obtaining erection during sexual intercourse or inability to maintain erection during the course of coitus. Occasional difficulties in obtaining erection are universal and should not be considered abnormal. The effect of age and physical health must also be kept in mind.

Many persons in their 50's or 60's presented with erectile difficulties because they cannot obtain erection as frequently as they used to have earlier. If they are able to have good erection after a suitable time period they should not be labelled as impotent.

Differential Diagnosis

Organic impotence should be differentiated from psychological impotence.

Psychological impotence (non-organic)	Organic impotence
Onset is usually acute	insidious (acute in traumatic impotence)
There could be morning erections and erection with masturbation	Erection is uniformly affected
Nocturnal penile tumuscence is usually present (N.P.T.)	Lost

FEMALE SEXUAL AROUSAL DISORDER

Though not many females complain of difficulties in arousal because it is often presented as hypoactive sexual disorder or aversion from sex yet various studies show that this disorder is quite common. Quite a few women loose sexual excitement during coitus. Hormonal factors may play a role but usually psychological factors are predominant. Any distraction during the sexual act may distract attention from sex and may lead to loosing of excitement. Marital difficulties and other psychological problems described earlier may also be contributory.

ORGASMIC DYSFUNCTION

In this condition, orgasm either does not occur or is too much delayed. This disorder is much more common in females. In males it is called retarded ejaculation which is quite uncommon.

Epidemiology

Inhibited female orgasm is quite a common condition. Primary anorgasmia (the female never had an orgasm) is infrequent. Various studies have shown that it's prevalence is around 5%. Secondory anorgasmia is much more common specially in the West. Nearly 50% of the sexual problems in females are comprised of difficulty or inablility to reach orgasm. It appears to be equally frequent in India though this is not a common complaint. It appears that due to cultural pressures most of the nonorgasmic women do not ask for help. This symptom is often hidden behind the mask of other somatic symptoms like headache, aches and pains of body, sleeplessness and dissociative symptoms.

,Etiology

Anorgasmia could be caused by endocrinal disorders like hypothyroidism, Diabetes mellitus and hyperprolactinaemia. Antihypertensives medications like propranolol, atenolol, antidepressants like fluoxetine and imipramine can affect the women's orgasmic capacities. Psychological problems have been described earlier.

Clinical Features

The patient should clearly present the difficulty in achieving orgasm inspite of adequate sexual excitement and adequate duration of sexual intercourse. This disability should present repetitively for a suffficient period of time. One will usually require interviewing skills for obtaining this information because most of our female patients avoid talking about sex or feel inhibited.

Once they are convinced that the doctor is trying to understand their problems, then they usually express themselves clearly.

Diagnosis

Repeated and persistent anorgasmia inspite of adequate sexual stimulation (consider the age and physical health also).

INHIBITED MALE ORGASM

This is a rare condition. This is characterised by the men's inability or difficulty to ejaculate in heterosexual coitus. A few may have primary problems when they have never been able to ejaculate in coitus while others who develop it after normal functioning are called secondary.

These patients are able to achieve ejaculation by masturbation or in nocturnal ejaculation.

Epidemiology — It is quite rare.

Etiology — It may occur after prostatic surgery when ejaculation may occur into bladder. It should not really be called retarded ejaculation because the ejaculation is occurring normally, but due to sphincteric disturbances it is occurring in bladder.

Drugs such as methyldopa, fluoxetine, tricyclic antidepressants and phenothiazines can cause retarded ejaculation.

Psychologically this may reflect the patients fear and hostility towards females. It may also result from marital conflicts. This problem is more common in obsessive compulsive individuals.

Clinical Picture and Diagnostic Guidelines

These paitents are unable to ejaculate during coitus or may take a very long time in ejaculation. This should be persistent and should not be a part of other pscyhiatric disturbances.

PREMATURE EJACULATION

This is characterised by ejaculation either before penile entry into vagina or soon after penetration. It has been defined in various ways ; few workers opined that if the person feels that the duration of sexual contact is too short then it should be called premature ejaculation. Masters and Johnson defined it as the inability of the male to control ejaculation to satisfy his partner in at least 50% of coitus. This definition presumes that the woman is a normal or a quick responder. However, for clinical purpose one can consider a person premature ejaculator if he ejaculates either prior to entry into vagina or soon after penetration.(within 30 secs. to 1 min.)

Epidemiology — This is a fairly common disorder. Premature ejaculation is the commonest complaint in sex clinics in India. In a general population survey this disorder is seen in around 15% to 20% of the population.

Etiology — Premature ejaculation is basically considered to be due to anxiety or due to faulty conditioning during adolescence by masturbation or quick sex. The author believes that quickness of ejaculation or delayed ejaculation may also have a constitutional determinant.

Clinical Picture and Diagnosis — The diagnosis is made on the complaint of repeated and persistent ejaculation either before entry into vagina or soon after penetration. One must consider the age, novelty of sex partner, and frequency of coitus before making diagnosis as all of these situations can effect dura-tion of coitus.

NON-ORGANIC VAGINISMUS

This is characterized by spasm of muscles that surround the vagina causing occlusion of the vaginal opening. Penile entry is either impossible or painful. Many women may also adduct their thighs at the time of coitus which makes penile entry impossible.

If this disorder is due to local painful condition then it should not be included here. The treatment of the local pathology will remove the difficulties in coitus.

This disorder is generally due to psychological reasons. The most prominent being the fear of damage and hurt by penile penetration. Other psychological factors enumerated earlier may also play a role.

The condition usually leads to non-consummation of marriage.

Diagnosis — The patient will not allow penile entry or may find it very painful. It may sometimes be difficult to differentiate it from situations when a woman completely rejects her husband or male partner and does not allow him to come near her. In typical vaginismus, the patient shoud be willing for sex but would find it impossssible to allow penile penetration due to pain or difficulty in penetration.

NON ORGANIC DYSPAREUNIA — This condition is characterized by pain during coitus. This can occur both in men and women. Local painful conditions in female and peyronie's disease in male should be excluded. Some time dyspareunia can also occur due to prolonged coitus.

For the diagnosis of non-organic dyspareunia all the above condition should be excluded. The pain shoud be repetitive and persistent.

EXCESSIVE SEXUAL DRIVE - Some men and women may complain of excessive sexual desire which may be uncontrollable. This increase in desire should not be due to drug intake (intoxicants) mania or dementia.

OTHER SEXUAL DYSFUNCTIONS, NOT CAUSED BY ORGANIC DISORDER OR DISEASE

Conditions which do not fulfil the criteria of disorders described above can be coded here.

INVESTIGATIONS IN MALE SEXUAL DYSFUNCTIONS

There is no substitute for a good and comprehensive clinical history which not only is of crucial significance in establishing the etiology but also helps in avoiding unnecessary, expensive time consuming investigations.

Pointers towards psychogenic origin in history are :

1. Situational or sporadic dysfunction
2. Acute onset
3. Presence of morning erections, nocturnal penile tumuscence, erection with masturbation
4. Presence of psychiatric symptoms preceeding dysfunction.

However, there are exceptions to these indicators. A person with a marginal penile vascular supply mat at times be able to attain and sustain erections or may have occasional morning erections. Physically caused dyspareunia may occur only in certain coital positions and not in others. Psychiatric symptoms and organic dysfunction can occur independently and concurrently.

Management

ALL MEDICATIONS (INCLUDING SUBSTANCES OF ABUSE) HAVE TO BE DISCONTINUED AND PATIENT EVALUATED AGAIN AFTER 3 — 4 WEEKS OF DRUG-FREE PERIOD

RECOMMENDED INVESTIGATIONS FOR SPECIFIED DYSFUNCTIONS

These investigations are not a battery of investigations to be invariably done in each and every case of male sexual dysfunction. They just represent a total armamentarium of tests from which appropriate specific tests are selected as and when indicated by the short-listed differential diagnosis history arrived at after careful screening from clinical history and examination. Only in a few patients in which the picture is very confused, a more comprehensive testing needs to be done.

I. INVESTIGATIONS FOR HYPOACTIVE SEXUAL DESIRE DYSFUNCTION

A) Biochemical Profile :

1. Blood sugar, Glucose tolerance test
2. Liver Function Tests
3. Thyroid Function Tests
4. Renal Function Tests.

b) Hormonal Profile :

1. Prolactin
2. Testosterone (Free and Bound)
3. Oestrogen
4. Leutinizing Hormone (LH)
5. Follicle stimulating hormone (FSH)
6. Cortisol.

II. **Investigations for Erectile Dysfunction**

A) Hormonal Profile :

1. Prolactin

2. Testosterone, free and bound
3. LH
4. FSH.

(Nocturnal Penils Tumescence)

There should be at least 3 — 4 episodes of tumescence lasting at least 15-20 minutes and showing an elevation of at least 20 units above baseline in the entire night. If NPT repeatedly shows abnormal results, then Ancillary Tests are indicated to elicit the exact derangements in the neurovascular erectile responses mechanism.

1. **Neurological :**

a) For somatic nerve dysfunction

Bulbo cavernosus and Ischio cavernosus reflex latency,

b) For autonomic nervous dysfunction

Prostrate urethra stimulation-response recording,

(Systemic ANS dysfunction such as heart beat-to-beat variability in deep breathing may also provide clues when systemic ANS involvement is present).

c) For sensory deficit - Penile sensory threshold recording,

d) For integrity of cerebral spinal cord neural circuits,

2. **Vascular :**

a) For penile pulse pressure and blood flow in dorsal and cavernosal arteries

Doppler's Examination at rest and after exercise to test for 'steal' (leading to loss of erection during thrusting)

b) For vascular efficiency

Diagnostic Intracavernosal Vasoactive Injection testing

c) Invasive tests

(i) Arteriography when stenosis is suspected and surgery is contemplated.

(ii) Cavernography when abnormal venous leakage is suspected.

INVESTIGATIONS FOR PREMATURE EJACULATION

None except expressed prostatic fluid examination when prostatis is suspected.

INVESTIGATIONS FOR RETARDED EJACULATION

Testing for local as well as systemic autonomic nervous system dysfunction may be done when required.

INVESTIGATION FOR DYSPAREUNIA

Examination and culture of expressed prostatic secretions, ejaculate and urine.

TREATMENT OF MALE SEXUAL DISORDERS

This can be divided into two broad areas :

I. Treatment of Male Sexual disorders of organic etiology, and

II. Treatment of Male Psychosexual disorders.

I. Treatment of Male Sexual disorders of organic etiology:

This depends on the etiology uncovered. Once the specific etiology is corrected the sexual derangement improves in the majority of the patients. However, in some patients, the resultant dysfunction is either of a permanent nature or is due to both organic and psychological causes.

When the sexual dysfunction has become permanent or irreversible then treatment modalities such as vasoactive intracavernous injections can be tried, and if found successful, employed on a regular basis. If these too fail, and if the patient is willing and can afford, then penile implants can be given. Penile implants are of various types :

a) Semirigid type, giving a permanent but flexible erection,

b) Reservoir type which are deflatable, using a pump (implanted in scrotal sac) to manoeuvre fluid (from a reservoir implanted in the abdominal wall) to mimic natural erection, and

c) Self contained type which again is deflatable but with an internal reservoir and pump instead of a cumbersome external reservoir and pump.

Penile implants themselves are not without problems, mechanical or otherwise. The patients require careful psychological screening and unrealistic expectations have to be clearly discussed and dealt with before doing implantation. Before and after the surgery is over the patients have to be given detailed psychological counselling, supplemented by follow ups.

In those patients where both organic and psychological etiologies co-exist and are jointly responsible for the sexual dysfunction, once the specific organic treatment has been instituted, the psychological treatment as detailed in the following section, is commenced. The psychological treatment can either be done simultaneously from the onset or after organic treatment is over and has affected partial improvement only.

II. TREATMENT OF MALE PSYCHO-SEXUAL PROBLEMS

A number of treatment approaches generally based on Master and Johnson's technique or behavioural therapy model, are practiced in the West. However, these techniques cannot be applied with many Indian patients due to the following factors :

(I) Many Indian patients are thoroughly convinced that their sexual problems are due to some organic derangement which could only be rectified by some specific drugs.

(II) Many patients are not married or when married their wives either do not cooperate or have already deserted them. In a significant proportion of cases, a husband may not be emotionally prepared to tell his wife about his sexual problems.

(III) Owing to ignorance, a large number of patients are not aware of normal physiology of sexual arousal and intercourse.

(IV) Due to cultural inhibitions, complete nakedness is sometimes anxiety producing.

Due to these limitations, sex therapy in India has to be modified for people belonging to different socio-cultural strata of society, according to their expectations and attitudes towards sex. Highly educated couples may very easily accept Master and Johnson's technique while illiterate villagers might be shocked by this approach.

(A) IMPROVEMENT OF MARITAL RELATIONSHIP

Marriages in India are generally very different than marriages in the West. Marriages in West usually have a period of engagement during which the couple learn to know each other. Their sexual relationship comes after the psychological relationship has developed. On the other hand, in most of the Indian marriages couples do not know each other before their marriage. The marital relationship starts with sexual union and psychological relationship develops later. In this situation, sex becomes the cornerstone of the marital relationship and if there are any deficiencies in sexual relationship the marital relationship might be jeopardized. Thus, both partners are usually very anxious to have proper sexual relationship in the initial encounters. If any problem is encountered, following type of reactions might occur :

(a) The partners who are more religiously inclined and conservative might feel that sexual happiness is not meant for them but as they have been married they should accept the relation without any external interference. In other words, they become resigned to their 'fate'.

(b) In the second type of reaction, the couple feels that once the basic purpose of marriage is not fulfilled there is no point in living together and they may go in for separation and divorce.

Under these circumstances, the therapist has to reassure the couple that sexual problems are quite common in early marital life and can be easily treated by proper guidance. In long standing marriages, secondary sexual problems are usually the result of marital incompatibility rather than the cause of it. Success of marital counselling largely depends on the motivation of both spouses and degree of mutual compatibility. Improvement of marital relationship is essential for therapy because the unmotivated will either not cooperate or try to sabotage the therapy.

Case History

A 35-year old man attended the clinic along with his wife with the complaint of having a poor erection. It was found that they were married nearly 5 years ago and had a rather infrequent sexual relationship in the first few months of their married life. Later, the husband more or less lost erection during sexual situation. His wife was very dominating while the husband was introverth. Wife's excessive demanding nature effected the patient's self esteem and he had become more and more unsure of himself. He ultimately avoided having any sexual contact with her.

In the early phase of the therapy it was observed that he was not very motivated. The first few interviews were mainly focused on the interactional problem of the couple. Once the couple started relating to each other in a more congenial manner, proper sex therapy was started. But as soon as the husband started having erections, the wife became remarkedly censoring and demanding with the result, the husband again withdrew from sexual relationship. Ultimately the therapy was broken off as the couple did not follow the therapeutic instructions. This case indicates that a grossly distorted marital relationship can adversely affect the therapeutic outcome of the sexual disorder.

(B) SEX EDUCATION

Proper sex education is essential especially in our country where either misinformation or ignorance about sexual matters is the rule even in highly educated classes. However, proper timing of sex education is very important. Often, the patients's concept regarding sex is diametrically opposite to that of the therapist. For instance, many patients believe that they have lost their sexual power because of excessive masturbation or passage of "Dhat". Excessive and premature insistence in the early phase of therapy on trying to correct this attitude may lead to of disruption of therapy as the patient feels that the therapist does not understand the disease. The authors prefer to provide sex education only after certain gains are evident to the patient. However, sex education regarding foreplay, proper technique of coitus and post-coital behaviour can be given in the beginning of therapy itself.

(C) DESENSITIZATION OF THE PATIENT FROM SEXUALLY INHIBITING STIMULI

Many of these patients have marked inhibitions and develop severe anxiety in the presence of the partner of the opposite sex. Once the marriage relationship is satisfactory , then the couple is advised to try to touch each other all over the body avoiding direct touch of sex organs like penis in male, breast and vagina in the female. The state of undressing is left to the choice of the couple. They should undress as much as possible but only upto the extent they do not feel uncomfortable. The purpose of this excercise is to make them aware of each other's body without the fear of performance. This excercise is continued till the couple is able to feel considerably relaxed and comfortable in each other's company.

(D) TREATMENT OF SPECIFIC SEXUAL PROBLEMS

(i) Failure of Genital Response :

After satisfactory completion of previously described steps, most men start having penile erections in a non-demanding sexual situation. Those who do not develop erection at this stage are advised to direct genital stimulation. The man is advised not to concentrate on erections but to try to relax and enjoy the sensation. Once the patient starts having erection, the wife is advised to take on the active role to avoid performance anxiety in the partner. The sexual intercourse in advised with female superior position. 50% to 60% of patient's do respond to this type of treatment.

Case History

A 24-year old man came to the clinic with complaints of marked general weakness, body pains, restlessness and inability to have proper erection. He was married two months earlier. When he approached his wife on the first night, a he had mild erection and ejaculated before he could have coitus. Since that day he became very anxious and apprehensive, and failed to develop sufficient erection whenever he approached his wife. Past history revealed that he was a shy and an introvert man with the history of frequent masturbation. About a year prior to his marriage, he developed intimacy with an elderly female in his family and when he tried to have a sex relation with her, he ejaculated early and could not perform the sex act satsifactorily. He developed marked fear and guilt and consulted a number of lay sex specialists with no improvement.

During treatment the patient was advised to lie down with his wife and not to attempt any sexual intercourse for a week and the couple was asked to touch each other all over the body without direct stimulation of genitalia. The husband started having erection and contrary to advice he attempted sexual intercourse and failed. This made him much more apprehensive. On subsequent visit, the couple was reassured of getting well, provided they strictly follow the given advice in a proper manner. This had a good effect and the husband started getting adequate and sustained erections. After few days, they were advised to have coitus in female superior position. They gradually started having normal sexual relationship.

(ii) PREMATURE EJACULATION (PME) :

For premature ejaculation, the aim of the treatment is to help the patient to develop some control over their ejaculatory reflexes. The patients are taught to discriminate between the following two sensations:

(a) When the patient feels that he is going to ejaculate shortly,

(b) When the patient knows that the ejaculatory reflex has started and nothing can stop the ejaculation.

The patient are asked to identify the first sensation

and stop the stimulation of penis at that time or apply squeeze technique to inhibit ejaculation. This exercise is repeated for a few times in the company of the wife and later coitus is allowed with the female on top position. The patient is advised to signal to his wife, whenever he gets the first sensation so that penile thrusting is stopped for a short while. With the help of this technique, many of the patients develop reasonably adequate control over their premature ejaculation.

Case History

A 24-year old male farmer of rural-background attended the clinic for complaints of general body weakness, loss of appetite and premature ejaculation. He had been married for 5 years and had two children. History revealed that he had been ejaculating immediately after penetration and sometimes even before penetration. It led to infrequent sexual intercourse which further aggravated premature ejaculation. During, therapy, this patient insistently demanded for some drug which could increase his potency. The patient was given a placebo and was advised ejaculatory control exercises which improved his performance substantially.

Psychopharmacological agents like fluoxetine, trazadone, thioridazine can be used for increasing the duration of ejaculation. Other male sexual disorders like lack of sexual desire, sexual aversion could be managed by psychotherapy. The aim of psychotherapy will be to analyse factors responsible for the problem and then adequately manage them.

Retarded Ejaculation : (Orgasmic Dysfunction)

The initial management is similar to as described earlier. The male partner is advised to masturbate to the state when he feels that ejaculation is inevitable and start coitus at that point. This will result in ejaculation inside the vagina. Later the duration of the masturbation is gradually reduced till the patient is able to have ejaculation during coitus.

MANAGEMENT OF FEMALE SEXUAL PROBLEMS

A detailed history to identify the exact disorder and its possible etiology should be obtained. A thorough physical examination should be done to rule out associated physical illness and local genital pathology.

Investigations may be required to rule out endocrinal disorders, vascular disorders and any chronic physical illness.

The rest of the investigation are the same as described under male sexual disorders, except those which are specific for male problems, e.g. N.P.T., study of penile vascularity, etc.

Psychological management is primarily aimed at the following :

Improve marital relationship,
Reduce fear of sex,
Improve sexual excitement,
Decrease inhibiting stimuli,

These can be done by the same steps as described under male sexual disorders.

MANAGEMENT OF SPECIFIC PROBLEMS

Lack of Sexual Desire, Sexual Aversion and Lack of Sexual Enjoyment

All these disorders are interelated and are symptomatic of fear of sex, sex partner or other psychological problems enumerated earlier. These have to be reduced or minimized by psychotherapy. The above enumerated steps should be able to improve sexual response in the majority of the patients.

Failure of genital response and orgasmic dysfunction may usually occur together but can also occur separately. They should follow steps A, B and C, as advised under male sexual disorders.

If the patient start showing adequate genital response by these steps then, couple may be advised to have coitus. However, if adequate genital response has not developed (wetting of genitalia by vaginal transudate and intense sexual excitement), then one may have to desensitise the patient for specific sexually disinhibiting stimuli which may be different in each case.

The male partner may also be advised to stimulate the female genital and breasts, if the female partner finds it pleasant. This direct stimulation may often produce adequate genital response.

Most of the females complain of delayed or absent orgasm. Very few females complain of early orgasm.

Delayed orgasm is usually due to psychological factors. These will have to be treated psychotherapeutically.

Dyspareunia and Vaginismus

The initial phase of treatment is the same (steps A,

B and C should be used). Once the patient feels comfortable and relaxed in a heterosexual situation, then desensitisation to the fear of painful penetration is done. The patient may be initialy asked to insert her own finger into the vagina if she is able to do that, then she may be asked to put two fingers. If vaginal dilaters are available then the patient may be asked to lubricate the dilator and then gradually introduce it into the vagina. Once the patient is able to do these exercises, then the same exercises may be repeated in the presence of the husband, because quite often the presence of sexual partner may lead to vaginismus. Later the husband may be asked to gently put his finger into the vagina. Later actual penile penetration should be tried.

Antianxiety drugs like alprazolam or diazepam may be helpful in reducing the anxiety.

CHAPTER 13

MENTAL RETARDATION

Mental retardation is characterized by incomplete or arrested development of intelligence during the development period and it is associated with difficulties in adaptation to requirements of daily life. Mental retardation develops either at birth or during the development phase (up to 16 years of age). Mentally retarded individuals may also suffer from any other psychiatric or physical disorders. The prevalence of other disorders is quite common in mentally retarded individuals.

Epidemiology

Mental retardation is quite common. Its prevalence is estimated to be around 1%. Severe and profound mental retardation are usually due to organic etiology while mild retardation may not show definite organic involvement. Moderately retarded can have clear-cut organic pathology or may be more akin to mild retardation.

Mental retardation with definite organic etiology is equally distributed in the population. Non-organic retardation which is nearly 75% is more commonly seen in families with borderline intelligence in rural areas and in socially disadvantageous groups.

Mental retardation. is more common in areas where adequate perinatal and natal care is not available for the mothers. Dietary deficiency and poverty may also have a contributory role.

Etiology

Mental retardation can occur due to a varied etiology. Some of the common factors are :

i) Factors operative during pregnancy :

— Malnutrition in mothers may effect development of fetus

— Uncontrolled diabetes in mother

— Placenta praevia, cord round the neck of the child may produce asphyxia

— Infections like Rubella, syphilis, cytomegalic inclusion disease and AIDS.

Drugs : Drugs taken during pregnancy can lead to brain damage. Thalidomide (hypnotic) produced damage in large number of children. Currently prescribed drugs are generally safe but caution should be observed. Lithium produces cardiovascular abnormalities.

Drug Abuse : Tobacco abuse leads to low birth weight child. Alcohol is known to produce retardation in the child. Other substances like opioids and cocaine may also have effect on the child.

ii) **Chromosomal Abnormalities :** Mental retardation has been seen in association with chromosomal abnormalities. Commonest disorder is Down's syndrome (Mongolism) but there can be many other chromosomal abnormalities which may give rise to mental retardation.

Down's Syndrome (Mongolism)

This is a common disorder. Its incidence increases with the increase in age of the mother. The older mothers have more chances of delivering children with Down's Syndrome. The risk of having such a child is around 1 in 100 in women above 32 years of age.

Other factors implicated in development of this disorder are higher age of the father and exposure to X-ray radiation during pregnancy.

Aetiology

— Common chromosomal abnormality seen in Trisomy of 21. These patients have an extra '21' chromosome and the total chromosomes are 47. The mother and the father have normal chromosome pattern.

— Translocations : In these patients one chromosome '21' fuses with chromosome 15. Thus, in spite of an extra chromosome '21' total number of chromosomes remains 46. This is an inherited disorder and translocation of chromosome can be seen in parents and siblings without extra chromosome 21. Thus, the total chromosome in mother are 45.

Clinical Picture

These patients exhibit mild to moderate mental retardation with following physical abnormalities:

— Palpebral fissures are oblique

— Mid-canthus distance is more (hypertelorism)

— Cheek bones are high

— Tongue is protruded

— Hands are broad and thick with single transverse crease. The little finger is short and curved inwards

— These children are usually docile and pleasant.

There are many other abnormalities described. These patients can now survive quite long and may start showing premature senesence and may develop picture similar to Alzheimer's disease. The pathological finding in Down's syndrome and Alzheimer's disease specially with regard to abnormal proteins are similar.

Treatment

There is no specific treatment. Training and rehabilitation is helpful.

There are many other chromosomal abnormalities associated with mental retardation. They are either rare or not well described.

Genetic Factors

Many genetic disorders are associated with mental retardation :

a) **Dominant Gene**

Tuberous sclerosis is due to a dominant gene. This disorder is characterized by adenoma sebaceum, epilepsy and mental retardation. Few children may not have mental retardation.

b) **Recessive Gene**

There are large number of disorders which develop due to recessive genes and they give rise to inborn errors of metabolism. The common amongst them are Phenylketonuria and Maple syrup disorder.

These disorders can be diagnosed at the time of birth or even during pregnancy by aminocentesis. In some of these disorders appropriate management may reduce the risk of development of mental retardation.

c) **Multiple Gene Effect**

Nearly 75% of the mentally retarded individuals do not show any specific pathology. Most of these individuals are mildly retarded and they usually come from families where other members also show mild mental retardation. This group is considered to be due to non-specific genetic influences and psychosocial deprivation. Other factors like poor diet and multiple infections may also play a part.

iv) **Natal Factors**

Obstetric complications are also responsible for large number of cases of mental retardation. Common complications are :

— Obstructed and prolonged labour

— Forceps delivery

— Neonatal asphyxia

v) **Factors During Childhood**

Diseases in the developmental phase can also give rise to mental retardation. Common conditions are :

— Head injury

— Infections : Various viral encephalitis and severe tubercular meningitis with involvement of brain parenchyma

— Severe nutritional disorders can also lead to mental retardation

— Poisons : Lead poisoning due to licking of paint in toys can lead to lead encephalopathy

— Brain tumours

— Severe Neonatal jaundice

— Thyroid deficiency (Cretinism).

vi) **Sociocultural Factors**

Sociocultural deprivation may play a part in development of mental retardation. It has been seen that mild mental retardation is more prevalent in deprived sections of the society. Poor environmental stimulation could be an important factor. Some studies in the West have shown that if children from deprived section are provided with more opportunities for interaction and are provided better emotional atmosphere it may lead to improvement in IQ.

Clinical Picture

Mental retardation is clinically divided into following subtypes on the basis of intellectual and adaptive functioning (I.C.D.X.).

Mild mental retardation
Moderate mental retardation
Severe mental retardation
Profound mental retardation

Mild Mental Retardation (IQ - 50 to 69)

These persons may be indistinguishable as children. The milestones of development are usually normal. There may be a minimal delay. Development of speech and understanding may be delayed.

The problem becomes manifest during schooling when such children may not show satisfactory scholastic performance. They may also have associated emotional immaturity which may lead to difficulties in adjustment.

As adults these people can perform well on semiskilled and unskilled jobs. They may be indistinguishable from other normal people. They might find it difficult to cope with stresses of marriage, parenthood etc.

These persons may show associated physical or psychiatric disorders. Their I.Q. is between 50-69. I.Q. (Intelligence Quotient) is calculated by finding out the mental age of the individual by giving him standardised tests which can provide information about his mental age. Common tests are Binet Kamath Test of Intelligence, Raven's Progressive Matrices, Bhatia's Battery of Intelligence and Wescheler Intelligence Test for children.

$$I.Q. = \frac{\text{Mental age}}{\text{Chronological age}} \times 100$$

$$\text{e.g.} \quad \frac{\text{Mental age} = 6}{\text{Chronological age} = 12} \times 100$$

$$I.Q. = 50$$

An I.Q. of 50 means that the individual's mental abilities are 50% of his age. Though with the increasing age the mental abilities will increase but generally the I.Q. will remain the same i.e at the age of 16 his abilities will be of 8 years.

Most of the intelligence tests assume a fixed age of 16 years for calculation of I.Q. If one is assessing an adult of 30 years his chronological age will be kept fixed according to that particular test.

MODERATE MENTAL RETARDATION (I.Q. 35 TO 49)

These patients may show delayed milestones as children. Their motor and speech development is delayed.

They usually cannot cope in ordinary school. They may be able to develop minimal skills needed for reading, counting, and simple calculations. They will find it difficult to adapt to demands of day-to-day life. As adults they may be able to do simple jobs under close supervision. They can do repetitive work which does not require intellectual involvement eg. they may be able to tighten screws in a vehicle, may be able to cut pieces of wood if the cutting place is marked. They will not be able to live independently, manage money or property. They can be married only if the spouse agrees to take all the responsibility of running the home. Their language development is limited and they communicate poorly.

SEVERE MENTAL RETARDATION (I.Q. 20 TO 34)

These children will show gross delay of milestones of development. They do not develop speech and language sufficient for proper communication. The control of bowel and bladder is delayed. Their motor movements are clumsy.

They cannot have formal education. They may be able to undertake simplest of tasks. They will require supervision all through their lives. They may be trained to attend to their basic needs like eating, cleaning and dressing.

PROFOUND MENTAL RETARDATION (I.Q. BELOW 20)

These individuals are severally limited in all of their activities. They may not be able to walk at all or may walk with difficulty. They do not have meaningful speech. They cannot save themselves from common physical dangers. They need close supervision all through their lives.

Diagnosis (I.C.D.X.)

Diagnosis of mental retardation is based on the following :

a) there should be reduced level of intellectual functioning

b) resulting in diminished ability to adapt to demands of the normal social environments; and

c) they may have associated physical disorders like epilepsy or psychiatric problems.

Levels of mental retardation is diagnosed on the basis of I.Q. and level of functioning as detailed earlier.

Aetiological diagnosis is made by history and investigations :

Detailed history and examination will provide indication for further investigation. Investigations are planned according to anticipated diagnosis.

Prognosis

Mental retardation once established is an irreversible condition. Only some errors of metabolism and hypothyroidism, if detected early, may be treated to prevent further increase in mental retardation.

However, with proper training, a large number of patients can be reasonably rehabilitated.

Management

Mental retardation cannot be reversed by any

drug. So drug management has no role to play. However, drugs may be prescribed for associated physical or psychiatric conditions.

Many such patients may develop behavioural disturbances or psychoses. They should be treated appropriately. Emphasis should be on training and rehabilitation. Useful literature for training has been developed by National Institute for Mentally Retarded at Hyderabad. They should be approached for procuring literature for guidance in training.

There are very few good schools for training the mentally retarded. These are generally situated in big towns. Thus, home management and local rehabilitation is the treatment of choice in India.

Prevention

Main emphasis should be laid on prevention of mental retardation.

Genetic Counselling — Genetic counselling may prevent some cases of mental retardation. Parents who have a child with trisomy should be discouraged to have more children. Patients exhibiting other genetic disorders should be appropriately counselled.

Proper Antenatal Management — All pregnant mothers should be properly evaluated during pregnancy. They should be treated for any pre-existing disease. They should be innoculated for diseases like German measles (Rubella).

— Nutrition should be maintained.

— Proper evaluation should be done whether this person can have a normal delivery or not, so that, unnecessary prolonged labour could be avoided.

Natal Care — Proper care at the time of delivery is essential to avoid neonatal asphyxia.

Post Natal Care — To avoid infection like tuberculosis or encephalitis and screening for inborn errors of metabolism at the time of birth or during pregnancy can be very helpful.

CHILDHOOD CARE — During childhood, child should be protected from head injury, infectious diseases can be avoided by inoculation. In our country tuberculosis, and some viral encephalitis are quite common. The child should be inoculated against them.

CHAPTER 14

DISORDERS OF PSYCHOLOGICAL DEVELOPMENT

Many children show certain developmental delays and others may show loss of already achieved abilities in early childhood. These disorders usually develop in infancy or early childhood. The developmental delays are often related to abnormalities or maturational delays in central nervous system. These disorders often show a steady course without fluctuation. A large number show improvement with age. Developmental delay is identified by conspicuous retardation of one ability in comparison to the general development of the child. There are a large number of disorders included under this category. Main categories are:

Specific developmental disorders of speech and language.

Specific developmental disorders of scholastic skills.

Specific developmental disorders of motor functions.

Mixed specific developmental disorders.

Pervasive developmental disorders.

Other disorders of psychological development.

Unspecified disorders of psychological development.

SPECIFIC DEVELOPMENTAL DISORDERS OF SPEECH AND LANGUAGE

These children can have difficulties in articulation of a particular word or sound eg. between T, Th. They may have difficulty in understanding spoken speech or difficulty in expressing themselves. They may have difficulty in identifying common objects in the early years and later they may not understand grammar or may not be able to differentiate negative from positive, etc.

Similarly, expressive language disorders are characterized by failure to speak simple 2 word phrases by 3 years of age. Later these children will show poor vocabulary and poor grammar.

These disturbances could occur alone or intermixed with other.

Epidemiology

These disorders are quite common and can be seen in 8%-10% of school-going children.

Etiology

Genetic factors seem to be important. Specific articulation disorders tend to run in families. All members of a family, may show similar articulation defects. Genetic factors may also be important in other disorders. Maturational delay of the nervous system are also involved in their development. Psychological factors may also play some role.

Prognosis

Majority of these disorders improve with time but some may persist life-long. Such children may develop emotional and relational difficulties which may make the prognosis worse.

Diagnosis (I.C.D.X.)

These disorders should be diagnosed keeping in mind the following :

1. The developmental delay should not be part of normal variation. The delay should be significantly more for that age and intelligence.

2. The delay should not be part of the intellectual retardation. It should be much more than expected in a child of that age.

3. It should not be explained by other neurological or physical disorder. Deafness, and other perceptual deficits like poor vision should be excluded. Articulation difficulties could be due to cleft palate or other neurological disorders.

Management

Most of these disorders require specific training programme. Speech therapists trained for such deficits should be helpful. If there are associated emotional problems like timidity and withdrawal, they should be handled psychologically.

SPECIFIC DEVELOPMENTAL DISORDERS OF SCHOLASTIC SKILLS

Some children may show specific disorders in scholastic performance. This delay should start in early childhood. Many students develop scholastic difficulties in later years due to lack of interest, difficulty of subject or poor training methods. Such problems are not included here. The scholastic difficulty should be out of proportion of general intelligence of the person. It should not be explained on the basis of other problems like deafness or specific neurological abnormalities.

Common problems included are specific reading disorders, specific spelling disorders and specific disorders of arithmetic skills. These children will show difficulty in reading, remembering, spelling or in arithmetic calculation.

Etiology

Most of these patients may have associated developmental disorders of speech and language. Often they may also have other neurological deficits or cerebral palsy. It is presumed that organic factors play a major role in the development of these disorders. Psychological difficulties are often associated and large number of such children may show emotional problems.

Prognosis

These disorders generally improve with time, but often some difficulties may continue. As adults they may have difficulties in spelling or expression of spoken speech.

Diagnosis (I.C.D.X.)

The scholastic difficulty should be clear cut and should be out of proportion to the age and intelligence:

— it should have started in early childhood,

— it should not be explained on the basis of mental retardation, deafness or gross neurological abnormalities.

Management

The basic management is by special training and emotional problems, if any, should be managed psychologically.

SPECIFIC DEVELOPMENTAL DISORDERS OF MOTOR FUNCTION

Some children show excessive clumsiness of movement which cannot be explained on the basis of any neuromuscular disorder or mental retardation. Such children may exhibit difficulty in speech (dysarthria), clumsiness in walking and examination and may show, choreiform and athetoid movements of body. They will show clumsiness while clapping, finger tapping or hopping on one foot.

Etiology

It is not well-known. It is possibly due to maturational difficulties or due to hypoxia at birth or malnutrition.

Epidemiology

Not well-known.

Prognosis

Many children improve in coordination with age but clumsiness may remain life-long.

Management

Special techniques to improve motor coordination are used.

PERVASIVE DEVELOPMENTAL DISORDERS

This group of disorders are characterised by generalised difficulties in communication, interest and activities. These disorders usually start in infancy but few children may show apparently normal development for 1-2 years and later develop symptoms. A commonly described syndrome under this group is childhood autism.

Childhood Autism

This disorder usually starts before 3 years of age. Usually, abnormalities are manifest from birth.

Epidemiology

Exact prevalence is not known because the diagnostic practices differ. Few people do not diagnose autism if there is any evidence of retardation, while majority of people do not use retardation as exclusion criteria and diagnose autism only on the basis of symptom pattern. Later workers report a much higher prevalence. Generally the prevalence is around .04% to .05% in children.

Etiology

It is now considered to be organic in etiology. It is associated with congenital anomalies and brain pathology. But no specific organic pathology has been identified.

Clinical Features

Autism — These children appear to be lost in their own world. They do not respond to their parents by smiling or recognition but deal with them as if they were inanimate objects. They do not react to being left alone but if strangers come to the house they may react by anger and hyperactivity.

Speech and Communication — Many autistic children may not develop speech till late. Those who develop speech do not speak in a manner which may be of communicative value. They may utter words and phrases without reference. Nearly fifty per cent will not develop useful speech. Many such children do not talk in first person. Instead of saying I want food, they say that "Mohan (his own name) wants food".

Emotions — These chilren may smile to themselves. There is no emotional relatedness. But they can show outbursts of anger and crying.

Sameness and Ritualistic Behaviour — These children get upset if their belongings are changed or disturbed. They will keep things in a particular way and any deviation makes them angry and fretful. They will deal with toys in their own fashion. They do not play with other children. They are attached to inanimate objects like toys, fur, clothes, etc. and usually cling to them all the time.

Intelligence — Majority of these children show mild to moderate retardation but a few may have normal intelligence. Their speech and communication skills are much below their intellectual level.

Behavioural Disturbances — These children may show continuous activity of a repetitive kind, repeating the same motor movement again and again (stereotype). They may exhibit aggresiveness, and may hurt themselves. Head banging and hair pulling may be seen.

Prognosis

The disorder develops at around 3 years of age. Children who have communicative speech and are of normal intelligence show good prognosis. Others may never develop meaningful speech and communication. Prognosis in general is poor.

Treatment

Children showing hyperactivity and abnormal behaviour may show response to Haloperidol 1.5 to 3mg/day. Other drugs are in an experimental stage. Behavioural management may be effective in some cases.

OTHER PERVASIVE DISORDERS

Some children may not show typical autism but may show different disturbances in communication, relationship and behaviour. These conditions have similar organic etiology and the prognosis is generally poor.

Chapter 15

Behaviour and Emotional Disorders with Onset Usually Occurring in Childhood and Adolescence

Young children and adolescents may show emotional disorders as seen in adults. There could be some differences in presentation. But there are some disorders which are specific to this developmental phase, their onset is in childhood and they may not lead to adult type of emotional disorders.

These are classified as under :

Hyperkinetic Disorder

Hyperkinetic conduct disorder
Other hyperkinetic disorders
Hyperkinetic disorder, unspecified.

Conduct Disorders

Conduct disorder confined to family context
Unsocialized conduct disorder
Socialized conduct disorder
Oppositional defiant disorder
Other conduct disorders
Conduct disorder, unspecified

Mixed disorder of conduct and emotion

Emotional Disorder with Onset Specific to Childhood

Separation anxiety disorder of childhood
Phobic anxiety disorder of childhood
Social anxiety disorder of childhood
Sibling rivalry disorder
Other childhood emotional disorders
Childhood emotional disorder unspecified

Disorder of Social Functioning with Onset Specific to Childhood and Adolescence

Elective mutism
Reactive attachment disorder of childhood
Disinhibited attachment disorder of childhood
Other childhood disorders of social functioning
Childhood disorders of social functioning, unspecified

Tic Disorder

Transient tic disorder
Chronic motor or vocal tic disorder
Combined vocal and multiple motor tic disorder (de la Tourette's syndrome)
Other tic disorders
Tic disorder, unspecified

Other Behaviour and Emotional Disorders with Onset Usually Occurring in Childhood and Adolescence

Nonorganic enuresis
Nonorganic encopresis
Feeding disorder of infancy and childhood
Pica of infancy and childhood
Stereotyped movement disorder
Stuttering (Stammering)
Cluttering
Other specified behavioural and emotional disorders with onset usually occurring in childhood and adolescence
Unspecified behavioural and emotional disorders with onset usually occurring in childhood and adolescence.

Hyperkinetic Diosrders

This disorder is characterized by hyperkinetic behaviour and poor attention span. It is also called Attention Deficit Disorder. The main feature is hyperkinetic behaviour eg. the patient is not able to sit still in any situation and may move from one place to another, may show movements of hands or may fiddle with objects. The second characteristic is poor attention span. These children do not concentrate on any task and leave most tasks unfinished. These patients may have many other associated symptoms like impulsivity, emotional lability, poor scholastic progress and anti-social behaviour.

Epidemiology — The prevalence of this disorder is estimated to be around 3.5% in prepubertal children. It is much more common in boys than girls. The onset is usually in early childhood but the problem is usually identified when the child starts going to school.

Etiology — Genetic factors seem to play some part. Monozygotic twins show a high concordance rate for this illness. The parents of such children may suffer from alcoholism. Minimal brain damage has been hypothesised. No direct evidence is available for this damage. Majority of these patients do show developmental delays. Soft neurological signs are common.

Others believe that the disorder occurs due to

maturational lag of the central nervous system. The condition improves with maturation. Psychosocial factors may play some part. This disorder is more common in orphanages where proper rearing atmosphere is not available.

Clinical Features : This disorder starts in infancy. Such infants are irritable and hyperactive and show excess of crying and poor sleep.

As children they are usually restless and cannot sit still. They will fiddle with everything around. They cannot concentrate on any given task. This leads to scholastic difficulties. They are emotionally excitable and may show episodes of rage or crying.

They are impulsive and cannot postpone their needs. If their needs are not fulfilled, they may show temper tantrums. They can have associated difficulties with learning, arithmetic, memorisation and disorders of speech or hearing.

On Investigation E.E.G. may show maturational lag.

Diagnosis (I.C.D.-X) — It is based on the presence of hyperactivity and poor attention span which is out of proportion of the age and intelligence of the child. Some children may show conduct disorder in form of truancy, lying, aggressiveness etc.

Course and Prognosis : Nearly three-fourths of such children improve by adolescence. Some may continue to have poor attention span. Others may continue showing both hyperactivity and poor attention. However, a small group may develop dissocial personality disorder and others may persist with difficulties in social adaptation.

Management

Pharmacotherapy

The CNS stimulants Dextroamphetamine and Methyl-phenidate are the drug of choice. (Unfortunately both are not available in our country). They are to be given in the morning and at noon because night time dose may produce sleep difficulty. Dextroamphetamine is given in a dose of 5-10mg./day. These drugs reduce hyperactivity and improve attention span.

Antidepressants like Imipramine are being used in our country. Their response is not uniform. They are more effective when this disorder is associated with depression. The dosage is from 50 mg to 150 mg/day. Clonidine has been also found effective. Dose may be started from .1 mg B.D. which may be increased gradually.

Psychological Treatment

These children are to be helped to understand that their hyperactivity and difficulty to concentrate are part of a disease which is likely to improve. They should be helped to integrate with their class so that they may not develop defiant and rebellious attitude. The parents and teachers are advised not to retaliate against the child but their hyperactivity could be channelised into outdoor sports and their poor attention can be improved by appropriate educational technology.

Hyperkinetic disorder could be associated with conduct disorder. The basic treatment is of hyperkinetic disorder which may improve the conduct disorder also.

Conduct Disorder

These are characterized by repetitive and persistent dissocial and aggressive or defiant behaviour. These children, may tell lies, steal, show cruelty to animals or other children, or may run away from school or home. This behaviour should be persistent and should not be limited to one or two situations.

Epidemiology : This is quite common in young children, 0.5 to 1% children may show conduct disorder before 18 years of age. It is four to five times more common in boys than girls. It is more often seen in families where parents also have dissocial behaviour.

Etiology : Definite etiology is not known. Following factors may be responsible :

i) Genetic Factors — Parents of such children do show more dissocial traits. Evidence for genetic influence in not very clear.

ii) Familial Factors — It is more or less accepted that the parenting of such children is not up to the mark. The parents may be inconsistent, negligent, or may indulge in child abuse.

iii) Sociocultural Factors — More conduct disorder children are brought up in localities where violence, crime and antisocial behaviour is rampant. The children are often brought up in situations of social deprivation.

iv) Psychological Factors — These children often feel neglected, unjustly punished or not given their due rights. This leads to development of rebelliousness against social norms. They identify with rebels, gangsters or antisocial persons. In a recent survey the children indicated ideals as Harshad Mehta (of the Security Scam fame) and Charles Shobraj (a repetitively convicted criminal). Movies with the emphasis on violence may also play a role.

v) Neurological Factors

Hyperactive disorders seem to have a close relationship with conduct disorders. Many children with conduct disorders may show developmental delays or other neurological abnormalities.

Clinical Features

These children may show any one or more of the following :

— excessive level of fighting or bullying;
— cruelty to animals or other people;
— severe destructiveness to property;
— fire setting;
— stealing;
— repeated lying;
— truancy from school and running away from home;
— frequent and severe temper trantrums;
— defiant provocative behaviour and persistent severe disobedience.

Conduct disorders can be further subdivided into the following :

a) Conduct Disorder Confined to Family Context — These children may show various dissocial acts described earlier only in relation with their family members while their behaviour outside home could be nearly normal. The prognosis of such children is good. They may show improvement by removing them from their families.

b) Unsocialized Conduct Disorders — These children find it difficult to develop enduring relationship with peers. They are usually isolated. These children usually have a poor prognosis and they are likely to develop dissocial personality disorder.

c) Socialized Conduct Disorder — These children become part of a delinquent group and indulge in antisocial activities as described earlier. Basically these children are able to form stable relationships with other children. They may establish relationships with normal children or with children from delinquent gangs.

The prognosis of these children is usually good. They give up their antisocial behaviour by the end of adolescence.

Management

Conduct disorders can coexist with emotional disorders or with hyperkinetic disorder. If such is the case then both the disorders should be considered in the management. Dissocial act could be part of mental retardation, pervasive disorders of childhood or schizophrenia. In such a situation, management should be of the primary condition.

Conduct disorders require psychological management. Following principle are to be kept in mind:

— If conduct disorder is associated with family disruption or poor parenting, the child may have to be shifted to some other place or a children's home;

— Family should always be involved and attempt should be made to help the family to provide consistent upbringing;

— These children may be involved with a group of normal children which may provide them proper role models to emulate;

— Behaviour modification with positive reinforcement may be helpful.

Medication may be needed to control aggressiveness or hyperactivity. Haloperidol in small doses may be helpful.

SEPARATION ANXIETY DISORDER OF CHILDHOOD

This disorder is characterized by acute anxiety and fear of being separated from parenting figures, close relatives and friends. The children may feel that something untoward is going to happen to himself or to close relatives. Separation anxiety is a normal feature of childhood, but when it becomes disabling or results in child's clinging to adults, then it requires treatment.

Epidemiology

Exact prevalence is not known. The disorder tends to become manifest between 10-12 years of age.

Etiology

Etiology is also not clearly understood so far, but genetic factors may play a role. Children of anxious parents tend to show this problem.

Clinical Picture and Diagnosis (I.C.D.-X)

The central feature of the syndrome is excessive anxiety about separation from parents or other dependent figures.

The symptoms may include :

a) Unrealistic worry that something untoward may happen to attachment figures;

b) Excessive worry that something bad may happen to him due to which he may be separated from his parents eg. accident, kidnapping etc;

c) Persistent refusal to go to school because of being away from the attachment figure and not due to fear of school; and

d) Any threat or actual separation may lead to intense anxiety and patient may develop symptoms like vomiting, headache etc.

This condition should be differentiated from other disorders where separation anxiety may be a symptom of other childhood disorders eg. pervasive developmental disorder.

Management

These children may respond to drugs like imipramine. This can be given in dose of 25 mg/daily which could be increased gradually.

The patient has to be shown that nothing untoward happens even if he stays away from his parents. Gradual distancing from attachment figure could be planned.

PHOBIC ANXIETY DISORDER OF CHILDHOOD

If children develop phobia as described in adults then they have to be treated as adult phobias. But some children may show phobia which is common in that developmental stage e.g. phobia of animals. If they show excessive anxiety in such situations, these are called phobias of childhood.

This disorder does not necessarily develop into adult phobias. Treatment is by behavioural psychotherapy.

SOCIAL ANXIETY DISORDER OF CHILDHOOD

Children are usually fearful of strangers, new and strange surroundings. When children show marked apprehensiveness while meeting strangers and this leads to undue clinging to parents, then this disorder could be diagnosed. This disorder should develop before 6 years of age. Management is mainly on behavioural principle.

SIBLING RIVALRY DISORDER

This disorder develops after the birth of a younger sibling. The older child shows marked jealousy toward the new child and the patient may try to hurt the younger child or may show temper-tantrum when others take care of the younger sib.

This disorder usually arises within months of the birth of the younger child and should be persistent for some time before it can be diagnosed.

Management

This problem should be prevented by preparing the child for the new arrival. He should look forward to the child's birth with positive expectation. Once the syndrome has developed then psychological management is required. The older child should be made to feel that he is not being neglected due to the new arrival. He should be given attention and should be involved with the care of the younger sibling.

DISORDER OF SOCIAL FUNCTIONING WITH ONSET SPECIFIC TO CHILDHOOD AND ADOLESCENCE

These children develop abnormalities in social functioning which develop in developmental phase. They differ from pervasive disorders by the social incapacity being circumscribed to specific areas. These disorders usually develop in response to disturbed environment. Common disorders included are :

ELECTIVE MUTISM

These children show mutism in selected situations while they can communicate normally at other times, common pattern being that child talks normally at home, but becomes mute at school. These children may show anxiety in social situations.

REACTIVE ATTACHMENT DISORDER OF CHILDHOOD

These children show hypervigilance and fearfulness. They cannot be comforted easily. This usually occurs in response to severe parental neglect or due to child abuse. They may respond to care-givers by turning their head in opposite direction (gaze avoidance).

These children appear miserable. They may show aggressiveness or temper-tantrums. The symptoms usually develop within first 15 years of life. These children loose most of their untoward behaviour when they are put in situation where normal and consistent pattern of care is provided.

DISINHIBITED ATTACHMENT DISORDER OF CHILDHOOD

This syndrome is characterized by diffuse

clinging behaviour which starts in first five years of life. Later the child may give up clinging to any adult, but may continue to show attention seeking behaviour. These children find it difficult to develop close relationship with peers. This syndrome generally develops in children who are reared in orphanages from early infancy. They do not develop one to one relationship and that is the reason they cling to all adults.

Management

Most of these disorders are managed by the following :

— providing stable care givers (parents or others);
— improving environemtal distortion; and
— helping the child to develop stable relationships.

TIC DISORDERS

Tic is an involuntary, rapid, recurrent, non-rhythmic motor movement or vocal production that is sudden in onset and serves no apparent purpose. There could be sudden eye blinking, neck jerking, hand movements or their could be vocal tics in form of clearing of throat or utterance of certain sounds or speaking obscene words.

Epidemiology

All type of tic disorders are estimated to be seen in 1 in 200 to 300 persons. Gilles de la Tourrette's syndrome is seen in around .05% population. It is more common in males. The onset is usually before 12 years of age.

Etiology

The etiolgy is not clearly known. Genetic factors seem to play a role. Family members of these children may show tic disorders.

Clinical Picture

The illness usually starts in childhood before 12 years of age. The children will show motor tics which may take the form of eye blinking, grimacing, hand movements or neck jerking. These occur abruptly. The patient may be able to control them for short periods.

Motor tics may be followed by vocal tics. These may take the form of repetitive throat clearing, uttering few sounds or uttering obscene words. The illness may take many forms.

TRANSIENT TIC DISORDER

These children will have tics for a period shorter than 12 months within which the tics will disappear.

CHRONIC TIC DISORDER

These children will have either motor tics or vocal tics (but not both) which may persist for long periods.

GILLES DE LA TOURRETTE'S SYNDROME

This disorder is characterized by development of both motor and vocal tics. The motor tics may become complex and the child may start hopping or jumping without any cause. Vocal tics develop later and will include obscene utterance. This disorder runs a chronic course and disease persist through adult life.

Management

Haloperidol in dose .25-.5 mg/day may be enough for younger children. Maximal dose is around 3 mg/day for 40 kg child. If the child shows side effects of Haloperidol like acute dystonia, then anticholinergics or diphenhydramine can be given.

Pimozide has also been found effective. The dosage is 1-2 mg/day.

Clonidine has also been found effective. The dosage is .1 mg twice a day.

Behaviour therapy in form of mass practice of tics has been found useful in mild cases.

OTHER BEHAVIOURAL AND EMOTIONAL DISORDERS WITH ONSET USUALLY OCCURRING IN CHILDHOOD AND ADOLESCENCE

This group contain certain symptoms which cannot be classified elsewhere. They do not have much relationship with each other.

NON-ORGANIC ENURESIS

Enuresis is characterized by involuntary voiding of urine by day or night. If it is caused by neurological or other organic factors then it is called organic enuresis. However, in majority of enuretics, no organic cause can be found.

Enuresis is divided into primary and secondary :

Primary Enuresis : These children do not develop control on passing urine. This is most common and nearly 70% to 80% enuretics belong to this group.

Secondary Enuresis : These children become dry at the age of 4-5 years and develop enuresis, couple of years later usually due to a psychological stress either after birth of a sibling or due to some other factor.

Epidemiology

Majority of children become dry by 4 to 5 years. Enuresis is seen in around 1% of children after this age.

Etiology

Definite etiology is not known. Genetic factors may play a role. Many enuretic children have a first degree relative who is also enuretic. Enuretics are said to have a bladder which reacts abnormally to small amounts of urine and leads to voidance of urine. Some children may have excessive production of urine due to reduced activity of Antidiuretic Hormone.

Psychological factors are more important in secondary enuresis. In primary enuresis, reactive psychological problems may lead to poor self image and familial tensions.

Clinical Picture

These children wet the bed at night or in the daytime. The frequency can be varying from daily to once or twice a week. These children usually become self-conscious and tense. They may avoid going to places where they have to pass the night. Family tensions may also develop.

Differential Diagnosis

Organic causes of enuresis like spina-bifida-occulta, cystitis, seizures etc. should be excluded.

Management

The children should be toilet trained more properly. They should be made to void urine before going to bed. Evening intake of fluid should be restricted. The child may be woken up in the middle of night and made to pass urine. Behavioural treatment has been found effective. The bell and pad method is in common use. The child is given a pad which is connected to a bell. When first drop of urine is voided the pad becomes wet and the bell starts ringing and the child is woken up. The child gradually starts waking up whenever the bladder is full.

Pharmacotherapy

Imipramine in dosage of 25 to 50 mg at bed time reduces enuresis. But many children relapse after stopping the drug.

Psychological Treatment

This is effective only in secondary enuresis. These children should be helped to overcome their anxiety and feelings of insecurity by providing them stable parental relationship.

NON-ORGANIC ENCOPRESIS

This is characterized by passing of stools at inappropriate places even after the age of bowel control has been attained (5 years). These children may pass stool in their underwear. This condition should be differentiated from organic encoperesis e.g. overflow incontinence resulting from constipation and, aganglionic megacolon (Hirschprung's disease). These children do not have any desire to defecate yet they may have incontinence.

Encoperesis is usually associated with some other psychiatric disorders like pervasive developmental disorders and conduct disorders.

Management

These children are usually very tense and families are disturbed. The tension should be eased out by explaining to them that this is a disorder and we should help the child to have change of underwears without much fuss. Behavioural training is useful. Treatment of associated psychiatric condition can be helpful.

FEEDING DISORDER OF INFANCY AND CHILDHOOD

Transitory feeding problems and food fads are common in children. But some children may show persistent refusal to eat and extensive degree of food fads (taking only specific foods) which may be detrimental to their health.

This condition is only diagnosed when other causes of food refusal like anorexia nervosa and other organic and psychiatric disorders have been excluded.

Management

The management is improving child-parent relationship. There should be limit setting to parental behaviour. Many parents want to feed the child excessively. Children are encouraged to eat with other children where social imitation can help overcome abnormal eating habit.

PICA OF INFANCY AND CHILDHOOD

This refers to intake of nonnutritious substances like soil, paint, wood pieces etc. This is usually seen in association with mental retardation.

Management is by behavioural techniques.

STEREOTYPED MOVEMENT DISORDERS

These children show rhythmic, voluntary, repetitive, non-functional movements that do not form part of any recognised neurological or functional disorder. They can be subdivided into non-injurious and injurious movement. Non-injurious movements include body rocking, head rocking, hair plucking, finger flicking and hand flapping. (Nail biting, thumb sucking and nose picking are not included). Injurious movements include repetitive head banging, face slapping, eye poking and biting of hands, lips or other body parts.

All these symptoms are indicative of disturbances in parent child relationship or of other environmental stresses.

Management includes improving parent child relationship and to encourage socially rewarding situations. Most such patients improve with increase in age.

STUTTERING

It is characterized by frequent repetition, or prolongation of sounds or syllables, or words, or by frequent hesitation or pauses that disrupts the smooth flow of speech.

Epidemiology — This is quite a common problem. Nearly 1% of adolescents and adults may show persistent stuttering while transitory stuttering is much more common. It is much more common in males.

Etiology — It is thought to be a disorder of brain development. Few consider it to be due to improper development of dominance of speech function in opposite hemisphere. It has also been shown that stutterers react to the negative feedbacks of their stuttering and if instead they are fed with white noise their stuttering is reduced.

Clinical Picture — Stuttering usually starts in childhood. Initially the child may stutter only when he is excited or emotionally upset. Later on, the disorder becomes more widespread and the child stutters in all situations. Most adults show stuttering only in specific situations or with specific words, sounds or adjectives. A stuttering adult tries to control stuttering by substituting words where he may not stutter. They may have long pause to overcome stuttering.

Course — It is usually a chronic condition. But majority of stutterers learn to overcome this difficulty and can get along in life reasonably well.

Management — Stuttering is managed by behavioural training and psychological support. The patient has to be helped to overcome his fear of stuttering and people's response to it. This will reduce his anxiety and decrease stuttering. The patient may be advised to speak slowly or may be asked to have a one second gap between words. Speech therapists are quite successful in helping these patients.

CLUTTERING

It is characterized by rapid rate of speech with breakdown in fluency, with no repetitions or hesitations but of a severity to give rise to reduced speech intelligibility. The speech is erratic and jerky, with inappropriate use of phrases. It is a rare disorder. Not much is known about its etiology and management.

CHAPTER 16

PSYCHO - PHARMACOLOGY

Psychotropic drugs are medications intended to affect the mental processes especially to modify the behaviour, thinking and mood.

The drugs included belong to following groups :

1. Antipsychotics
2. Antidepressants
3. Antianxiety drugs
4. Miscellaneous
   Lithium
   Calcium antagonists
   Anti-epileptics

Antipsychotic Drugs

This group includes following drugs :

1. Phenothiazines
   Aliphatic chain - Chlorpromazine
   Piperazine ring - Prochlorperazine
   Trifluperazine
   Fluphenazine
   Piperidine ring - Thioridazine
2. Butyrophenone
   Haloperidol
3. Diphenylbutylpiperidines
   Pimozide
4. Thioxanthene
   Thiothixene *
   Flupenthixol
   Clopenthixol *
5. Dihydroindolone
   Molindone *
   Oxypertine *
6. Dibenzodiazepine
   Clozapine *
   Loxapine
7. Benzamide derivatives
   Sulpiride *
   Tiapride *
   Remoxipride *
8. Dihydroisoquinolone
   Piquindone *
9. Benzisoxazol
   Risperidone *

* Not commercially available in India at present.

Pharmacology

1. Dopamine blockade
Therapeutic effect
Parkinsonian side effect
2. Anticholinergic effect
Autonomic side effect
3. Antinoradrenergic effect
Orthostatic hypotension and sedation
4. Antihistaminic effect
Sedation
5. Antiserotonin effect
Antihallucinogenic
Improve Negative symptoms

Pharmacokinetics

1. Absorption from gastrointestinal tract affected by food, anta acids and presence of anticholinergic drugs.

2. High lipid solubility resulting in wide tissue distribution, passes across the blood brain barrier, placental barrier and into the mothers milk.

3. Wide intra and inter individual variations of plasma concentration.

4. Elimination from body follows multiphasic pattern. Rapidly eliminated from blood. Concentration in brain higher than in blood. Half life in blood variable from 10 to 20 hours. Biological effect lasting up to 24 hours. So single dose is possible.

Relation Between Plasma Concentration and Clinical Effect

Not yet certain for most antipsychotic drugs.

Some evidence of therapeutic window for blood haloperidol concentration and beneficial clinical effects. Therapeutic effect present in a narrow range of plasma concentration. The therapeutic effects remain as long as the narrow range of plasma concentration is maintained and the therapeutic gain decreases below or above that range.

Long Acting Antipsychotic Drugs

Drugs with prolonged elimination time (Diphenylbutylpiperidine group)

Pimozide-plasma half life 53 hours.

Fluspirilene | remain biologically

Penfluridol | active up to 2 weeks

Depot preparation are made by esterification of active drugs and dissolving them in an oily vehicle — enanthate or decanoate forms have therapeutic effect

for 1 to 2 weeks or 2 to 4 weeks duration, respectively.

ADVERSE EFFECTS

A wide range of side effects have been reported.

1. Dermatological — Not severe and disappear on discontinuation.

Dermatitis

Urticaria

Maculopapular rashes

Skin pigmentation (due to enhaced sensitivity to sunlight).

2. Hepatic — Allergic or immunological

Nonspecific increase in gamma-glutamyl-transpeptidase (GGT), SGOT and SGPT

Jaundice may be present — usually obstructive type.

Most cases develop this complication during 2nd to 4th week.

3. Haematological

Mostly appear in 4th to 19th week

Leukopenia

Agranulocytosis (< 3200/cmm)

4. Autonomic effects — Due to anticholinergic and antinoradrenergic effects

Blurring of vision and pupillary dilatation

Dryness of mouth

Constipation and urinary retention

Orthostatic hypotension and sedation

Tachycardia

5. Endocrine Effect

Rise in prolactin levels

6. Effect on Sexual Functions

Decreased libido and orgasm

Priapism (Thioridazine)

7. Immunological Side Effects

Increase in autoimmune antibodies may lead to systemic lupus erythematosus.

8. Increase in body weight

Due to increased appetite and diminished motor activity.

9. Neurological

Epileptogenic potential — lowering the seizure threshold.

Extrapyramidal symptoms

Acute — Acute dystonia

Akathisia (inability to sit at one place)

Parkinsonism (Tremors, rigidity and bradykinesia)

Chronic — Tardive dyskinesia

Neuroleptic malignant syndrome (syndrome characterised by markedly raised temperature, hyperreflexia with high incidence of mortality.)

CHLORPROMAZINE

Dimethylamine derivative of aliphatic group of phenothiazines.

Pharmacokinetics

Readily absorbed from gastrointestinal tract. Absorption decreased by food, antacids and anticholinergic drugs

First pass metabolism : Bioavailability by perenteral route increases many fold.

T_{max} (time taken to achieve maximum serum concentration) — 2 to 4 hours.

Metabolites — More than 100 metabolites identified.

Extensive plasma protein binding (up to 97%)

Widely distributed and crosses blood brain barrier to achieve higher concentration in brain than in plasma. It also crosses placental barrier and is excreted in milk.

Therapeutic Indications

Management of psychotic conditions (200 mg to 800 mg daily orally)

Nausea and vomiting (10 to 25 mg, every 4 to 6 hours orally)

Acute intermittent porphyria (25 to 50 mg TDS orally for several weeks)

Intractable hiccups (25 to 50 mg TDS or QID orally for 2-3 days; if no response 25 to 50 mg (IM)

Severe behavioural problem in children.

Adverse Effects

Discussed in section on antipsychotics in detail.

Sedation during 1st or 2nd week

Postural hypotension — momentary fainting and dizziness

Management — Keep patient in head low position, foot end raised; norepinephrine in cases of severe hypotension.

Haematologic — Agranuocytosis, eosinophilia, leukopenia

Jaundice —

~ Laboratory features of obstructive jaundice

Severe exfoliative dermatitis

~ Contact dermatitis in nursing personnel

Skin pigmentation — Rare. In female patients on dosage of 500 to 1,500 mg daily for more than a year; restricted to exposed areas of body; darkened skin to grey color; fades on discontinuation

Ocular Change —

More frequent in patients receiving 300 mg daily for two years or more; Deposition of fine particulate matter in lens and cornea; nature of this matter not defined; epithelial keratopathy and pigmentary retinopathy; lesions regress on stopping the medication

Fever following large intramuscular doses may occur

Peripheral edema reported

Systemic lupus erythematosus-like syndrome may occur

THIORIDAZINE

Phenothiazine derivative of Piperidine group

Pharmacokinetics

Orally absorbed from gastrointestinal tract

* T_{max} = 1½ to 4 hours (Time to achieve peak blood concentration)

t1/2 10 to 40 hours (Plasma half life)

Active metabolites are mesoridazine and sulforidazine.

Plasma protein binding — 99%

Uses — Psychoses — 50 to 100 mg (up to 800 mg can be given)

Side Effects

Pigmentary retinopathy (decreases visual activity in night)

Change in electrocardiogram

Sexual function (Ejaculatory failure and priapism)

Oedema (due to increased activity of antidiuretic hormone)

TRIFLUOPERAZINE

Phenithiazine derivative of piperazine group

Pharmacokinetics

Absorbed readily from gastrointestinal tract

T_{max} = 1.5 to 4.5 hours (Time to achieve peak blood levels)

t1/2 = 12.5 hours (plasma half life)

Plasma protein binding 90%

Uses

Psychoses — 2 to 5 mg twice daily orally (increased upto 15 to 20mg)

Nausea and vomiting (1 to 2 mg)

Anxiety — (1 to 2 mg)

Adverse Effeccts — Same as discussed with phenothiazines

CLOZAPINE

A dibenzodiazepine derivatives.

Pharmacology

Dopaminergic antagonism (greater affinity for D_1 than for D_2 receptor)

5 HT_2 Antagonism

Noradrenergic antagonism

Histaminergic (H_1) antagonism

Muscarinic (acetylcholine) receptor antagonism

Pharmacokinetics

Bioavailability 50-60% of oral dose

T_{max} - 2 hours (Time to achieve peak blood levels)

Plasma protein binding extensive

Extensively metabolised by liver and a high first pass effect

t1/2 - 12-16 hours (Plasma half life)

Plasma concentrations do not correlate with clinical response or adverse effects

Clinical Use

Initiate with 25 mg twice a day schedule (Escalate by 25-50 mg every day until the target dose of 300-500 mg per day).

Useful equally for positive and negative symptoms

In refractory or resistant schizophrenia

Adverse Effects

Haematological — agranulocytosis (monitoring of complete blood counts in patients on a weekly basis). Incidence 0.6%

Leukopenia in 1.8% Time of appearance — First 6 months. Recovery within one to three weeks of stopping treatment.

Sedation, tachycardia, constipation, dizziness, hypotension and sialorrhoea.

Weight gain (present in one third patients)

Seizure threshold lowered

Tremor, syncope, restlessness, nausea, diaphoresis, hyperthermia and delayed micturition.

Advantages

Minimal extrapyramidal symptoms

Little sexual dysfunction

Improvement — in negative symptoms

Effective in resistant cases.

RISPERIDONE — Benzisoxazol derivative

Pharmacology

affinity for dopamine D_2 receptors

high affinity for $5HT_2$ receptors

reduced propensity to induce extrapyramidal adverse effects

Therapeutic Efficacy

Risperidone produced significantly more response than haloperidol and did not produce significantly higher ratings for extrapyramidal adverse effects than placebo.

No significant difference in efficacy when compared with clozapine.

Advantages over clozapine appears to be lower risk of agranulocytosis with risperidone.

Adverse Effects

Concentrations difficulties, asthenia and sedation

Weight gain and orthostatic hypotension

Dose — 4 to 8 mg/day in two divided doses

REMOXIPRIDE

Substituted benzamide derivative

Pharmacology

Weak but relatively selective D_2 antagonist and appears to have affinity for extrastriatal D_2 receptors

No effect on muscarinic, histamine and serotonin receptors

Therapeutic Efficacy

Similar efficacy to haloperidol

Produces less sedation, few autonomic or cardiovascular effects and relatively few extrapyramidal symptoms

Adverse Effects

Tiredness

Insomnia

Concentration difficulties

Dose — 150 to 300 mg/day

Antidepressants

Classification

I. Tricyclic antidepressants
   - Imipramine
   - Amitriptyline
   - Nortriptyline
   - Clomipramine
   - Amoxapine

II. Tetracyclic antidepressants
   - Mianserin
   - Maprotiline*

III. Monoamine oxidase inhibitors*
   - Hydrazine — Iproniazid*
   - Phenelzine — Isocarboxazid*
   - Nonhydrazine — Tranylcypromine
   - Newer antidepressants — Moclobemide*
   - Selegiline (Available for indication in Parkinsonism)

IV. Atypical antidepressants
   - Trazodone
   - Fluoxetine
   - Bupropion*
   - Fluvoxamine*
   - Paroxetine*

* Not commercially available in India at present.

TRICYCLIC ANTIDEPRESSANTS

Pharmacology

Inhibit uptake of monoamines (norepinephrine, serotonin, dopamine) from synaptic cleft into neurons.

Anticholinergic action - mild atropine like

Antinoradnergic action (alpha$_1$ blockade)

Pharmacokinetics

Absorbed rapidly in gastrointestinal tract

Time to achieve maximum concentration varies from one to four hours

Extensively bound to plasma proteins and widely distributed in body tissues

Plasma half life is generally prolonged and single time dosing possible

Drugs metabolised in liver and excreted in bile and urine

Steady blood concentration vary considerably amongst patients and this difference may be as high as 40-fold

Relationship between plasma concentration and therapeutic responses for most antidepressants not yet established. Some evidence to suggest therapeutic window for nortriptyline and a linear relationship for amitriptyline and imipramine

Clinical Use

Major indication-depressive disorders

Initial 6 to 8 weeks full dosage is recommended. Dose varies for individual drugs

Two to three weeks are required for antidepressant effect to appear

During maintenance phase lower dosage may be given and recommended mean duration is six months but may be as long as one year.

There is enough evidence to suggest effectiveness of antidepressants in preventing depression in patients with recurrent depressive episodes and full therapeutic dose may be required for long periods.

Adverse Effects

Autonomic effects —

Dryness of mouth, difficulty with visual accommodation. Difficulty in micturition and constipation

Cardiovascular Effects —

Electrocardiographic changes T-wave flattening and prolonged PR and QT intervals

Conduction defects leading to bundle branch block

Postural hypotension

Central nervous system effects —

Fine tremors

Toxic confusional state

Delirium

Haematologic

Agranulocytosis

Weight gain has been reported

Delay in orgasm in women and men

Impotence

Drug induced mania or hypomania

Over Dose —

Not uncommon especially in patients with suicide risk

Prominent anticholinergic effects are present— mydriasis, flushed dry skin, dry mouth, arrhythmia.

Most urgent need is to support the vital functions at this time.

Usual course of severe poisoning — the comatose phase passes in 1 to 3 days followed by a period of excitement and anticholinergic signs. The risk of dangerous arrhythmias persists for several days and patients should be closely monitored during this period of recovery.

Physostigmine can sometimes help, especially when the vital functions are stable but anticholinergic effects are prominent.

Cardiac toxicity and hypotension can be difficult to manage. The QRS complex is prolonged to over 100 msec in acute overdosage. Cardiac glycoside and procainamide are contraindicated but phenytoin may be helpful.

IMIPRAMINE

A tricyclic antidepressant

Pharmacology

Blocks the reuptake of norepinephrine and serotonin and down regulates their receptors.

Pharmacokinetics

Absorbed rapidly orally

T_{max} (time to achieve peak concentration) 4 hours

Plasma half life 18 to 25 hours

Metabolised in liver. Active metabolite desipramine. Antidepressant effect due to combination of imipramine and desipramine.

Clinical use

Major depressive episode

Panic attacks

Enuresis

Dose — 100-300 mg in divided doses or in single dose

Side effects — (Discussed above in detail)

Dryness of mouth, blurring of vision, micturition difficulties in elderly, constipation and tachycardia,

Postural hypotension,

Fine tremors, confusional states and seizures.

AMITRIPTYLINE

Tricyclic antidepressant

Pharmacology

Blocks the reuptake of 5-hydroxytryptamine predominantly at the nerve terminal. But also affects norepinephrine reuptake. Potent muscarinic cholinergic blocker.

Pharmacokinetics

Absorbed rapidly when administered orally

T_{max} (time to achieve peak blood levels) 4 to 6 hours

Plasma half life 16 to 22 hours

Metabolised in liver — nortriptyline is active metabolite.

Plasma protein binding up to 98%

Clinical use

Major depressive episode

Dose

150 to 300 mg per day in divided dose or in single dose.

Side effects

Burring of vision, dryness of mouth, constipation

and tachycardia,

Postural hypotension.

MONOAMINE OXIDASE INHIBITORS (MAOI)

Non-hydrazine —

Tranylcypromine *

Hydrazine

Phenelzine *

Isocarboxazid *

Iproniazid *

Newer

Selegiline

Moclobemide *

Drugs marked as "*" not commercially available in India.

Pharmacology

Monoamine oxidase (MAO) inactivates catechol amines (dopamine, norepinephrine and serotonin) in the synaptic cleft and thereby MAO inhibition increases concentration of monoamines

MAO exsits in two forms, A and B. The antidepressant effect appears due to MAO-A inhibition, although majority of MAOI inhibit both.

Reversibility of these MAOI has important clinical implications.

Pharmacokinectics

Rapidly absorbed from gut

Widely distributed throughout all parts of body including brain

Metabolism — through acetylation and metabolites are inactive

Clinical Use — They have been found useful in :

Major depressive disorder

Anxiety state

Phobic anxiety states

Obsessional state

Adverse Effect

The side effects of MAOI can be either due to interaction with other drugs or food content or due to drugs alone

Foods containing high tyramine content could produce hypertensive crises presenting with headache confined to occipital or parietal region, sweating, pallor, chest pain and palpitation. In some cases cerebral haemorrhages have been reported. (Cheese reaction)

Drug induced mania

Hepatocellular damage resulting in jaundice (especially with hydrazine MAOI)

Insomnia

Hypertensive crises may develop even in absence of drug or food interactions

Rashes on skin and a lupus-like reaction has been reported

FLUOXETINE

Mechanism of Action — Selective serotonin reuptake blocker

Pharmacokinetics

Absorption — From gastrointestinal tract

— Peak plasma conc. in 4-8 hours

Metabolism — In liver to active metabolite norfluoxetine

Half-life — 2-3days (cf norfluoxetine 7-9days)

Excretion — Kidney

Indication

1. Treatment of depressive episodes
2. Dysthymia
3. Obsessive compulsive disorder
4. Reducing appetite and weight

Dosage

— 20-80 mg/day

— Usually 20 mg is effective. Therefore start with 20 mg/day and only if no improvement occurs in 3 weeks, increase dose by 20 mg

— For Obsessive Compulsive Disorder starting dose is 40 mg/day

Side Effects — (Antidepressants with least side effects which occur in only 15-20% of cases)

1. Insomnia — Therefore, do not give bedtime dose of fluoxetine
2. Headache
3. Drowsiness
4. Anxiety
5. Nausea
6. Diarrhoea
7. Weight loss

TRAZODONE

Pharmacology — Specific serotonin reuptake blocker

Pharmacokinetics

Absorption — Rapidly absorbed from gastrointestinal tract, peak plasma concentration in 1-2hrs.

Metabolism — Liver

Half life — 6-11 hours

Excretion — Kidney

Indications

1. Depression — Especially for improving sleep quality

Does not decrease stage 4 sleep (which is reduced by imipramine)

2. Some cases of panic disorder

Dose — 200-600 mg'day in divided doses

Side-effects — Almost no anticholinergic side effects

Most common side effects — Sedation
— Orthostatic Hypotension
— Dizziness
— Headache
— Nausea

Serious Side Effect — Priapism (prolonged erection in absence of sexual stimulation)

Patients should be advised to report if erection become more frequent and prolonged. If it occurs Trazodone, should be replaced by another antidepressant.

In case priapism does occur it should be treated with an intracavernosal injection of 1mg/ml solution of epinephrine.

NORTRIPTYLINE

Pharmacology — Norepinephrine reuptake blocker

— It loses its efficacy below plasma levels of 50 ng/ml and above 140 ng/ml

- These plasma levels are achieved between doses of 75-150mg/day

Side-effects — Nortriptyline differs from other tricyclics as it very infrequently causes — Orthostatic hypotension, therefore can be used safely in patients with pre-existing cardiac disease or in older patients.

AMOXAPINE

Pharmacology — 5 Hydroxtryptamine (5-HT) and norepinephrine reuptake blocker

Its metabolite — 7 Hydroxyamoxapine is a dopamine receptor blocker.

Specific Indication — Due to presence of antipsychotic properties, it is effective in the treatment of psychotic depression.

Side Effect — Extrapyramidal symptoms

— Tardive dyskinesia. If amoxapine is continued for more than six months chances of this side effect are greatly increased. In psychotic depression, need for antipsychotic is very brief, only till the resolution of psychotic depression, after which antipsychotic medication should be stopped. With the availability of modalities such as ECT and combination of tricyclics and antipsychotics, amoxapine has doubtful role.

MIANSERIN

Tetracyclic antidepressant.

Pharmacology

Blocks presynaptic autoreceptors (alpha-adrenoreceptor)

Blocks post synaptic 5HT receptors

Potent histamine antagonist

Pharmacokinetics

Rapidly absorbed on oral administration

Peak plasma levels achieved in 3 hours

Plasma half life 10 to 17 hours

Some evidence for therapeutic window (15 ug.ml to 70 ug/ml). The efficacy is lost above and below this range.

Adverse Effects

Epileptogenic potential

Blood dyscrasias - agranulocytosis

Dose

30 mg to 200 mg'day orally in single dose

MOCLOBEMIDE

Pharmacology — Inhibits MAO-A (Moclobemide converted to an adduct which is tightly but reversibly bound to MAO-A). Structure of adduct not defined.

MAO-activity restored within 24 hours of stopping medication.

Pharmacokinetics

Rapidly absorbed

Extensively distributed

Entirely metabolized in body (Metabolites not active)

Rapidly eliminated, half life 1-3 hours.

Clinical Use

100 to 150 mg dose in patients of endogenous depression (up to 300 mg in divided doses)

Efficacy from good to very good in 70% patients.

Adverse Effects

Gastrointestinal — nausea

ANTIANXIETY DRUGS

Main groups are :

1. Benzodiazepines
   Chlordiazepoxide
   Diazepam
   Nitrazepam
   Oxazepam
   Lorazepam
   Clonazepam*
   Triazolam*
2. Azaspirodecanediones
   Buspirone

Drugs marked as '*' are not commercially available in India.

1. Benzodiazepines

Pharmacology —

Facilitate GABA transmission in central nervous system

(Antianxiety action)

Antiagression effects

Anticonvulsant effects

Skeletal muscle relaxant action

Pharmacokiectics —

Rapidly absorbed from gastrointestinal tract and clinical effects appear within 1 hour and peak plasma levels by 2 hours.

Rapidly distributed all over the body.

Bound extensively to plasma proteins.

Plasma half lives vary and is the basis to divide them into three groups :

Long acting : Plasma half life more than 30 hours

Diazepam

Chlordiazepoxide

Nitrazepam

Medium acting : Plasma half life 10-30 hours

Lorazepam

Flurazepam

Short-acting : Plasma half life less than 10 hours

Oxazepam

Triazolam

Temazepam

Excretion is through liver and in liver disease this is delayed.

Older patients are more sensitive.

Clinical use

For relief of pathological anxiety

As anticonvulsant especially clonazepam is used for this purpose only.

Intravenously diazepam in cases of status epilepticus.

In anaesthesia as premedication before surgical and dental operations. Benzodiazepines have advantage of anterograde amnesia and this may be useful in anxiety about an operation

As muscle relaxant in cases of tetanus

Agoraphobia and social phobias.

Hypochondriacal states

Drug and alcohol withdrawal.

Adverse effect

Remarkably free of serious toxic effects

Sedation

Impairment of psychomotor functions, impair reaction time..

BUSPIRONE

Pharmacology — Partial agonist of serotonin type 1A receptors.

Pharmacokinetics

Absorption — through GI Tract unaffected by food.

— Peak plasma conc. 1½ hours after ingestion.

Half life — 2-11 hours

Generalised anxiety disorder (not panic disorder)

Advantage of buspirone 1. Non addictive

2. Non sedating

3. No withdrawal phenomenon

Disadvantage of Buspirone : Takes 2-4 weeks for clinical response to appear. Benzodiazepines have immediate action.

Dose

15-60 mg/day

Side effects

Mild Headache, dizziness and nausea.

ALPRAZOLAM

Indication

1. Panic disorder
2. Mixed anxiety with depression

Doses

2 to 6 mg/day. It should be given 2-3 times a day as half-life is short.

Advantages over imipramine

1. Has few side effects
2. Quick onset of action

Disadvantages over imipramine

1. Short half life necessitates use of multiple doses.

2. Rebound increase in anxiety a few hours before next dose.

3. Withdrawal syndrome leading to dependence.

LITHIUM

Lithium is third element in periodic table and a monovalent alkaline metal.

Pharmacology

Lithium increases the retention and turnover of noradrenaline in both acute and chronic administration.

Chronic administration stimulates turnover of 5-HT possibly by inducing tryptophan hydroxylase activity.

Lithium decreases acetyl choline synthesis

It also affects metabolism of GABA

Inconsistent effects on dopamine

~ DA synthesis inhibited

~ Pretreatment with lithium prevents DA receptor sensitivity induced by chronic administration of haloperidol

Lithium inhibits the formation of cyclic AMP in brain, kidney and thyroid-indirectly reduces the responsiveness of target cells to hormones.

Pharmacokinetics

Only administered orally and is rapidly absorbed. Mostly absorbed in small intestine

Distribution in the tissue is slower than the absorption. It passes into every compartment.

Elimination half life from 5 to 42 hours (a mean of 13 hours)

Concentration in CSF is usually one third of lithium concentration in serum.

Steady state CSF levels are reached somewhat later than in serum. Elimination from CSF is also slower than the serum.

Elimination — 90% is excreted through kidneys. Five per cent is lost in faeces. A small amount is found in sweat and saliva (<1%).

Optimal Serum Levels

— 0.6 to 1.2 meq/L in acute phase

— 0.4 to 0.6 meq/L in maintenance phase

Clinical Use

In manic phase of Manic Depressive illness

In prophylaxis of bipolar disorder

Precaution

1. # Sodium depletion leads to lithium accumulation

~ With thiazide diuretics

~ Chronic diarrhoea

~ With ulcerative colitis

~ Sweating in hot weather or an acute attack of diarrhoea

2. Cardiac disease

Associated with heart failure, arrhythmias sino-atrial and atrio-ventricular block and ventricular ectopic beats

ECG change — usual therapeutic dose may cause flattening of T wave in ECG

3. Epilepsy

An increase in fits as a result of therapy in patients with existing epilepsy

EEG pattern may change

4. Parkinsonism

Parkinsonism can become worse or can appear as toxic phenomenon

5. Thyroid disease —

Hypothyroidism can be worsened

6. Psoriasis —

Rashes may appear

Psoriasis may be precipitated or aggravated.

7. Pregnancy

An excess of Ebsteins anomaly and cardiovascular malformations. So avoid lithium in first trimester. Fetal thyroid gland is at risk.

Side effects

Early side effect — usually present within one week

* Abdominal discomfort
* Loss of appetite
* Nausea
* Loose stool
* Thirst and polyuria
* Fine tremors of hand

Later side effects — From one week of initiation up to 5-6 weeks of therapy

* Lethargy
* Muscle weakness
* Tiredness
* Emotional blunting
* Polyuria and thirst may appear for the first time or may persist from early on
* ECG — Flattened T wave

Broadened QRS complex

Long term maintenance

After 6 weeks other symptoms may appear

* weight gain — can be due to

— oedema

— gain in solid tissue 'fat'

* Hypothyroidism with or without goitre

* Skin — rashes, exacerbation of psoriasis and acne

Lithium Toxicity

— Therapeutic index of lithium is low

— Toxicity develops slowly due to delay in entry of Lithium into brain

— Lithium toxicity may appear even though plasma levels are within therapeutic range — Plasma levels, therefore, are not a reliable guide to toxicity. Appears above 1.3 or 1.4 meq./l

INITIAL SYMPTOMS

Decreased appetite

Nausea, vomiting

Diarrhoea

LATE SYMPTOMS

impairment of consciousness, incoordination ataxia, dysarthria, and coarse tremor of hands

acute brain syndrome leading ultimately to coma

fasciculation of muscles, myoclonus, hyperreflexia, nystagmus and fits — signs of neuromuscualr excitability

urinary output may drop as a result of direct toxic effects on kidney

cardiac arrhythmias may appear

ANTICONVULSANTS

1. Hydantoins — Phenytoin
2. Barbiturates — Phenobarbitone
3. Deoxybarbiturates — Primidone
4. Iminostilbenes — Carbamazepine
5. Succinimides — Ethosuximides
6. Benzodiazepines — Clonazepam
7. Miscellaneous — Valproic acid

Pharmacology

1. Increase the effectiveness of GABA (Gamma-amino butyric acid) thus enhancing neuronal inhibition (Benzodiazepines).

2. Blocking of picrotoxin receptors. This receptor reduces the action of GABA (Barbiturates and phenytoin).

3. Phenytoin prevents propagation of epileptic discharges, but not excitability of the primary focus whereas phenobarbitone decreases general neuronal excitability (therefore phenytoin is effective in grand mal but less so in preventing minor seizures originating from a focal discharge).

4. Elevation of cerebral 5-HT levels

5. Inhibition of enzymes catabolising the inhibitory neurotransmitter GABA and prevention of its uptake by neurons (Valproic acid).

PHENYTOIN

Pharmacology

Stabilises all neuronal membranes (excitable and nonexcitable)

Pharmacokinetics

— Intestinal absorption variable

— Saturation kinetics make it invalid to calculate plasma concentration and enzyme saturation because rate of elimination depends on plasma concentration and enzyme saturation

— After single dose t 1/2 is 10-17 hours

— After multiple dose t 1/2 as long as 140 hours

— Therapeutic plasma concentration 10-20ug/ml

— Extensively metabolised in liver (elimination impaired in liver disease)

— Plasma protein binding 90%.

Clinical Use

— Drug of choice in treatment of grand mal epilepsy

— Shown to reduce excitement and hostility (to be used as adjunct to neuroleptics)

— May also be used in psychomotor epilepsy (temporal lobe)

— Dose 300 mg/day in a single dose, dose increment 50 mg at a time and no more frequently than every 4-6 weeks.

Adverse Effects

1. Nervous system (ataxia, nystagmus, tremor, dysarthria and psychological disturbances)

2. Allergic rashes (hypersensitivity) hepatitis and drug fever

3. Collagen change — coarse facial features, gum hypertrophy

4. Haematological Megaloblastic anaemia (responds to folate); rarely aplastic anaemia, lymphadenopathy

5. Fetus — Increased perinatal mortality, cleft palate, hare lip microcephaly, congenital heart disease.

ETHOSUXIMIDE

Pharmacokinetics

Well absorbed orally

Plasma half life is 70 hours in adults but only 30

hours in children (single time dosing preferred).

Steady state levels achieved in seven days

Effective concentration 40 to 120 ug/mi.

Clinical Use

Treatment of choice for petit mal epilespy

Daily dose = 0.5 to 2 g per day

Adverse Effects

Dizziness, nausea, epigastric discomfort

TRIMETHADIONE

Alternative drug for the treatment of Petit Mal

Pharmacokinetics

— Main metabolite dimethadione is active

— Plasma half life of active substances 16 hours

— More than 700 ug/ml produce toxic effects.

Adverse Effects

— Sedation

— Blurring of vision in bright light

— Scotomata

— Rashes

— Blood dyscrasias (neutropenia, agranulocytosis)

— Nephrotic syndrome

— Hepatitis

CLONAZEPAM

Benzodiazepine

Mechanism of action

Potentiates the GABA mediated inhibitory pathways

Pharmacokinetics

Well absorbed orally

Plasma half life 30 hours

Therapeutic plasma levels 30 to 60 ng/ml

Clinical Use

* Petit mal epilepsy and infantile spasm

* Reduces excitement, negative symptoms in schizophrenia (to be used as adjunct to neuroleptic)

* Neuroleptic related myoclonus, oculogyric crisis, akathisia and blepharospasm.

* Psychomotor and myoclonic epilepsy

* Status epilepticus

* Dose — 4-8 mg/day in divided doses.

Adverse Effects

Lethargy and somnolence

Dizziness

Muscular incordination, ataxia, hypotonia and muscle relaxation.

CARBAMAZAPINE

Structurally related to tricyclic antidepressants

Mechanism of Action

Facilitates the GABA-ergic neurons

Pharmacokinetics

slowly but well absorbed following oral administration

plasma level fluctuates widely during absorption (? due to direct effect of gastric mobility)

plasma half life 25 to 60 hours after single dose but falls to 10 hours after chronic dosing (Twice a day dose suggested)

therapeutic drug level — 4 to 10 ug/ml

Clinical Use

Grand mal and temporal lobe epilepsy

trigeminal neuralgia

manic depressive psychoses as monotherapy also

starting dose 100 to 200 mg twice daily. Dose increments to be done slowly

Maximum dose — 1,200-1,600 mg/day

sedation, ataxia and giddiness

Nystagamus

leucopenia initially is common but usually transient

Hyponatraemia

Water intoxication — may lead to (due to antidiuretic action) therapeutic failure

induces hepatic enzymes

SODIUM VALPROATE

Pharmacology

Inhibition of GABA transaminase resulting in increased GABA concentration in synaptic regions.

Pharmacokinetics

well absorbed orally (95%-100% bioavailability)

plasma half life — 7 to 10 hours

therapeutic plasma levels — 40 to 80 ug/ml

Clinical Use

It is effective against several forms of epilepsy - grand mal, petit mal, psychomotor epilepsy (but not other forms of partial epilepsy) and myoclonic epilepsy.

Dose — 600 mg daily in divided dose (8 hourly). Dose increment every 3 days by 200mg/day until control achieved.

Dose range — 1,000 to 1,600 mg/day.

Adverse Effects

nausea, vomiting, diarrhoea, abdominal pain

temporary hair loss

teratogenic effects
hepatic necrosis rarely
acute pancreatitis

PHENOBARBITONE

Pharmacology

It reduces the spread of seizure activity and elevates the seizure threshold.

Reduces the excitatory effects of glutamate and enhances the inhibitory effects of gamma-aminobutyric acid.

Pharmacokinetics

well absorbed (80-90%) after oral and intramuscular administration
peak blood levels achieved in 6 hours.
therapeutic drug levels — 15 to 40 ug/ml
plasma protein binding 50%
metabolised in liver (55-75% of dose)
plasma half-life adults — 100 hours
children — 40 hours
(Drug given once daily)

Clinical Use

grand mal and partial seizures
it may exacerbate petitmal.
Dose — 60 to 180 mg daily
those increments not more frequent than every 3 weeks
should not be withdrawn suddenly — dose should be slowly reduced over the course of months.

Adverse Effects

nystagmus on lateral gaze
ataxia
tremor
dysarthria
allergy, rashes
haematological — folate deficiency anaemia, apalstic anemia
congenital abnormalities
hepatic enzyme induction leading to drug interaction

CALCIUM ANTAGONISTS

(CALCIUM CHANNEL INHIBITORS)

These are chemically and functionally heterogenous compounds.

The WHO classification is given below

Group I — (derivatives of phenylalkylamine)

Verapamil
Gallopamil
Emopamil
Tiapamil

Group II — (1, 4 dyhydropyridine or DHP derivatives)

Nifedipine
Nimodipine
Nicardipine
Nitrendipine

Group III — (Benzothiazepine derivatives)

Diltiazepam

Pharmacology

Ca_{++} is a second messenger linking cell membrane excitation with subsequent intracelluair enzymatic processes. There appear to be four different voltage sensitive channels designated as L, T, N and P. Only the L-type channel, in the nervous system located primarily on neuronal cell is considered to be sensitive to calcium channel inhibitors. These could be responsible for particular behavioural process and are under study.

They suppress the development of neuroadaptive changes in the course of chronic neuroleptic therapy. Recently these drugs have shown increased reinforcing properties for alchohol, cocaine and morphine also.

Pharmacokinetics

Verapamil can be considered as a prototype of calcium antagonists. It has been demonstrated that drug is well absorbed orally.

Bioavailability is low (20%) due to extensive hepatic first pass metabolism and only one fifth of the dose administered reaches the systemic circulation.

Extensive plasma protein binding.

Clinical Use

They exhibit antidepressant, anxiolytic, neuroleptic, anticonvulsant and sedative effects.
Calcium antagonists suppress alcohol and morphine tolerance/addiction.
These protect against dopaminergic supersensitivity brought about by neuroleptic treatment.
Verapamil is the most widely used calcium channel inhibitor for psychiatric indications.
There are wide differences in the effectiveness of various calcium antagonists. These differences could be due to varying bioavailability within the central nervous system.

CHAPTER 17

PSYCHOTHERAPY

Mental disorders were earlier considered to be a result of degeneration of brain and were not considered amenable to treatment. This approach resulted in development of large mental hospitals outside the city to segregate insane persons from the sane and thus protecting both from each other. Twentieth century saw a marked shift from this earlier position and all mental disorders were considered psychological in origin and amenable to psychological treatments. This shift has largely occurred due to the pioneering effort of Sigmund Freud and his followers. They developed a system of psychology which provided a theory of human psychological development, a method of treatment and investigation. It was called psychoanalysis. Simultaneously, Pavlov developed a theory of conditioning which explained psychological development from learning perspective. These theories were refined and further developed by large number of scientists.

Few decades later other workers emphasised the role of interpersonal and social factors in human development and they emphasised the role of social factors in mental disorders.

Till late sixties the psychological methods were considered essential for treatment of mental disorders. Large number of workers developed various methods of therapies and each emphasised the effectiveness of their methods.

Another evolution started in psychiatry during early sixties when researchers started looking critically at claims of improvements by these methods. Simultaneously, newer psychopharmacological agents produced marked relief in various mental disorders and the effect of various psychotherapies was more critically evaluated. At the same time the development in investigative techniques provided more information regarding neurophysiological dysfunctions in various psychiatric disorders.

Current evaluation seems to indicate that psychoanalytic psychotherapies are no better than placebo. Cognitive, behaviour and interpersonal therapies are more effective and in certain situations as effective as drug therapies. Common sense psychotherapy is also quite useful.

Definition

Psychotherapy is a treatment by psychological methods for problems of psychological origin or with psychological symptoms or dysfunctions by a trained therapist with the aim of minimizing or modifying or removing the symptoms or altering the person's response to them. Following are main factors of this definition :

a) treatment by psychological methods —

Psychological methods include psychoanalytic and behavioural methods and other psychosocial intervention.

b) problems of psychological origin or with psychological symptoms —

This method can be applied to all situations where disorders may have a presumably psychological origin or may have psychological symptoms. This will include not only mental disorders but also physical disorders with psychological symptoms like anxiety, depression, irritability etc.

c) by a trained therapist —

This is an essential ingredient of the definition. The psychotherapist requires training in the art and science of psychotherapy before he can conduct psychotherapy.

d) with the aim of minimising, modifying or removing the symptoms or altering the patient's response to it.

This covers the broad framework of aims of psychotherapy. It may not necessarily aim at removing the symptom, but aim at modifying or minimising it or may change the person's response to it. Ultimate aim is to make the patient more comfortable despite the limitation imposed by the disorders, personality of the patient and limitations imposed by psychosocial circumstances.

Different theoretical schools have developed their own theory of human development and methods of treatment. Some of the prominent are described below:

Psychoanalysis — This is a school of psychology developed by Sigmund Freud. The theoretical constructs of this school are as under :

1. Psychic determinism — Freud believed that

every event of psychic life is determined by previous psychological experiences. Nothing occurs accidentally. So-called slip of tongue or forgetting were explained on the basis of influence of unconscious psychic life.

2. Unconscious- Freud postulated an unconscious mind about which the individual is not aware. The unconscious is a repository of instinctual desires, and various conflicts which have been repressed. The unconscious tries to become conscious but it is kept in check by ego according to the demands of reality (reality principle).

Freud divided mental functioning into three area : id, ego and super ego.

Id — This is the repository of instinctual demands. He postulated that all human activities are due to two basic instincts i.e. life instincts or sexual instinct and death instinct or aggressive instinct. The first instinct is related to growth and development and the latter to death and destruction. The instinctual demands are part of the Id and are relegated in unconscious. Their conscious experience is only permitted when they have been modified enough to follow the reality principle.

Ego — This is a hypothetical construct. It is also known as self. The ego modifies the instinctual demands according to the reality principle as well as to the demands of the super ego. e.g. Ego functions through defense mechanisms.

Super ego — The child internalises the moral principles of the society by identifying with his parents and these moral principles become his own and he scrutinises each of his actions through these moral principles.

Ego defense mechanism — Defence mechanisms are methods employed by the ego to ward of the anxiety which develops from unacceptable demands of the id and to keep them in conformity with super ego and reality.

These defence mechanisms are divided into following :

Immature defences

Denial — The person denies the existence of painful reality. This may help in healthy adaptation if it is minimal. But it may lead to psychotic behaviour if reality is totally denied and in its place new reality is assumed.

Projection — The person projects his own unacceptable desires and fantasies on to others and then react to them as if they have their wishes. e.g. if a person hates his father, he may instead project this feeling to his father and may feel that his father hates him.

Introjection — An external object may be introjected within the self. If the object is desirable one feels comfortable with this process and may take on the qualities of the introjected good objects. If the introjected object is bad then one may direct the hostility towards the object on the self and it may lead to self punishment.

Identification — The person may identify with the loved object.

Regression — The person may regress to earlier level of adjustment in face of a conflictual situation.

Schizoid fantasisation — These individual retreat into fantasized world to escape the difficulties of the real life.

Repression — This implies the repression of primary instinctual wishes from reaching conscious awareness as well as suppression of painful and conflicting events. The latter leads to selective forgetting.

Displacement — The aim of the wish or desire is changed to a more acceptable one, yet the content of the wish remains the same. One may wish to hurt his father but may instead hurt the horse of the father.

Dissociation — There is dissociation of certain part of psychic functioning to avoid the pain of conflict. It is often seen in dissociative disorders in form of fits and fugue states etc.

Intellectualisation — The impulses are controlled by finding intellectual solutions about them and this reduces the force and makes them inocuous.

Isolation — There is intra-psychic splitting of affect from an idea e.g. I wish to kill my mother is an idea associated with strong feeling of anger. By isolation the idea becomes devoid of the effect and thus becomes inocuous. This defence is seen in obsessionals.

Reaction formation — Here the unacceptable wish is changed into its opposite and thus made acceptable. The person may change his sexual desires into excessive religiosity etc.

Undoing — The person tries to undo an already performed act by some imaginary act or magical thinking. A desire of hurting others may be undone by doing some repetitive magical act e.g. touching the object etc. It is seen in obsessionals.

Rationalisation — The unacceptable impluse is changed into acceptable activity.

Somatisation — Psychic anxiety is converted into somatic symptoms.

Mature ego defense mechanisms —

Sublimation — The forbidden sexual impulses are desexualised and the energy so freed is utilised in constructive work.

Suppression — The conscious decision to postpone gratification of wishes.

Humour — The instinctual wishes are presented in a pleasant way which does not hurt others or self.

Altruism — The inner desires and wishes are converted into acts of service to others.

Psycho-Sexual development

Psychoanalysis presumes that sexual instinct has an aim and organ through which it is fulfilled and these aims and organs change with age and this development occurs in a specific sequence.

Oral stage — In this stage the organ of gratification is the mouth and it lasts up to 18 months of age. This involves gratification initially by sucking and later by biting. The proper development of this stage leads to development of trusting dependence on the mother and other adults. If the oral stage does not develop normally it may lead to excessive dependence, demandingness and such children are usually envious and jealous of others. Such individuals when confronted with stress may revert back to oral character traits.

Anal stage — In this state the libidonous organ is the anal area and satisfaction is obtained by controlling defecation. The conflict in this stage centers around toilet training and the infant starts developing feelings of independence from the parents. At the same time he also feels that he can control the parents as he can control defecation. Successful resolution of this stage leads to development of autonomy; lack of ambivalence and a capacity to cooperate with others. Disturbances in the resolution of this phase may lead to sadism, ambivalence, and defiance.

Phallic stage — The organ of libido becomes the penis and the genital area. It leads to infantile masturbation and sexual fixation on the other sex parent. This is also known as Oedipal complex. The Oedipal complex is suppressed by castration fear (i.e. the genitals may be cut due to child's unacceptable fantasies of loving his mother). This suppresses the infantile sexuality and leads the person into latency stage.

In females, the development is slightly different. The female child develops sexual desires for the father. The fear of this unacceptable desire as well as her awareness of lack of penis (penis envy) suppresses her sexuality.

The successful resolution of this phase provides a sense of mastery of instinctual urges and the person develops his sexual identity. There are no feelings of shame or guilt. Improper resolution may lead to feelings of insecurity about sexual desires and later sexual attraction may reawaken oedipal anxieties.

Latency phase — This phase is characterised by suppression of sexual drives and it is utilised in learning and playing activities. The child develops inter-personal skills and develops a sense of mastery. If the inner controls have not developed properly then the child may find it difficult to accomplish the above-mentioned psychological tasks. This stage lasts from 5-12 years approximately.

Genital Stage — This stage starts around 12 years and continues till a person becomes a mature adult. This stage is characterised by fully developed sexual identity and by development of mature heterosexual object relation. The dependency of child should give way to autonomy of the adult. The sexual phantasy or object relations should not be contaminated with incestuous desires. Successful development will lead to a mature independent adult, who can make heterosexual relationship without anxiety and deal with various situations appropriately.

Psychoanalysis is also a method of investigation. The major techniques used for investigation are :

a) Free association — The subject is asked to speak out everything that comes to his mind without censoring anything. This may help to unravel the unconscious material.

b) Dream analysis — Dreams are said to be manifestations of unconscious life and their analysis is said to be the royal road to unconscious.

c) Analysis of slips of tongue — These may also give an idea about the unconscious life.

Psychoanalysis as Treatment Method

Psychoanalysis aims at analysing the origin of the mental disorder by unravelling the unconscious by analysing transference and resistance.

The treatment requires 5 sessions per week of 40-50 minutes. The patient lies down on a couch and the therapist sits behind him so that he does not inhibit the patient's free association. Treatment may take 3-5 years.

Brief Psychodynamic Psychotherapy

These are practised more often these days. The aim of these psychotherapies are more modest and they tend to focus only on certain specific aspects.

Critical Evaluation of Psychoanalysis

Freud was a genius and was well ahead of his time. He revolutionised psychiatry by his contributions. Unfortunately Freud has been converted into a demi-god by his followers. However, every individual works within the frame of reference of the time when he was working. Freud's contribution to psychiatry may be conceptualised as under :

1. Freud's emphasis on effect of earlier psychological experiences on later behaviour is universally accepted .

2. Freud's concept of unconscious process is acceptable to the extent that many of our behaviours might originate from the past experiences which are not in our direct awareness.

3. His concept of psychological treatment for emotional disorder is also largely acceptable.

4. The concept of transference and resistance in therapy is also generally accepted. His theoretical explanations for these phenomenon are not acceptable to many.

5. Concept of defense mechanism — enumerated by the psychoanalyst are acceptable to many.

6. Freud's concepts of instincts, his division of psychic life into id, ego and super ego and other theoretical explanations are not generally accepted now.

In conclusion it can be said that Freud was an astute observer of human behaviour. His observations are still valid but his explanation for these observations were dependant on the philosophical ethos of his times and are no longer valid.

Behaviour Therapy — This is an approach to treatment which is based on learning principles. It presumes that all behaviour is learnt whether normal or abnormal and it can be modified according to learning principles.

Following are common learning paradigms.

Classical conditioning — This method was first described by Pavlov. He demonstrated that salivation in the dog which occurred at the sight of food could be conditioned to other stimuli if it is paired with food. The dogs were presented with food soon after a bell was rung. After few practice sessions the bell became a signal for food and produced salivation. If the bell is rung repetitively without presenting food then this response is extinguished which leads to unlearning of the response.

This model is used in modifying physiological response of the body in various psychophysiological disorders.

Operant Conditioning — This paradigm states that occurrence of a response is dependent on the nature of reinforcement. If a child says 'Ma' and the mother responds positively then the sound 'Ma' gets learned and becomes associated with mother.

On the other hand if the child uses an abusive word and he is punished, he gives up usage of that word and it is called negative reinforcement. Most of the learning occurs by providing positive reinforcement for desirable behaviour and negative reinforcement to undesirable behaviour.

Based on these observations the following techniques are used by the behaviour therapist.

The behaviour therapist defines the problems and treatment methods before the treatment is started. As behaviour therapy focusses on observable behaviour the progress of treatment can be monitored. Many modern-day behaviour therapists emphasise that the difference in behaviour and other therapies is only in their abitity to monitor progress by their method.

The behaviour therapist starts therapy using the following steps :

1. Identification of precise behaviours to be modified and measure them by some method. e.g. a person has repetitive hand washing as a symptom. The behaviour therapist will measure the frequency and time spent in this behaviour.

2. What are the environmental or personal reinforcer that are maintaining these symptoms.

3. Based on the above the therapist decides which strategies can be useful.

Following techniques are generally used.

Relaxation technique — The aim of this exercise is to help the patient to develop motor and psychic relaxation.

The patient is advised to contract a group of muscles e.g. in the hand and asked to experience the tension of the muscle. Then he is asked to relax the muscles of the hand and feel the difference. Similarly, he is progressively asked to contract the muscles of forearm, upper arm, shoulder, head, face, neck, chest, abdomen, back, thighs, calf and foot etc. Once he has experienced tension and relaxation in each group of muscles on both sides, he is asked to contract all of them together and then relax the whole body and brain slowly. He may also be asked to focus attention on any neutral object like flickering flame of a lamp. This will help him to drive out conflicting thoughts. This process will help the patient to experience a feeling of well-being and release of tension. The patient is advised to do it twice a day. Once he becomes proficient in this exercise he may do so whenever he experiences tension or anxiety.

Ancient Indian system of yoga has a specific posture which produces the same effect (*Shavasana*). Many other methods of meditation also produce relaxation.

Pharmacological relaxation : — Relaxation can also be produced by I. V. Sodium pentothal given slowly. This can hasten the process of treatment.

Systematic Desensitization

This is usually indicated in patients of anxiety and phobias. Initially the therapist makes a list of hierarchy of anxiety-provoking situations. The situation which produces least anxiety is put first and that produces maximum anxiety should be put last. The patient should agree with this list.

Systematic desensitization is started with relaxation training. Once the patient is able to relax properly, he is advised to imagine least anxiety provoking situations. If he can tolerate it without getting anxious then he is exposed to next higher situation. This process is repeated till the patient can remain anxiety-free in maximum anxiety provoking situations.

Later on the patient is exposed to real situation in the same order. It is hoped that after some time the person will be able to go into the anxiety provoking situation without any difficulty. Initially the therapist may accompany the patient in actual situations.

This treatment is effective in phobias, obsessions and sexual disorders.

Graded Exposure — This is similar to above except that there is no relaxation and desensitisation in imaginary situations. The patient is directly exposed to real life situations in graded fashion.

Flooding — In this process the patient is exposed to maximum anxiety-provoking situation instead of doing so gradually.

He is encouraged to stay in the situation and advised that the anxiety will subside with time. This treatment must be used with full consent of the patient.

It is used in phobias and obsessions.

Aversion Therapy

In this therapy an aversive stimulus is paired with the behaviour to be extinguished. The aversive stimuli can be a mild electric shock, nausea-producing drugs, bad odours, punishment etc.

For instance in the treatment of alcoholism, apomorphine is given first and then the patient is asked to take his favourite drink. As soon as he takes the drink he develops nausea due to apomorphine and alcohol intake becomes associated with nausea and thus the desire to take alcohol is inhibited.

Positive Reinforcement

Behaviours which are desirable are rewarded and it increases the chance of their persistence. This is usually done in children and schizophrenics. Whenever the child does a socially acceptable behaviour he is rewarded with a toffee or some other thing which he likes. Similarly, schizophrenics are rewarded if they clean their teeth, wash face, take bath properly etc. It is important to reinforce a specific behaviour. If one rewards general behaviour, proper reinforcement may not occur.

Modelling

The person is exposed to role models which are

desired. The patient gradually develops confidence by seeing other people behave without anxiety and will be able to do so himself. This technique has been used successfully in phobias and other behavioural problems.

Assertiveness and Social Skill Training

This is taught to those patients who lack assertiveness and social skill. Such training is important for many patients of personality disorders and schizophrenia.

One must identify the skills to be learned (e.g. to talk positively with opposite sex) and to devise methods for its learning (modelling and positive/negative reinforcement).

Critical evaluation of behaviour therapy :

1. Biggest strength of behaviour therapy is its ability to demonstrate observable change.

2. Major drawback of behaviour therapy is that it does not take into consideration the autonomy of the individual. The symptoms are considered in isolation which is often not acceptable to many patients.

3. Success of behaviour therapy is largely dependent on motivation. If the person is not motivated he will not cooperate in treatment and the treatment will fail.

Behavioural therapies have been found useful in a large number of psychiatric disorders.

Cognitive Therapy

Psychotherapy emphasise mainly on emotions, motivations, desires (intrapsychic process) or effect of social interaction (inter-personal process), but the process of cognition was largely left unstudied or unemphasised. Beck postulated that depressive disorders could be due to faulty cognitions and these may be equally important in many other disorders also.

Cognition refers to the ability to know about reality accurately. If a person has a faulty cognition e.g. he feels that he is useless, inferior, and incompetent; this may lead to changes in his behaviour and may lead to depression.

Cognitive approach has been well studied in depression. According to Beck the depressives have a cognitive triad :

a) Negative view of self —

Self is perceived as incompetent, useless and undesirable.

b) Negative view of the world —

The world is experienced as demanding, censoring and demeaning.

c) The person expects continuous hardships and failures.

Similarly, obsessives have faulty cognition of self-doubt and fear of unforeseen happenings.

Treatment Strategy

The therapist has to be energetic, optimistic and should have the ability to empathize. The technique of treatment can be divided into following :

Didactic : The patient is explained the basis of treatment, how faulty cognitions and wrong assumptions are affecting his life. He is further told that he need not take the therapist's world on face value and the therapist and the patient will together test the correctness or otherwise of these assumptions.

Cognitive Techniques

The patient is helped to elicit his automatic thoughts and assumptions and to test their validity.

Testing and identifying autonomic thoughts — The patient is asked about an event of the previous day e.g. what happened when he had to take bath? He may state that he felt weak because of which he was not able to take bath. The automatic thought is, patient's view that he was too weak. He is encouraged to take bath which may not produce any difficulty. Thus, he can test the faultiness of his assumptions.

Testing and Identifying Faulty Assumptions

The patient will soon be able to identify many faulty assumptions. If I cannot get that particular promotion I cannot be happy. The patient is helped to understand that happiness and promotion may not go hand in hand.

Behavioural Methods — The patients are provided graded tasks and he has to divide his whole day into distinct periods. The task of each period is specified and the patient is encouraged to do simplest of tasks initially. As he is able to do this he will experience a feeling of pleasure and mastery. Gradually more difficult tasks are undertaken. These tasks must be recorded. The records also help to correct the faulty assumptions and help to regain confidence. Many other behavioural techniques can be used.

This technique has been found useful in mild non-bipolar depression and obsessions. It is now being used for panic and anxiety disorders.

Most therapists now use a combination of behaviour and cognitive therapy which is called cognitive behaviour therapy.

Interpersonal Psychotherapies

This type of psychotherapy is based on assumption that the psychological problems arise due to interpersonal miscommunications and due to familial and other social stresses. Therapist aims at changing interpersonal communication by marital and family therapy. The focus could also be on modifying other areas of functioning like job, social interactions etc.

These therapies are useful in those patients where social problems are initiating or maintaining psychiatric disorders eg. marital problems leading to sexual dysfunction and in adjustment disorders.

Integrated Psychotherapy

Each individual can be presumed to have following characteristics :

a) Genetic influences : These will determine the range of his cognitive, social and interpersonal behaviour. In some person the genetic influence may alter the patterns of thinking and experiencing. One will need to delineate the basic personality and cognitive style of the individual eg. patients of schizophrenia may have severe limitations in thinking and relating. The psychotherapy will need to be planned acordingly.

b) Effect of life experiences : Life experinces tend to modify and shape one's personality and way of relating with the world. It is important to analyse the type of experiences this individual has undergone and what is their influence on him.

c) Symptomatology : Decide whether it is directly related to —

i) genetic influences

ii) life experiences

iii) cognitive styles

Before starting psychotherapy following questions should be answered :

a) What are the patient's problems ?

i) diagnosis

ii) symptoms

iii) psychosocial problem

b) What is the patient's personality ?

c) Are there any organic deficits ?

d) What is the management plan ?

i) Drugs

ii) Psychotherapy

e) What are the aims of psychotherapy ?

Symptom removal

Symptom amelioration

Improvement in interpersonal relationship

Modification in personality.

f) What are the methods to be used ?

Much will depend on the diagnosis, symptoms, education, psychological mindedness of the patient and his expectation, as well as on the expertise of the therapist. The therapist and the patient should agree on the goals of treatment. Psychotherapy is an essential part of psychiatric treatment. One need to decide the method on the basis of one's training and needs of the patient.

Chapter 18

ECT AND OTHER THERAPIES

Electroconvulsive therapy (ECT) is an extremely effective therapy when used for those psychiatric disorders where it is indicated. Unfortunately, a lot of bad publicity by the lay press and even by a section of mental health specialists, has led to a lot of misconceptions in the public, leading to understandable fright and perturbation in the patients and their families. The commonest myths are that ECT leads to permanent brain damage and even death. While all options and the risk - benefit ratio should be explored when recommending ECT to a patient, it is necessary to recognize that the major alternatives — pharmacotherapy or psychotherapy have their own risks and benefits, a fact which is often forgotten when making an impassioned plea against the use of ECT.

HISTORY

It was von Meduna who, in 1934, first reported successful treatment of acute schizophrenic symptoms, including catatonia, with pharmacologically induced seizures, using intramuscular injections of camphor in oil, which he soon replaced with intravenous Phenylmetrazol. This use had stemmed from the prevailing belief — now known to be erroneous — that schizophrenia and epilepsy could not coexist in a single patient. Cerletti and Bini modified this initial therapy and administered the first electroconvulsive therapy in 1938 in Rome, then known as Electroshock therapy (EST). This was followed by the introduction of muscle relaxants to avoid convulsion (which has resulted in fractures), and, as generalized muscle relaxation led to respiratory distress, it was used together with General Anaesthesia to prevent the occurrence of cerebral anoxia. Since its introduction in 1951, succinylcholine (Scoline) has been the most popular relaxant used for the purpose. Recently, the work of Max Fink and two American Task Force reports (1978, 1990) have provided updated information regarding the use of ECT in modern psychiatry.

CLASSIFICATION OF ECT

ECT can be classified according to various parameters —

I) According to the use of Anaesthesia :

When ECT is given under general anaesthesia with premedication and a muscle relaxant, it is termed as modified ECT (M-ECT). ECT given without anaesthesia and pre-medication is called Direct ECT (D-ECT). While this is not an issue in the West currently, and the 1990 American Task Force Report does not recognise the use of D-ECT at all, this procedure is still widely used in a country like India where the average patient commonly cannot afford the cost of anaesthesia and pre-medication associated with the complete course of ECT. It seems cruel to deny such patients the obvious benefits of ECT just because they do not have adequate funds. More over D-ECT seems to have less complications.

II) According to the placement of electrodes :

Placement of electrodes may be bilateral (introduced first) or unilateral. While the 1990 Task Force Report is ambiguous on the choice of electrode placement, current consensus opinion is that, while both placements are equally effective in treatment of depression, unilateral non-dominant electrode placement is associated with less cognitive impairment.

III) According to the shape of the electric current (Stimulus Waveform) :

The electric current waveform, as visible by an oscilloscope is the basis of dividing ECT devices into sine-wave and brief-pulse types. Brief pulse stimulus delivery is reportedly associated with less energy delivery, and thus, less cognitive impairment. This is an issue which has received less importance in India and a present survey of Indian psychiatrists showed that a good 23.7% did not know the nature of stimulus waveform of their ECT devices while 55.8% employed constant voltage sinusoidal waveform ECT devices. While the 1994 Task Force Report recommends sinusoidal wave ECT only for refractory patients, the credibility of this form of ECT is being re-established due to its superior therapeutic efficacy.

WHEN SHOULD THE PATIENT BE REFERRED FOR ECT

ECT should be administered only by qualified mental health professionals well versed in its use. Non psychiatric physicians may refer patients for ECT on the following grounds :

1. PRIMARY USE :

— when a rapid, definitive response is essential;

— when the risk of other treatments outweighs the risk of ECT; and /or

— when there is a previous history of poor drug response and good response to ECT in the past.

2. SECONDARY USE :

— when an alternative primary treatment fails; and/or

— when primary treatment is associated with more adverse effects than estimated with ECT.

MAJOR DIAGNOSTIC INDICATIONS

1. Major Depression—The most common indication. ECT is effective in

— all subtypes of Unipolar Major Depression and

— all subtypes of Bipolar Major Depression

It is probably as efficacious as drugs in depression, with possibly a quicker onset of action. While presence of delusions has now been shown not to indicate a better response to ECT, such patients respond poorly to drugs hence there is strong case for primary use of ECT in delusional depression. ECT is not, however, used usually for prophylaxis of depression and the role of maintenance ECT is controversial.

2. Mania — Effective in all subtypes of Acute Mania, it has been shown to be probably as effective as lithium and possibly with more rapid improvements. However, since drug therapy of mania is equally effective, and can be advantageously continued for prophylaxis, ECT is preferred only in cases of acute excitement or when, for some reason, drugs are contraindicated.

3. Schizophrenia : ECT is used for specific indications : presence of catatonic schizophrenia

— presence of affective symtomatology

— past history of a favourable response to ECT

It is effective in about 10% of chronic schizophrenics and should not be used as primary treatment for this indication.

4. Other functional psychoses (1990 Task Force Report)

— Schizoaffective disorder

— Other Atypical Psychosis

When clinical features resemble those described under indications 1-3.

OTHER INDICATIONS

Other disorders, where the use of ECT has been shown to be of benefit in a few cases resistant to the primary treatment, are being listed to complete the list.

MENTAL DISORDERS

— Functional psychoses other than those listed above

ORGANIC MENTAL SYNDROMES

— Severe organic affective and psychotic conditions showing clinical features similar to the major indications

— delirium of various etiologies (e.g. toxic and metabolic)

MEDICAL DISORDERS

— Catatonia secondary to medical conditions

— Hypopituitarism

— Intractable seizures

— Neuroleptic malignant syndrome

— Parkinson's on-off phenomenon

It is important to note that usage of ECT in all the above diagnoses should be considered experimental and should be documented in the clinical records with clear justifications for its rather unusual use.

CONTRAINDICATIONS

1. Absolute :

Contrary to traditional teaching, the 1990 Task Force Report has listed no absolute contraindications.

2. Relative :

Specific situations asociated with increased risk are listed, in which ECT must be undertaken for a life-threatening indications in which ECT has proven benefit. Further, a full medical evaluation must be undertaken prior to the procedure and necessary precautions taken to modify the risk level. Such conditions include :

— conditons with raised intracranial tension eg. space-occupying lesions

— recent myocardial infarction

— recent intracerebral haemorrhage

— bleeding/unstable vascular aneurysm or malformation

— retinal detachment

— phaeochromocytoma

— anaesthetic risk.

PROCEDURE

1. Informed consent :

This must be taken after providing sufficient information of the benefits, risks, procedures and alternative treatments available. It should always be in writing, for a specified number of ECT sessions, with the understanding that consent can be withdrawn whenever wished, and should be appended to the clinical records.

2. Pre-ECT investigations :

This should include, at a minimum, a thorough medical history and physical examination. Urine and blood chemistry, chest and spine X-ray, and an ECG may be done specially in the elderly patients. Relevant special investigations should be done according to each individual patient's needs.

Possible concurrent drugs which raise the seizure threshold, should be looked for and discontinued - eg. benzodiazepines and anti-convulsants. MAOI's and lithium may alter scoline metabolism, increased post-ECT sequeale in patients on lithium have been reported. Low to moderate doses of antipsychotics may even be helpful early in the course of ECT's.

3. Pre-anaesthetic precautions :

— nil orally at least since 6 hours prior to a treatment

— ask patient to void urine

— check hair for pins and such objects that may cause injury, and for hair oil which impedes the passages of electrical current

— remove jewellery, glasses, contact lens, hearing aids and dentures and check mouth for loose teeth, paan, chewing gums and other foreign bodies.

— record vitals and establish venous and airway access.

4. Premedication, anaesthesia and muscle relaxant :

— anticholinergic (usually atropine) intramuscularly (0.3-0.6 mg) 30-45 minutes before treatment to minimize secretions and prevent ECT-induced bradycardia. It can also be given at time of treatment intravenously (0.4-1.0 mg) though routine use has been discontinued in some centres, except in patients on β-blockers and with ventricular ectopics.

— methohexital or thiopentone is usually used as a short-lasting intravenous anaesthetic. The former is associated with fewer ECT-induced cardiac arrhythmias. Ultra brief, light anaesthesia is preferable.

— scoline, the ultra fast acting depolarizing muscle relaxant — is administered within a minute of the anaesthetic agent after ensuring complete anaesthesia and patency of airway. Dosage should be adjusted according to body weight and degree of relaxation required, 0.5-1.0 mg/kg being the usual IV dose. Complete relaxation is preceded by muscle fasciculations, which can be observed moving from head to toe, with the naked eye.

— oxygenation should be maintained from onset of anaesthesia, using positive pressure ventilation (100% oxygen at a flow rate of at least 5 litres/min) until spontaneous respiratory movements are established.

5. Electrode placement :

— bifrontotemporal: centre of each electrode approximately one inch above the midpoint of a line drawn from the tragus to the outer canthus of the eye. This is the traditional electrode placement.

— unilateral placement: one electrode over the non-dominant frontotemporal area and the other placed on the non-dominant centro parietal scalp, about an inch ipsilateral to the midline vertex, in the position suggested by D'Elia.

— other placements, though suggested have only historical value.

6. Duration of seizure :

The stimulus dose is usually adjusted according to the duration of seizures, which should last at least 25 seconds. A seizure duration of about 30-60 seconds, occurring bilaterally symmetrically is usually considered optimum.

7. Seizure monitoring :

— Ictal motor activity : The cuff method is commonly used (inflating the BP cuff above the systolic blood pressure in an arm to impede flow of relaxant distally), and the longest duration of seizure-related activity noted. If unilateral placement is used, the occluded limb should be on the same side as the stimulating electrode.

— Ictal EEG activity. This is highly recommended at least on a one-channel basis.

— Ictal ECG : should be carried out, at least on a one- channel basis, from anaesthesia induction to resumption of spontaneous respiration .

— Cardio vascular vital signs : include BP and pulse rate, should be monitored until stabilization of ECT induced changes.

8. Special Issues :

— Missed seizures: restimulate the patient with a 25% - 100% increase in stimulus dose, after ensuring proper oxygenation and a 20 - 40 second delay between restimulation, to a maximum of 4 per session.

— Abortive seizures: Modality of seizure monitoring used should be specified. Re-stimulate at a higher dosage after a 60-90 seconds' delay.

— Prolonged seizures: seizures persisting more than 180 seconds are dangerous, and should be terminated pharmacologically by

intravenous anaesthetic agent used, or

intravenous fastacting benzodiazepine, with adequate ventilation, and

repeat muscle relaxant if ictal motor activity presists.

— Difficulty in generating seizures:

Check for seizure - threshold raising medication hyperventilate.

Use smaller dose of thiopentone with additional use of stimulating agents (e.g. caffeine and sodium benzoate) hydration of patient should be adequate change anaesthetic agent, using one with less effect upon seizure threshold e.g. ketamine

NUMBER AND SPACING OF ECT SESSIONS

While there are no fixed number of ECT's to be given in each patient, certain guidelines are suggested:

1. The clinical response should determine the number of ECT sessions.

2. Most physicians employ a bi- or tri-weekly schedule of ECT administration on non-consecutive days, although some prefer 2-3 consecutive ECT sessions in the initial phase of treatment.

3. Prolonged consecutive every day ECT can lead to severe cognitive dysfunction and is best avoided.

4. An ECT course usually consists of 6-12 ECT's, and cases referred for reason of refractoriness to pharmacotherapy may require more, some schizophrenics may require up to 20 ECT sessions.

5. Target symptoms should always be identified and monitored for improvement, and ECT discontinued when a significant improvement is found. Use of a rating scale to monitor improvement objectively is recommended.

6. Post - ECT maintenance therapy is a must, and is usually done pharmacologically. Controversy surrounds the use of ECT as maintenance treatment. Whether 1-2 'prophylactic' ECT sessions, after complete remission, prove beneficial, is also still debatable.

MECHANISM OF ACTION OF ECT

Some clinical observation and many hypotheses have been proposed, but the issue is still far from being satisfactorily resolved.

— generalized, symmetric tonic-clonic seizures, lasting at least 25 seconds, are considered essential for the ECT response.

— change in the neurotransmitter function is seen as a result :

down regulation of post-synaptic Beta adrenoreceptors,

change in the post-synaptic serotonic receptors: the exact direction of change has been variously reported.

* down regulation of acetylcholine muscarinic receptors.

* decreased synthesis and release of GABA.

* increased activity of endogenous opioids.

* — a compromised theory suggests that it is the balance of effects on some, or all of the above, that leads to the beneficial effects of ECT.

— advanced neuroradiographic techniques have shown an immediate post-ECT metabolic hypoactivity in regions hitherto hyperactive.

— the exact correlation between the above neurochemical observations and therapeutic effects of ECT has evaded the workers so far .

ADVERSE EFFECTS

1. Mortality — usually from cardiovascular complications, especially in the presence of compromised baseline cardiac functions. Mortality from ECT (1 per 10,000) is comparable with that from brief general anaesthesia.

2. Confusion and cognitive impairment — This is of great importance and has been minimized by use of unilateral non-dominant brief-pulse ECT. Memory function should be regularly monitored prior to starting the course, and then, at least weekly, by using brief bedside cognitive screening instruments 24 hours after the last ECT session. Memory functions return to the base line usually within 6 months but in some, they may persist for longer periods. If memory impairment is demonstrable, following steps may be taken :

* change over to unilateral, non-dominant electrode placement
* decrease electrical stimulation intensity
* increase time intervals between sessions
* alter medications
* if all fail, consider terminating the ECT course.

3. Cardiovascular — Transient cardiac arrhythmias are occasionally seen, especially in presence of pre-existing cardiac dysfunction.

4. Prolonged apnoea — maintain airway and intubation, with ventilation, until patient begins spontaneous respiration.

5. Prolonged seizures — has already been dis-

cussed.

6. Emergent mania — should be differentiated from organic euphoria. Discontinuation of the course may have to be considered.

7. Allergic reactions — to drugs or anaesthethic agents used in the ECT procedure are occasionally reported.

8. Minor problems — include post-ECT headache, backache, nausea and muscle soreness. Usually they subside with symptomatic treatment. In rare cases, these may be severe enough to warrant termination of the ECT course.

ECT IN SPECIAL POPULATIONS

1. Children — While age is not a contraindication for ECT, in children the issue of permanent cognitive impairment is still not disproved. Hence, ECT should be used in children only when alternative therapies fail, in the presence of proven indications, and by a team experienced in giving ECT's to children. It may be best to take the objective opinion of another psychiatrist in writing, before proceeding with ECT in this group.

2. Elderly - No age is a contraindication to the use of ECT, and ECT is not less effective in the elderly. While ECT, like any other somatic therapy, may be associated with increased risk in this group, it is usually considered a less risky alternative to pharmacotherapy. Certain points are worth remembering:

* physiological changes associated with aging necessitate smaller doses of pre-medications anaesthetic agent;

* seizure threshold increases with age; and

* cognitive dysfunctions may be greater in this group.

3. Pregnant women:

No trimester of pregnancy is a contra-indication to ECT, but up to eight weeks, the anaesthetic agents carry a teratogenic risk, which is comparable to that of other psychopharmacological agents. In the first trimester, ECT may be a less risky alternative to pharmacotherapy. Some points to be remembered are:

* the risk of teratogenesis should be included in the informed consent form;

* obstetric consultation prior to ECT, and during ECT in high risk cases, is recommended; and

* if the patient is not in the first trimester, it may be prudent to monitor foetal heart rate during ECT and in the post ECT recovery period.

4. Medical illness :

specialist consultation and relevant laboratory investigations are imperative. The risk-benefit ratio must be weighed and suitable modifications in the ECT procedure may be necessary to decrease post-ECT morbidity.

ECT is an effective somatic treatment for certain specific psychiatric indications, in which it has undoubted efficacy. While administering ECT for other indications may be considered experimental, and even unethical by some it should be borne in mind that withholding ECT where it is clearly indicated is even more unethical. If the treating psychiatrist has personal reservations against the use of ECT, he would do well to refer the case to another, more objective, colleague.

PSYCHOSURGERY

Psychosurgery is considered as a last-resort treatment when all rational alternative therapies fail to provide succour, in psychiatric (e.g. Depression, OCD) and neurological (e.g. epilepsy, chronic pain) patients. It is a means of surgical modification of certain brain areas or their connecting association areas or tracts, with the specific aim of modifying certain resistant, distressing symptoms of the patient. Moniz and Lima are credited with performing the first psychosurgery in 1935. Moniz won the 1939 Nobel prize for his work in this area, but ethical concerns and appearance of effective neuroleptics in the 1950's led to a loss of interest in this technique. Better diagnostic and surgical techniques, fewer risks, and research on treatment refractory patients have led to a renewed resurgence of interest in this technique.

INDICATIONS:

The major indication is the presence of a debilitating, chronic psychiatric disorder, refractory to other alternative treatments, present for at least 5 years. Disorders include:

1. Recommended:
— chronic intractable major depression
— obsessive compulsive disorder
2. Possibly effective:
— extreme, intractable aggression
3. Controversial:
— resistant mania
4. Not recommended currently:

— schizophrenia.

BENEFITS AND PROBLEMS

— up to 70% of patients selected with specific indications, may show benefit;

— benefit may continue till a few years after the procedure;

— there is an increased ability to attend to cognitive tasks, leading to improved IQ scores;

— no known undesirable personality changes reported;

— about 3% or less become worse. This risk should be explained and documented in the informed consent form;

— about 1 in 100 patients may develop post-operative seizures but usually respond well to traditional anticonvulsants;

— mortality rates are not reported and possibly vary with expertise of the treating team and individual patient characteristics.

OCCUPATIONAL THERAPY

The use of occupational therapy probably dates back to the early part of this century. A modern definition of occupational therapy was given by Fine in 1972 : The application of goal-directed, purposeful activity in the assessment and treatment of individuals with psychological, physical or developmental disabilities. Occupational therapists are required to work in close coordination with mental health specialists. Unfortunately, the full potential of this highly effective therapeutic modality is yet to be realized in India.

When a patient is referred for occupational therapy (OT), information regarding the problem, for which the referral has been made, is gathered from all possible sources. On the basis of this, the problem is identified, areas for intervention identified and specific procedures with specific short and long-term goals are planned. The aim is basically to encourage the development of group interaction and group skills.

Under the general heading of occupational therapies are included a large number of specialized sub-activities :

— social skills education

— social activities

— task activities

— activities involving communication between patients e.g. drama therapy.

Thus, it is imperative to recognize the important role of this specialized therapy in therapeutics and rehabilitation, and therapists require special training. It is certainly not a diversion activity for bored inmates of psychiatric hospitals and should not be considered as such.

CHAPTER 19

PSYCHIATRIC EMERGENCY

Emergency is a sudden development which can threaten the life, psychological or physical well-being of the individual, or of people around him or may lead to loss of property unless immediate remedial measures are taken.

Psychiatric emergencies are quite common and most of them are not properly treated as there are very few psychiatric hospitals in the country. Majority of psychiatric emergencies are treated by general hospital emergencies or by private practitioners. It is of utmost importance that the general practitioner should learn to deal with these problems. Common psychiatric emergencies are :

1. Violent and aggressive patient
2. Suicidal patient
3. Patient in stupor or semicoma
4. Panic/anxiety
5. Drug related problems
6. Drug induced dystonia and extra pyramidal syndrome
7. Psychosocial crisis.

1. **VIOLENT AND AGGRESSIVE PATIENTS** : These patients are brought for emergency consultation because of the following reasons :

a) patient is trying to assault others or is destroying property

b) he is abusive, talks incoherently

c) he is not eating anything

d) sleep is lost

e) may harm himself

Diagnoses and Management

Obtain basic information from the accompanying person regarding the duration of the problem, main symptoms any history of previous physical or psychiatric illness, any history of recent head injury or drug abuse. Also ascertain from the informants whether they suspect that the patient is carrying a weapon.

The physician should try to interview the patient. While interviewing four people should be kept around so that the patient can be restrained if need arises. If the patient is amenable to interview he should be informed that the doctors are trying to help him and he should tell his problems without fear so that proper help can be provided. In case he cannot be properly interviewed and he is markedly excited then he should be restrained with minimum but sufficient force. His hands and feet should be tied. While restraining the patient, care should be taken to restrain by wide gauge rolls and cotton should be kept below the gauge. Keep watch for any evidence of cyanosis beyond the site of restraint.

Once the patient is restrained then he should be examined.

Differential Diagnosis of Acute excitement:

1. Organic Causes

— History of head injury

— Any evidence or history of Diabetes, Hypertension

— History of seizures

— Any neurological symptoms

— Pupils

— Cranial nerves

— Motor weakness

— Aphasias

History of drug abuse e.g. alcohol, cannabis, barbiturates, cocaine, steroids, antidepressants, amphetamine, L Dopa, I.N.H.

Investigation

Blood — Hb TLC DLC

Blood Sugar Random

Urine — Routine and for acetone

X.Ray Skull — AP and Lateral views, other views if needed

CT Scan if needed

Any other specific investigation

Management

The patient can be sedated with Haloperidal 5 mg or Chlorpromazine 50 mg given by intra muscular route if there is no contra-indication.

In case of head injury, sedation should be avoided, and patient should be kept under watch.

Other neurological conditions should be treated appropriately.

In case of drug intoxication sedation should be used judiciously. Appropriate treatment for drug intoxication should be started without delay.

B. **OTHER PSYCHICATRIC DISORDERS**

If there is no evidence of organic involvement or

drug abuse then diagnosis is based on following :

Acute psychoses and schizophrenia will present with history of change in behaviour from last few days or gross psychotic symptoms from quite sometime. Common symptoms are delusion (fear of being poisoned, or killed, police being after them), hallucinations (voices talking) thought disturbances (speech being incoherent and irrelevant). These symptoms should be present now as well as few days earlier.

Such patients can be sedated with Haloperidal 5mg IMI, which can be repeated if needed. Patient's nutrition should be maintained.

Mania — These patients will give history of excessive talking, grandiose delusions (false belief that he is very rich or powerful) excessive spending and quarrellsomeness. Past history of similar episode or episode of depression can be helpful..

Management

These patients may require a higher dose of haloperidol and 10 mg IMI can be given. It could be repeated after few hours.

Dissociative Disorders —

These patients will give history of a conflict or stress which has led to the aggressive behaviour. They will not show evidence of thought disorder. Their aggressiveness may vary from moment to moment.

Management

They may be calmed down by simply listening to them. In severe cases Diazepam 10 mg can be given intravenously.

DISSOCIAL PERSONALITY DISORDER

These patients will have a history of life long pattern of dissocial behaviour (repeated lying, aggressiveness etc.). They may become violent when opposed or when faced with a difficult situation.

Management

These patients can be sedated with Diazepam 10 mg IMI. After a short sleep they may loose their aggressiveness.

PSYCHOSOCIAL DIFFICULTIES

Few persons may become aggressive and violent due to psychosocial conflict. Persons faced with exposure in public, or cornered in a tight situation may react violently eg. after sudden death of close relatives, caught in a scam or a demoralising act. Such person will usually show momentary excitement with periods of despair. They will not show any thought disorder, hallucination, or delusion. Neurological examination will be normal. They can be managed by talking to them sympathetically and drugs like diazepam 5 mg or more can be given to induce sleep which may help them to overcome immediate crisis.

STUPOR AND COMA

Stupor and coma must be differentiated. Stuporose patient does not respond to commands but he is not unconscious. He may respond to painful stimuli. His eyes may appear alert.

Comatose patient is fully unconscious. His mentation is not clear. He may respond to deep pain. Comatose patients are to be managed by medical or surgical experts.

Stuporose patients should be dealt with by psychiatrists.

Functional stupor is characterized by:

— Mutism

— Not moving body parts

— Eyes open, may follow objects

— Patient may be able to recognise others

— Physical examination normal

— Investigations normal

Possibility of catatonic,
depressive,
dissociative or
manic stupor and
malingering should be considered.

Differential diagnosis

Catatonic stupor — History of earlier episodes of schizophrenia. The stupor usually follows a period of abnormal behaviour characterized by irrelevant talking, suspiciousness, hallucinations etc. It should be differentiated from organic stupor by the following:

— Not responding to stimuli

— Presence of neurological symptoms

— Physical examination reveals neurological signs

Investigations

— Blood sugar

— Urine sugar

— Ketone

— Evidence of liver damage

Management

Inj. Haloperidol 5 mg daily or twice a day. Maintain nutrition by I.V. drip. If patient does not start eating within 3 days, ECT should be considered

DEPRESSIVE STUPOR

There will be a history of sadness of mood, accompained by negative thinking, apprehensiveness, excessive tiredness, sleeplessness, which has gradually led to complete immobility and mutism or patient may talk in whispers.

Management

Patient should be persuaded to talk and eat. If he does not agree, then ECT may be the treatment of choice. If patient starts eating then oral antidepressants can be given. (Imipramine 75-150/day).

MANIC STUPOR

These patients will give history of excitement, high and grandoise talks, sleeplessness and excessive spending for many days prior to the onset of stupor.

Management

The patient should be put on Haloperidol 5-10mg I.M.I. It could be repeated in the evening. If the patient does not respond within 3 days he may be given ECT.

DISSOCIATIVE STUPOR

These patients will give a history of stress or conflict prior to the onset of stupor. There may be history of dissociative symptoms in the past. On examination the stupor will be quite variable and the patient may become normal for short periods.

Management

The patient should be encouraged to talk. The doctor may need to give him time so that he can overcome inhibitions and he is able to communicate. In case he is not able to talk Pentothal Sodium 2.5% sol (.5 g dissolved in 20 cc distilled water) can be given slowly and the doctor should try to talk to the patient and he may also give a suggestion that the patient will be able to talk now. Most patients will respond.

MALINGERING

These patients will be under demonstrable stress eg. imminent prison sentence, severe difficulties in job or with family. These patients will show normal behaviour when they think that they are not being observed. Any attempt of movement of any body part may be met with resistance.

Management

These patients will require skillful interviewing. They should be helped to face the situation and they should be provided with legitimate help.

PANIC DISORDER

These patients usually present with a severe feeling of apprehension, and they may feel they are going to die. They usually present with the fear of having a heart attack or difficulty in breathing.

They generally approach a cardiologist or medical emergency room.

These patients do not require any emergency medication because the panic symptom disappear within 30 to 60 minutes. They should be treated for panic disorder as described earlier. Emergency medication will make them ask for the same drugs whenever panic occurs again. They need to be counselled. All relevant investigations should be done in the first episode. Later the investigation should not be repeated.

DRUG RELATED PROBLEMS

Large number of patients may come for emergency consultation after excessive intake of intoxicants like alcohol, opium, barbiturates. The management of overdosage is described in chapter on Drug Dependence.

DYSTONIA, AKATHESIAS AND OTHER EXTRAPYRAMIDAL SYNDROMES

Many patient may present with phenothiazines induced dystonias, extrapyramidal syndromes and neuroleptic malignant syndrome.

Clinical Picture

Dystonia — The patient will present with neck turning to one side or the body twisting, or tongue becoming protruded. These may occur in any combination.

Management

Immediate relief can be obtained by injection promethazine — 50 mg IMI or IVI.

Injectable anticholinergics can also be given. Phenothiazines and haloperidol can be reduced and antiparkinsonian drugs e.g. Trihexyphenydyl can be added (2 - 6 mg/day).

EXTRAPYRAMIDAL SYNDROME

This is characterized by coarse tremors of hands and feet, marked rigidity of body, patient may not be able to eat because of difficulty in chewing. There will be history of phenothiazines intake.

Management

Anticholinergics like Trihexyphenyldyl 2-6 mg. day.

NEUROLEPTIC MALIGNANT SYNDROME

This is characterized by hyperpyrexia, rapid pulse, increased blood pressure and confusion. There will be history of phenothiazine intake. Investigations will reveal increased white cell count, increase creatinine phosphokinase (CPK) and increase myoglobin.

Treatment

Discontinue phenothiazines. Patient should be given cold sponging. Vital signs to be monitored. Bromocriptine 1.25 mg twice a day may be useful.

PSYCHOSOCIAL CRISIS

Many patients may seek emergency consultation because of a crisis situation. Crisis is a situation in which if proper measures are not taken may lead to long term difficulties. Common crisis situations are :

— Marital crisis

— Job crisis

— Imminent exposure of certain immoral acts

— Sudden failure or losses (bereavement)

All these situations can lead to suicidal attempts, start of legal proceedings, resignation from job etc. which can effect the individual's life adversely.

Management

The aim of management is to help the patient to tide over this situation so that he can take proper decisions when he is in a more stable frame of mind.

SUICIDE

Suicide is an act of self destruction. It has been variously defined. The major components of suicide are :

a) an act to destroy one self which is consciously planned.

b) The individual considers suicide to be the best solution for the problem confronting him.

Suicidal act if successful leads to destruction of life, if not the person may escape with or without injuring himself. Unsuccessful act is called attempted suicide.

However, some people make attempt to end their lives which are really not meant to kill them, but to attract the attention of others towards their sufferings or to alter the existing pattern of life. Such attempts usually do not lead to cessation of life e.g. taking two tablets of tranquilizers, wrist slashing etc. Such attempts are called parasuicide and are more common in females. However, such attempts may accidentally lead to death.

Epidemiology

Suicide is a universal phenomenon and it is seen almost in all societies. Worldwide prevalence of suicide varies from 5 to 30/100,000 population. Highest suicide rates are seen in Japan and former communist countries of Eastern Europe (Hungary, Austria, Eastern Berlin) while lowest rates are seen in the Middle East countries.

The variation of rates may reflect the religious acceptance of suicide in that country and rigourousness of reporting practices. Official rates as published by Govt. of India each year put the suicide rate between 5 to 7/lakh population. However, these rates should not be taken as the correct rate because there is too much under reporting, and often suicidal attempts are hidden because Indian law considers suicide to be a crime till recently. The actual suicidal rate would be around 10-12/100,000 population in India.

Sex

Suicide rate is higher in males in the West. Indian studies also indicate that males tend to commit suicide more often, but there is an excess of suicides in females between 20-30 years.

Age

Suicide is infrequent in children. Adolescent exhibit suicidal behaviour usually in response to failure in examinations or due to failure in love. Females in the age group of 20-30 exhibit high suicide risk. Elderly males have a higher suicidal risk.

Method of Commiting Suicide

In India most common methods of committing suicide are, taking poison, hanging, drowning and burning. Amongst the poisons insecticides are commonly used. Jumping in front of running train is another common method. Use of fire arms, tranquilisers and hypnotics are not that common as in the West.

Etiology

Suicidal act is a deliberate decision of an individual to end his life as the best course available to him under the existing circumstances. Such decisions will depend on the following :

a) personality of the individual and his level of frustration tolerance.

b) availability of social support which can help him tide over the present crisis e.g. psychological help from family and friends, monetary support, medical support, support from state in form of disability pension etc.

c) Religious Beliefs — If the religion accepts suicide as an honourable way of exit from this world then the suicide will become more frequent as seen in Japan. Even in India Sati Pratha (self immolation of wife on the husbands funeral pyre) or *Jauhar* (self immolation of women folk after defeat in war seen in Rajputs) or giving up life by ascetics were permitted by religion.

d) The type of stress will also influence the decision to commit suicide. If an honourable man is threatened by exposure and dishonour he may take recourse to suicide to avoid humiliation. If a person has severe painful condition from which no relief is expected he may decide to end his life.

Following are the common etiological factors responsible for suicide :

1. Genetics — Suicidal behaviour may have a genetic predisposition. It has been observed that suicide is much more frequent in some families. It is usually seen as an expression of heritable depressive disorder.

2. Biochemical Factors — It has been shown that low level of 5-HIAA (5 hydroxy indole acetic acid) is common in people who commit suicide specially with violent means.

3. Sociological Theories — Durkheim divided suicide into three types on sociological basis :

a) Egoistic Suicide — This type of suicide occurs when individual is not properly integrated into society — This type of suicides explain high suicide risk of the old, lonely, widow/widower.

b) Altruistic Suicide — This type of suicide occurs in those who have excessive integration with society and they consider their groups well-being much above their own. It was seen in Japan during World War II when Japanese soldiers committed suicide for the welfare of the state. It was also seen in India during freedom struggle when people gave up their lives for the welfare of the country.

c) Anomic Suicide — These suicide occurs in those persons where integration with the society is disturbed e.g. a person who suddenly loses fortune may attempt suicide. It is also seen in societies with break-down of social norms and values. This could be the reason for higher suicide rates in former East European communist countries.

4. Psychiatric Disorder — Psychiatric disorders are a major cause of suicide. Suicide rates in psychiatric patients are 10-12 times more than the general population. Common disorders leading to suicide are:

a) Depression — Nearly 15% of depressives end their lives by suicide. Depressives perceive themselves to be a burden on others and feels that they will never be able to get well and will suffer all through their life. This perception of life leads to the decision of committing suicide. Depressives who have experienced good recovery may loose much of the suicidal intent. On the other hand depressives with delusions of poverty and hopelessness are more likely to commit suicide.

b) Schizophrenia — Schizophrenics usually commit suicide for the following reasons:

— During recovery phase when they understand that they may never be able to lead a normal life.

— They may commit suicide to escape the persecution or due to hallucinations commanding them to end their life.

— Post-psychotic depression may also lead to suicide.

c) Obsessive Compulsive Neurosis — These patients become severly depressed because of their obsessions and compulsions and may decide to end their lives to escape misery.

d) Drug Abuse — Chronic drug and alochol abusers often commit suicide to escape the misery of withdrawal symptoms and to avoid social ridicule.

e) Other Disorders — People with personality disorders sometimes commit suicide.

5. Physical Illness —

Suicide is often resorted to by people who have incurable or painful illness. Patients with cancer, AIDS and painful conditions like Herpes Zoster often try to end life by suicide.

6. Psychosocial Factors —

Psychosocial factors often lead to suicide. Common factors are :

a — failure in examination
b — failure in love
c — marital difficulties
d — illegitimate pregnancy
e — job problems

f — loneliness and despair
g — loss of love object by death or by other means.

The above list is by no means comprehensive. There could be many other situations which may produce despair of such a magnitude that the person may decide to end his life.

Clinical Picture

Most of the suicidal patients consult physicians few months prior to suicidal act. It is important to elicit suicidal intent whenever such a possibility exists. Whenever any psychiatric patient or persons with chronic painful conditions or untreatable conditions like cancer or AIDS are being evaluated it is imperative to elicit the patients views regarding the illness and its impact on the quality of life.

One should assess the suicidal intent on the following parameters:

a) Does the patient feel that life is a burden or not worth living ?

b) Has he ever thought about ending his life ?

c) Has this thought persisted or has he given it up as a ridiculous idea ?

d) Does the idea still persist, has he made any attempts ?

e) Does he still plan to end his life ?

Previous attempts and persistent suicidal wish with plans to commit suicide will indicate serious suicidal risk. Following factors are generally indicative of high risk :

1. Old age
2. Males
3. Females in 20-30 year age group
4. Severe depression
5. Previous suicidal attempt
6. Recent loss or bereavement
7. Single, widow or divorced
8. Poor physical health
9. Severity of the condition leading to suicidal intent

All of the above require validation in Indian context. As a rule of thumb every suicidal ideation should be taken seriously.

Management

Majority of suicides are preventable if identified in time. Most persons may not attempt suicide again if the immediate impulse passes off. The management of suicide essentially revolves around prevention, as once the act has been committed and it is successful nothing can be done. For prevention, following strategies are important :

1. If a patient or relative communicates that the patient has suicidal intent don't ignore it.

2. Disorders which are associated with high suicidal risk, should include assessment of suicidal risk.

3. General practitioners should be sensitized for assessing suicidal risk in all chronic painful conditions and depressions.

4. Self help group can provide round the clock help for people who have suicidal intent. Such services require wide publicity.

5. Conditions associated with suicidal risk should be promptly treated.

6. When a patient has been identified with high suicidal risk following steps should be taken :

a) It should be decided whether the patient requires hospitalisation. Decision to hospitalise depends on the following:

i) Patients who are lonely and have no support should be hospitalised.

ii) Patients who have treatable acute conditions like depression or schizophrenia should be hospitalised.

iii) If the family members can provide good care at home then the patient can be treated at home.

iv) Before hospitalisation of a patient one should also assess the facilities available in the hospital for round the clock surveillance. When such facilities are not available, hospitalisation may be counter-productive.

b) If the patient is suffering from a physical or psychiatric disorder it should be effectively treated. Severe depressives can be treated by ECT. Patients with painful conditions should be given enough analgesics to reduce pain.

c) Patient should be helped to develop hope about future. His immediate problems should be realistically tackled. Family or other agencies should provide psychological support. He should be ensured continuous support till he needs it.

In spite of all measures suicide may still happen and the physician should not feel disheartened by the failure of his treatment. If suicide does happen the support is needed for the surviving family members.

Concluding one can say that suicide is a multifaceted problem and will require attention of different specialities. Though majority of suicides can be prevented yet best preventive measures have not succeeded in eliminating suicide.

SUICIDE AND LAW

Section 209 of Indian Penal Code considers suicide to be a crime. This section state " whoever attempts to commit suicide and does any act towards committing such an offence, shall be punished by simple imprisonment for a term which may extend to one year, or with fine or with both." Due to this act majority of people try to hide suicidal acts. Though few high courts in the country have found this act anachronistic and struck it down. Yet it is still part of the law. It is essential for prompt and better treatment of these patients that this law should be removed from the statute book which is also the recommendation of 42nd report of Law Commission. Section 305 and 306 prescribes penalties for abetment of suicide by insane persons and by normal individuals, respectively. The penalties are stiff.

Section 209 has now been repeated by the Supreme Court of India.

Recent legislation on Dowry death states that if any woman commits suicide within seven years of marriage and the inlaws are found to be harassing or torturing her, they will be held guilty and can be imprisoned for 3 years. This act has also lead to many negative consequences. If any married female shows depression or suicidal behaviour the inlaws try to send her back to her parents to avoid these penalties. This often lead to aggravation of depression. This law also requires a careful reappraisal.

CHAPTER 20

PSYCHIATRY AND LAW

Mental illness may often effect the sufferer's capacity to make decisions due to which he may not be able to take care of himself or may find it difficult to handle his affairs. Each country has made certain laws to protect the individuals with disorders of mind.

The law relating to mentally ill can be divided into the following categories: .

1. Laws relating to treatment and care of the mentally ill.
2. Laws relating to the criminal responsbility of the mentally ill.
3. Laws relating to the civil responsibility of the mentally ill.

LAWS RELATING TO THE TREATMENT AND CARE OF THE MENTALLY ILL

Treatment and care of the mentally ill, till recently was being regulated by the Indian Lunacy act of 1912.

Mental Health Act was passed by Indian Parliament in 1987 and the Act has come into force from 14.4.93 in all the States and Union Territories vide Notification No. S.0. 43 (E) dated 11-1-93.

This Act replaces the older Indian Lunacy Act. The main feature of this Act are the following.

Chapter I of the Act deals with definitions. Important definitions for clinical purposes are :

'Mentally ill person' means a person who is in need of treatment by reason of any mental disorder other than mental retardation. This definition explicitly excludes persons with mental retardation from the definition of mentally ill. The Act also provides that mentally retarded will be kept at separate place other than a mental hospital.

The definition of mental illness is not quite satisfactory because it will include many minor mental illnesses like anxiety, depression, obsession etc. Such patients are competent to take care of themselves and their affairs and hence are not in need of protection from law. It would have been better if an additional clause of "incapacity to look after themselves or their affairs due to mental illness or disorders" was added.

"Psychiatric hospital" or "Psychiatric nursing home" means a hospital or as the case may be, a nursing home established or maintained by the Government or any other person for the treatment and care of mentally ill persons and includes a convalescent home established or maintained by the Government or any other persons for such mentally ill person; but does not include any general hospital or general nursing home established or maintained by the Government and which also provides care for the mentally ill.

This clause is not clear about non-government owned general hospitals or nursing homes which may also cater for psychiatric patients.

Chapter II

This chapter deals with creation of Central and State Mental Health Authority. Ministry of Health and Family Welfare vide notification No G S R 1004 (dated December 29, 1990 published in the Gazett of India Extra) Part II Section 3(i), dated 29th December 1990 has framed rules regarding constitution and functioning of these authorities. The authority shall:

a) be incharge of regulation, development, direction and coordination with respect to mental health services under the Central (State) Government and all other matters which, under this Act are the concern of Central (State) Government or any officer or authority subordinate to the Central (State) Government;

b) supervise the psychiatric hospitals and psychiatric nursing homes and other mental health service agencies (including places in which mentally ill persons may be kept or detained) under the control of the Central (State) Government;

c) advise the Central (State) Government on all matters relating to mental health; and

d) discharge such other functions with respect to matters relating to mental health as the Central (State) Government may require.

This chapter provides for the supervision and planning of mental health services in the states and under Central Government.

Chapter III

This provides for the establishment or maintenance of psychiatric hospitals or psychiatric nursing home.

This chapter provides that separate hospitals will be established for those who are under 16 years of age, for persons addicted to alcohol or other drugs and for criminal lunatics.

This chapter provides the details regarding who can establish such hospitals and the procedure for obtaining licence.

Chapter IV

It deals with procedure for admission and detention in psychiatric hospitals.

Part I

Section 15 — Request by major for admission as voluntary patient — Any major person who considers himself to be mentally ill may request the medical officer incharge of the hospital for admission.

Section 16 — Request by guardian for admission of a ward — where the guardian of a minor considers such minor to be mentally ill and desire him to be admitted in a psychiatric hospital, he may request the medical officer incharge of the hospital for the same.

Section 17 — Admission of and regulation with respect to voluntary patients — The medical officer incharge of the hospital after receiving request under Section 15 or 16 will make such enquiries as he deems fit to assess that such person requires admission and he can admit such person if in his opinion they require admission. This decision should be made within 24 hours.

Section 18 — Discharge of voluntary patients. The medical officer incharge of psychiatric hospitals will discharge a voluntary patient when the patient himself makes the request for discharge and in case of minor when his guardian makes such request.

In case of minors who attain majority during voluntary admission the medical officer incharge should inform them that they should give voluntary consent for hospitalisation within a month. Otherwise they have to be discharged.

However, if the medical officer incharge of the hospital is satisfied that discharging such a patient will not be in his interest; he can within 72 hours constitute a board of two medical officers and seek its opinion whether such voluntary patients needs further treatment. In case the board consider that further treatment is required the said patient can be further hosptalised for a period of 90 days at a time.

Part II

Admission Under Special Circumstances

If a mentally ill person is not willing for admission, in such a case his close relations can apply for admission in prescribed form. Such an application should be supported by certificates from two medical officers, one of whom should be in the service of the Government. However, if the incharge of the psychiatric hospital feels it proper or needed he may cause such person to be examined by two doctors working in that hospital. Such patient will not be detained for more than ninety days. Judicial review of such admission is possible.

Part III

Reception Order

Application for reception order can be made by :

a) the medical officers incharge of a psychiatric hospital

b) by the husband/wife or other relatives.

a) the medical officer incharge of a psychiatric hospital can apply for a reception order where the patient is undergoing treatment under a temporary treatment order and the doctor is satisfied that the patient requires longer treatment either for his own well-being or of others and the treatment needs to be continued for more than six months.

Husband/wife of the mentally ill or other relatives can also apply for reception order. Other relatives should specify why they are applying for the patient's admission. The person applying for reception order should have seen the patient in previous fourteen days.

The application for reception order should be made in a specific form and should be accompanied with two medical certificates, one of which should be from a doctor in Government service. The medical certificate given by doctors should clearly state the following.

a) That the doctor has examined the patient independently and has formed his opinion on the basis of his observations and from the particulars communicated to him.

b) That the person is suffering from mental disorder of such a nature and degree as to warrant the patient's detention in a psychiatric hospital either for his own safety or health or for the protection of others.

On production of such an application for reception order the magistrate may either pass the order on documentary evidence or may examine the patient himself and then decide whether such an order is needed or not. Patient will be admitted in a hospital prescribed for the area.

Reception order on production of mentally ill before magistrate :

Every officer incharge of a police station can take any person in police custody when he thinks, that due to mental disorder he is not able to take care of himself or who is dangerous to others.

Such person should be produced before a magistrate who will decide whether a reception order can be directly issued or he may order such person to be examined by a medical officer.

Order in case of mentally ill person cruelly treated or not under proper care and control :

Any person or police can apply to the magistrate that a mentally ill person is either being cruelly treated or is not under proper control. The magistrate after due inquiry either can ask the persons responsible for the patient to take proper care or can admit such a person in a psychiatric hospital.

Admission as in-patient after inquisition

Persons who are found mentally ill on inquisition can also be admitted in a psychiatric hospital if the District Court finds it necessary in the interest of the patients.

Admission and Detention of Metally Ill Prisoners

Any mentally ill prisoner may be admitted to a psychiatric hospital after proper proceedings.

DETENTION OF ALLEGED MENTALLY ILL PERSON PENDING REPORT BY MEDICAL OFFICER

Magistrate can order an alleged lunatic to be kept under observation in a psychiatric hospital or in an observation ward of a general hospital for 10 days. This period can be extended for another 10 days if required. But the total period of detention shall not exceed 30 days.

Discharges

The medical officer incharge of a hospital can discharge a patient from the psychiatric hospital after being recommended for discharge by two medical officers, one of them should preferably be a psychiatrist. This does not apply to mentally ill persons being treated as voluntary patients. After discharge a copy of discharge certificate should be sent to the appropriate authority under whose order the patient was admitted.

Discharge of Mentally ill Persons on Application

If the person who has applied for the admission of the patient applies in writing for the discharge of the patient then the patient can be discharged provided that the medical officer incharge is satisfied. If he thinks that the person is dangerous and unfit to be at large, then such request can be refused.

Discharge of a Person on his Request

Any mentally ill person who feels that he has recovered can apply to the magistrate for his discharge. Such an application should be supported by a certificate from the medical officer incharge of the hospital where he is undergoing treatment.

Leave of Absence

Leave of absence can be granted up to maximum of 60 days by the medical officer incharge to patients admitted on reception order, if their relatives apply in writing and execute a bond guaranteeing the safety of the mentally ill. It can be refused if the officer incharge feels that it will not be in the interest of the patient or of others.

Magistrate can also grant leave of absence to mentally ill person if he is satisfied that it is necessary to do so.

Application for Judicial Inquisition

If a person who is possessed of property is thought to be unable to manage his property due to mental illness, an inquisition proceedings can be started by the district court. The court will determine whether this person is suffering from unsoundness of mind of such a degree or extent that he cannot manage his estate. If the court is satisfied that the person is suffering from mental disorder of such a degree that he cannot manage his affairs the court can appoint a manager for his property. Such patient may also be ordered to be admitted to a psychiatric hospital if it is considered necessary.

Chapter III Protection of Human Rights of Mentally ill Persons

It provides for treatment with dignity and protects the patient's human rights.

(1) No mentally ill person shall be subjected during treatment to any indignity (whether physical or mental) or cruelty.

(2) No mentally ill person under treatment shall be used for purposes of research unless :

i) such research is of direct benefit to him for purposes of diagnosis and treatment ; or

ii) such person being a voluntary patient has given his consent in writing or where such person (whether or not voluntary patient) is incompetent by reasons of minority or otherwise to give valid consent, the guardian or other person competent to give consent on his behalf, has given his consent in writing, for such research.

(3) Subject to any rules made in this behalf under Section 94 for the purpose of preventing vexation or defamatory communications or communications prejudicial to the treatment of mentally ill persons no letter or other communication sent by or to a mentally ill person under treatment shall be intercepted, detained or destroyed.

CHAPTER IX OF THE ACT DEALS WITH PENALTIES UNDER THIS ACT

Comments — This Act has made the procedure of admission and discharge of the mentally ill person easier. However, the Act has not kept pace with the recent development in the field of psychiatry. The Act does not understand the ground realities of Indian situation. If every mentally ill who is dangerous to himself or to others is to be detained in psychiatric hospitals then we will need few million hospital beds and we have only 25,000 hospital beds in the country.

There should be a provision of out patient treatment where the patient may be kept under care of relatives or social agencies and who should be responsible for their welfare.

Criminal Responsibility of Mentally Ill

Criminal responsibility of an individual is judged on the following :

a) That the Act was voluntary,

b) That there was a guilty intent.

If a mentally ill person is suffering from such a disorder due to which he can neither control his action nor has a guilty intent then he will not be considered responsible for his action.

Indian Penal Code Section 84 deals with defense on grounds of insanity and follows the McNaughten Rule. These rules state that:

— it is the duty of the defense to establish,

— that the person was suffering from unsoundness of mind of such a degree or extent,

— that at the time of committing the act by reasons of unsoundness of mind the person was,

— incapable of knowing the nature of the act

— or that he was doing what is either wrong or contrary to law.

Insanity defence is usually put forward when the person is charged with murder and it is the duty of defense to prove that the person was insane at the time of commiting the act. The medical officer is often asked to give evidence of insanity in such cases.

The medical officer should observe the following

a) Was he suffering from a mental illness prior to the commitment of the Act ?

b) What was the nature of the illness ? Did he have delusions that people are trying to defame or harm him. Did he act on these delusions ?

c) Was the act planned ? The act of mentally ill may not be planned.

d) Was there an accomplice ? Mentally ill will not usually have an accomplice.

e) There will be no attempt at secrecy.

f) His behaviour before and after the act will be abnormal.

g) There may be a lack of motive and senselessness in the act.

In spite of all care it is often impossible to categorically state that the person was mentally ill at the time of committing the act.

INSANITY DUE TO INTOXICATION

If insanity is due to voluntary intake of alcohol or other drugs it cannot be taken as defense against a criminal act.

However, if intoxication has been taken unknowingly then it can be taken as a defense.

If insanity has occurred due to continuous intake

of intoxication e.g. delirium tremens then it will be accepted as defense against criminal acts.

COMPETENCY TO STAND TRIAL

A medical officer is often called upon by a court to decide whether the accused is competent to stand trial.

In these cases the doctor has to be satisfied of the following :

a) Can the patient understand the court proceedings e.g. does he know that he is standing a trial, what are the charges against him ?

b) Can he instruct his lawyers properly ?

If a person cannot do so due to unsoundness of mind then he can be certified that he is incompetent to stand trial :

CIVIL RESPONSIBILITY

1. Contract — For making a valid contract the parties at the time of making a contract should be of sound mind.

It has to be established that one of the parties to the contract did not understand the nature of the contract or its consequences due to unsoundness of mind.

Lucid interval is often invoked as defense in such a case. The law recognises that mentally unsound person can be sane for short intervals and these periods are called Lucid intervals. Any contract made during this period is valid.

MARRIAGE

Section 5 (ii) introduced by Act 68 of 1976 states that at the time of marriage neither party

a) is incapable of giving valid consent (due to) unsoundness of mind.

b) though capable of giving consent, has been suffering from mental disorder of such a kind or to such an extent as to be unfit for marriage and the procreation of children; or

c) has been subjected to recurrent attacks of insanity or epilepsy.

Any of the above conditions can be a ground for declaring marriage as null and void. If the marriage has been solemnized by concealing the fact of mental illness then it can also be considered as suppressing valid information.

Divorce can be granted if the other party "has been incurably of unsound mind or has been suffering continuously or inter-mittently from mental disorder of such a kind and to such an extent that the petitioner cannot reasonably be expected to live with the respondent'.

In Muslim law also the woman can seek divorce if the husband has been insane for a period of two years.

The diagnosis of any mental illness is not relevant for dissolution of marriage but the emphasis is laid on reasonable capacity to fulfil marital duties and responsibilities.

TESTAMENTARY CAPACITY

This relates to a person's competency to make a valid will to dispose of his property. It is assumed that the testator is of, 'sound and disposing mind' at the time of making the will.

A medical expert may be called to certify this capacity of the testater at the time of making the will. In assessing a person's ability to make a valid will following points are to be kept in mind ;

1. Presence of a psychiatric illness does not make a person unfit for making a will. A mentally sick person or a person suffering from disease of the brain (stroke etc.) can make a valid will provided he fulfils the necessary conditions required to make a will :

a) The person should understand that the documents he is preparing is for the disposition of his property.

b) He should be able to clearly recall all the properties he possesses and their value.

c) He should know all the natural heir. If he is planning to dispose any one or all of them he should be able to provide understandable reason for the same.

d) He should not be under influence of intoxicants or other mind altering drugs at the time of making the will.

e) The person making the will should be examined alone so that one may be able to exclude the undue influence of one or more family members.

d) In case of a person who is usually suffering from a mental illness but fulfils all the above conditions, he will be said to be in a lucid interval and he can make a valid will.

CHAPTER 21
MEDICAL ETHICS

Medical men exercise enormous powers over their patients and the doctor's decisions can largely affect the well-being of their patients. Most of the patients know very little about medical diagnosis and treatment due to which they have to accept the advice of their physician. In ancient times medicine was considered to be a calling and not a profession due to which the doctors put the patient's well-being before their own but with the changing pattern of life while medicine is being perceived as an industry the ethical codes appear to be crumbling.

Ethics must be differentiated from morality and law though ethical principle cannot contravene either of them. Morality requires one to observe certain set of rules which are considered universally true and are based on religious principles. Any transgression of morality leads to guilt and anxiety. Law, on the other hand, is formulated by the State to maintain law and order and any transgression of these rules is punishable. Ethical code is decided by a professional group which can regulate activities of the members of the group. It neither has the rigidity of the morals nor a fear of punishment as envisaged in the legal codes. Ethical codes can be changed with changing situations and they usually act as guidelines to improve the standards of the profession.

Medical ethics has an ancient origin. Hippocrates and Sushruta have enumerated ethical principles. Indian Medical Council also has enunciated an ethical code. But most of them have not been updated. The following are the common ethical guidelines for medical practitioners.

Do no harm

"Do no harm" is the basic principle of medical practice. This is a very important principle which is often ignored. Whenever a doctor undertakes treatment of a patient without proper diagnosis or when he does not have enough expertise to treat the patient in such a situation he is likely to do harm to the patient. "Only treat those patients where you are certain of your expertise" is the basic principle of medicine. In other cases where the doctor is unsure of himself he should refer to a colleague who is competent in treating such patients. In our own set-up where specialist may not be available for every disorder it is mandatory that the primary care physician should develop minimal expertise of treating all kinds of disorders. Moreover, he should use only those drugs of methods on which he has sufficient mastery. Many doctors out of their anxiety to please the patient or to treat them quickly prescribe a number of drugs, hoping that any of the prescribed drugs may turn out to be useful. This is a pernicious practice and does more harm than good in several ways.

Confidentiality

The patient may communicate many things to his doctor which may be harmful to him if the obtained information is passed onto other persons. The doctors should, therefore respect the confidence of the patients and should not divulge any thing which they come to know during the course of the professional relationship.

This concept of confidentiality is not absolute and it may be violated in certain situations such as under :

a) When a court of law orders the physician to provide certain information.

b) When keeping the confidence of the patient may lead to harm to others or to himself. For instance, if a patient communicates to the doctor that he is going to kill Mr. X, it is the duty of the doctor to take suitable action so that Mr. X could be protected. Similarly, if a patient suffering from AIDS refuses to take necessary precautions it may be essential for the doctor to inform his spouse or others.

Consent

The patient or his relatives should be informed of the nature of the disorder, possible management, likely side-effects and probable outcome. The patient should give consent for the treatment planned.

The informed consent is especially important whenever an unconventional treatment is being proposed. In our country often the patients have no option to refuse treatment because either no other doctor is available or due to economic constraints the patient cannot seek help elsewhere. In such a situation the responsibility of doctor is increased manifold. The doctor has to be extra careful to protect the interest of the patient.

Medical ethics in our country is guided by paternalistic model where the doctor takes on the role of the parent and does what he thinks is best for patient. With changing times this pattern is giving way to contractual medicine where medical treatment is a contract between two parties.

Both these patterns have been criticised. Paternalistic ethics provides the doctor unbridled freedom which may be misused while the contractual medicine may lead to not only unnecessary investigations but also affects doctor-patient relationship and the whole process of therapeutic management in a substantial manner.

Involuntary treatment

Many patients may refuse treatment because they are not mentally competent to decide for them selves. In such a situation the following is to be kept in mind.

a) Is the patient not able to decide as to what is good for him because of the effect of the mental illness?

b) Whether the relative of the patient or the court of law has permitted the doctor to treat such a patient ?

If the relatives consent is available then the patient can be treated against his will.

Charging of fees

Most doctors charge fees for the services rendered to the patient others get paid by the government or other agencies for the services offered. The fees structure varies from doctor to doctor as well as from place to place. So there could not be any fixed fee pattern. However, it is important that the fee structure should be transparent and charges should be fixed for the type of services and not according to the income of the client. In India where poverty is rampant, every doctor also need to provide help to many patients free of charge.

Sexual relationships with the patient

Doctors are usually perceived as desirable and rather ideals especially by the opposite sex patients and as a result of this the patients are likely to become enamoured by their doctors. Such a situation is likely to be more often countered in the practice of psychiatry as it primarily relates to interpersonal problems. The doctor should not take advantage of this situation. If the doctor and patient feel strongly attracted to each other then the patient should be transferred to some other therapist.

Referral

Any patient who is not getting better by one's treatment should be referred without much delay to other more competent doctor or a second opinion may be obtained. The referring doctor should provide care till such time that the referred doctor accepts the patient.

In India most patients consult a number of doctors without referral and as it is the prevalent practice it may be continued.

Death, dying and suicide

Many a times a doctor is in dilemma as to how long life-sustaining measures may be continued once irreversibility of dying process is established. Modern life sustaining devices may be able to keep a dying patient alive for long period of time. There is a raging controversy on this issue and it is still for from settled. One must follow the law of the land. Some patients who are interminably ill and are in severe agony may request their doctor to hasten death for helping them to avoid the suffering. Should a doctor assist them is again a controversial issue which needs to be further debated. At present Indian law does not permit the doctors to do so.

Cost effectiveness of treatment

Money very often is a crucial factor which may decide whether a particular treatment is feasible in a given patient or not. If the cost of treatment cannot be comfortably borne by the patient and the advantages are few or minimal then such treatments should be avoided. This also includes costly and unnecessary investigation. Only those investigations should be done which are crucial for the diagnosis or management. Investigation having low probability of providing meaningful advantage should be avoided. Similarly, unnecessary medication needlessly increases the cost of treatment.

Aforementioned are the guidelines which could imporve medical practice and restore patient's confidence in their doctor. Today the doctors have lost their credibility and it can only be restored by our own actions. Often the unethical acts are a result of ignorance. It is essential that all doctors should keep themselves abreast with scientific advances in their area. Once they are uptodate the chances are that their practice will also be ethical. Simple test of ethical practice is to keep yourself in the patient's place and decide whether you will like to have the treatment which is being offered.

SUGGESTED READING

1. American Psychiatric Association Task Force Report on Electroconvulsive Therapy. 1990. American Psychiatric Association, Washington, D.C.
2. Child and Adolescent Psychiatry — II edition. Rutter, M., Hersov, L. (Eds.), 1985. Blackwell, N.Y.
3. Cognitive Behaviour Therapy for Psychiatric Problems : A practical guide. Hawton, K., Salkovaskis, P.M., Krik, J., Clark, D.M. (Eds.), 1989. Oxford Medical Publications, Oxford University Press.
4. Comprehensive Textbook of Psychiatry. V edition. Kaplan, H.I., Saddock, B.J. (Eds.), 1989. Williams and Wilkins, Maryland.
5. Electroconvulsive Therapy. Abrams, 1988. Oxford University Press, New York.
6. Fish's Clinical Psychopathology : Signs and Symptoms in Psychiatry. II edition. Max Hamilton (Ed.), 1985. Wright, Bristol.
7. Handbook of Affective Disorders — II edition. Paykel, E.S. (Ed.), 1992. Churchill Livingstone, London.
8. Handbook of Mental Illness in the Mentally Retarded. Menolascino, F.J., Stark, J.A. (Eds.), 1984. Plenum, N.Y.
9. Human Sexual Inadequacy, Masters, W.H., Johnson, V.E., 1970. Little, Brown, Boston.
10. Human Sexual Response. Masters, W.H., Johnson, V.E., 1970. Little, Brown, Boston.
11. ICD–10 Classification of Mental and Behavioural Disorders — Clinical Descriptions and Diagnostic Guidelines. 1992. WHO, Geneva, Oxford University Press, New Delhi.
12. Oraganic Psychiatry — II edition. Lishman, W.A., 1986. Blackwell, London.
13. Oxford Textbook of Psychiatry. II edition, Gelder, M., Gath, D., Mayou, R. (Eds.), 1989. Oxford University Press, Oxford (ELBS).
14. Pocket Handbook of Psychiatric Drug Treatment. Kaplan, H.I., Sadock, B.J., 1993. B.I. Publications, New York.
15. Pocket Handbook of Emergency Psychiatric Medicine. Kaplan, H.I., Sadock, B.J., 1993. B.I. Publications Pvt. Ltd., New Delhi.
16. Postgraduate Psychiatry. Vyas, J.N., Ahuja, N. (Eds). 1992. B.I. Churchill Livingstone Pvt. Ltd., New Delhi.
17. Recent Advances in Addictive Disorders. Miller, N.S. (Ed.) Psychiatric Clinics of N. America, March 1993. W.B. Saunders Company, Philadelphia.
18. Schizophrenia. Powchik, P., Schulz, S.C. II (Eds.) Psychiatric Clinics of N. America, June 1993. W.B. Saunders Company, Philadelphia.
19. The Life and Work of Sigmund Freud. Jones, E. Vols. 1–3, 1953–57, Basic Books, New York.
20. The Mental Health Act 1987 (Act. No. 14 of 1987). Law Publishers (India) Pvt. Ltd., Allahabad.

SUGGESTED READING

1. American Psychiatric Association Task Force Report on Electroconvulsive Therapy 1990. American Psychiatric Association, Washington, D.C.
2. Child and Adolescent Psychiatry — II edition, Rutter M., Hersov L. (Eds.) 1985, Blackwell, N.Y.
3. Cognitive Behaviour Therapy for Psychiatric Problems. A practical guide. Hawton K., Salkovskis P.M., Kirk J., Clark D.M. (Eds.) 1989. Oxford Medical Publications, Oxford University Press.
4. Comprehensive Textbook of Psychiatry, V edition. Kaplan, H.I., Saddock, B.J. (Eds.) 1989. Williams and Wilkins, Maryland.
5. Electroconvulsive Therapy. Abrams R. 1988. Oxford University Press, New York.
6. Fish's Clinical Psychopathology — Signs and Symptoms in Psychiatry, II edition. Max Hamilton (Ed.), 1985, Wright, Bristol.
7. Handbook of Anxiety Disorders — II edition. Tyrer, P.J. (Ed.) 1992. Churchill Livingstone, London.
8. Handbook of Mental Illness in the Mentally Retarded. Menolascino, F.J., Stark, J.A. (Eds.) 1984. Plenum, N.Y.
9. Human Sexual Inadequacy. Masters, W.H., Johnson, V.E., 1970. Little, Brown, Boston.
10. Human Sexual Response. Masters, W.H., Johnson, V.E., 1970. Little, Brown, Boston.
11. ICD-10 Classification of Mental and Behavioural Disorders — Clinical Descriptions and Diagnostic Guidelines, 1992. WHO, Geneva. Oxford University Press, New Delhi.
12. Organic Psychiatry — II edition. Lishman, W.A., 1986. Blackwell, London.
13. Oxford Textbook of Psychiatry, II edition. Gelder, M., Gath, D., Mayou, R. (Eds.) 1989. Oxford University Press, Oxford (ELBS).
14. Pocket Handbook of Psychiatric Drug Treatment. Kaplan, H.I., Sadock, B.J., 1993. B.I. Publications, New York.
15. Pocket Handbook of Emergency Psychiatric Medicine. Kaplan, H.I., Sadock, B.J., 1993. B.I. Publications Pvt. Ltd., New Delhi.
16. Postgraduate Psychiatry. Vyas, J.N., Ahuja, N. (Eds.) 1992. B.I. Churchill Livingstone Pvt. Ltd., New Delhi.
17. Recent Advances in Addictive Disorders. Miller, N.S. (Ed.) Psychiatric Clinics of N. America, March 1993. W.B. Saunders Company, Philadelphia.
18. Schizophrenia. Bogerts, B., Schulz, S.C. II (Eds.) Psychiatric Clinics of N. America, June 1993. W.B. Saunders Company, Philadelphia.
19. The Life and Work of Sigmund Freud. Jones, E. Vols. I–3, 1953–57. Basic Books, New York.
20. The Mental Health Act 1987 (Act No. 14 of 1987). Law Publishers (India) Pvt. Ltd., Allahabad.